HOPE *or* HYPE

The Obsession with Medical Advances and the High Cost of False Promises

RICHARD A. DEYO, M.D., M.P.H.
DONALD L. PATRICK, PH.D., M.S.P.H.

AMACOM

Special discounts on bulk quantities of AMACOM books are available to corporations, professional associations, and other organizations. For details, contact Special Sales Department, AMACOM, a division of American Management Association, 1601 Broadway, New York, NY 10019. Tel.: 212-903-8316. Fax: 212-903-8083. Web site: www. amacombooks.org

Library of Congress Cataloging-in-Publication Data

Deyo, Richard A.

Hope or hype : the obsession with medical advances and the high cost of false promises / Richard A. Deyo, Donald L. Patrick.—1st ed.

p. cm.

Includes bibliographical references and index.

ISBN 0-8144-0845-1

1. Medical innovations—United States—Evaluation. 2. Medical technology—United States—Evaluation. 3. Medical care—Technological innovations—United States—Evaluation. 4. Medical care—United States—Evaluation. 5. Medical innovations—Economic aspects—United States. 6. Medical technology—United States—Cost effectiveness. 7. Medical care—Technological innovations—United States—Cost effectiveness. 8. Medical care, Cost of—United States. I. Patrick, Donald L. II. Title.

RA418.5.M4D49 2005
610'.28—dc22

2004022295

Printing number
10 9 8 7 6 5 4 3 2 1

TO LYNDA AND SHIRLEY

CONTENTS

PART IV

Crossing the Threshold: Improving the Transition from "Experimental" to "Standard Care"

PREFACE: DISILLUSIONED INSIDERS

This book isn't intended to be an anti-technology rant, although some people may read it that way. We're great fans of many medical innovations, and we are definitely not Luddites, opposed to technological change. We don't long for the bad old days before antibiotics, anesthesia, cataract surgery, joint replacements, or Prozac. Indeed, we're happy consumers of medical products, old and new.

Both of us are hopelessly nearsighted, and without spectacles would have been seriously disabled since about the second grade. Rick likes his soft contact lenses and Donald his photosensitive glasses. Maybe some day both Rick and Donald will even have a Lasik procedure, but for now we're chicken. Rick also likes his antihistamines for allergies and his inhaled cortisone drugs that prevent both runny nose and wheezing. His eighty-two-year-old mother has benefited tremendously from cataract surgery in both eyes and from hip replacements on both sides.

Donald maintains his cholesterol at a normal level with a remarkable statin drug, and he has a family member with chronic illness who benefits hourly from assistive technology and drugs. He's waiting for advances in affordable wheelchair technology that will permit going up stairs and wheeling on the beach. We're not reflexively opposed to new technology, and we would be hypocritical if we were.

On the other hand, we've witnessed disturbing practices that seem designed to maximize someone's income, regardless of whether there was benefit or harm to patients. Those practices include aggressive marketing of new products with high costs but only modest (or no) advantages over older alternatives. They include performing operations with the rationale that "it may not be necessary, but if I don't do it, somebody else will." They include writing guidelines to ensure that one medical specialty doesn't lose patients or income to another with a competing approach. They include selling more newspapers or ad time by exaggerating medical advances and making catastrophes out of health risks. They include medical promises that seem only to replace one problem with another. The reality is that most medical advances are incremental, and true breakthroughs are rare. Our hope is to inject some healthy skepticism into the way medical advances are received.

Our Own Conflicts of Interest

We'll describe some questionable practices that involve the drug industry, device manufacturers, professional interests, the media, advocacy groups, and even regulators. Aggressive drug marketing, for example, permeates medical education and medical practice. Conflicts of interest by researchers, faculty, and practitioners are almost ubiquitous because of honoraria, consulting fees, grants, gifts, travel, and other incentives from industry. We're not lily-white ourselves, and we feel obliged to disclose our own real and potential conflicts of interest. The list of things we've done and haven't done may be instructive in itself.

The health-care industry pushes enticements on doctors from the first day of medical school. Rick turned down the black leather medical bag that was offered by a drug company to every first-year medical student in his class. He's not had any grants or contracts from a drug company or been on their "speaker's bureaus." He's turned down all-expenses-paid trips with his wife to the Caribbean and to five-star hotels in major U.S. cities—offered for "educational opportunities" or to serve on ad hoc "consultant's boards." He doesn't own any pharmaceutical or biotech stocks (or stock options), except as they're included in many general mutual funds.

But the longer he's in the business, the harder it is for him to avoid entanglements with industry. The entanglements are almost a byproduct of the way medical care is organized. For example, Rick may benefit in the near future from a gift for research provided to the University of Washington by Synthes, a manufacturer of surgical instruments and devices. Furthermore, he's been wined, dined, flown, consulted, and handed honoraria at drug company expense on too many occasions to list. As a resident and faculty member, he's eaten countless glazed donuts and pizzas on drug reps' tabs while attending noon conferences or grand rounds. For many of these activities, the money was "laundered" through professional societies, educational institutions, or other organizations that actually wrote the checks, making Rick feel better. But the source of the funds was clear.

He's provided a few hours of consultation regarding research design to companies such as Parke-Davis Pharmaceuticals, Merck, Sanofi-Synthelabo, Medtronic Corporation, Procter & Gamble, Premera Insurance Company, and probably others that he's forgotten. He recently lectured for a surgical research group in a luxury box at Safeco Field before a Seattle Mariners baseball game—courtesy of Pfizer. He has lectured or consulted on back problems for General Motors, Innovative Health Solutions, Time-Life Medical, MediaLogic, State Farm Insurance, and Safeco Insurance. He once had a research grant funded by the John Alden Insurance Company. He's been to editorial meetings for medical journals and lectured at continuing education courses for which expenses were covered by Sofamor Danek and Aesculap, manufacturers of surgical devices.

He's also consulted for government agencies such as the Agency for Health Care Policy and Research, the Federal Trade Commission, and the FDA—all of which have their own agendas. He's consulted with nonprofits such as Group Health of Puget Sound and the Kaiser health-care system, multiple universities, and others—again, with their own agendas.

Donald has received numerous contracts and grants from companies in the drug industry, including Abbott, Aventis, Astra/Zeneca, Bayer, Johnson & Johnson, Lilly, Merck, Novartis, Pfizer, Serono, and others. With these funds, some of which were through contracts with the University of Washington, he has developed patient-reported outcome measures used in the approval and marketing of drugs and devices, but also to evaluate non-pharmacologic treatments. He has testified on behalf of industry to the FDA, giving his opinion on the evidence for certain product claims. He has participated in FDA advisory committees evaluating new drug approvals, when there was no conflict of interest. This past year he spent his sabbatical as a Special Government Employee working with the FDA on patient-reported outcomes. In fairness, his work in "quality of life" measurement couldn't have progressed without industry support, given the generally low level of government funding for outcome assessment.

Over our entire careers, though, most of our research support has come from federal agencies and private foundations like the Robert Wood Johnson Foundation, which funded our effort on this book. By way of full disclosure, we should note that the Johnson Foundation was created from the estate of a Johnson & Johnson CEO whose father and uncle founded the company. So even though the foundation is independent of the Johnson & Johnson company, profits from the pharmaceutical industry at least indirectly supported this book.

White Hats, Black Hats, Gray Hats

Throughout our exploration of medical innovations, we've encountered what we'd call atrocities—stories of people who were attacked because they got the "wrong" results, publicized damaging information, or simply challenged the conventional wisdom. In many cases, the attacks came from commercial interests, but sometimes they came from professional groups, advocacy organizations, or political sources. Some of these attacks have been publicized, and their newsworthiness makes them seem unusual. Our thesis, though, is that such events are simply business as usual, and that most of the elbows are thrown where the referees can't see them—outside the public spotlight. The development of clinical policy (how new treatments get used) is as much a contact sport as the development of public policy.

We tend to see the embattled researchers in these stories as the "white hats" and the source of the attacks as the "black hats." The reality is more complex, of course, and nearly all hats are some shade of gray. We secretly think that our own hats are more nearly white than everyone else's, but we assume that everyone feels the same way. Rather than thinking of white hats and black hats, good guys and bad guys, it may be more helpful simply to consider who's profiting and who's paying in any given scenario. We must then decide whether we're happy with the way health is affected and money is distributed.

Our Hopes for This Book, and Some Writing Conventions

Ultimately, our goal isn't to vilify special interests, but to identify them and the tactics they use, many of which are poorly visible. We also want to celebrate individuals who have the courage of their convictions, and the successes of scientific inquiry that have sometimes overcome tall obstacles.

The flip side of special interests is the insatiable demand for new medical technology among us all. We all have a tendency to think that "newer is better" and "more is better" when it comes to medical care. We want to believe the marketing and media hype that describes many modest scientific steps as "lifesaving new technology." The drug industry, doctors, and hospitals want us to believe it, too. We want every medical test or treatment that we even imagine may be helpful, and we expect to pay nothing for it. Insurance should cover it. Then we wonder why medical costs are rising so fast and why fewer and fewer people can afford health insurance.

Many consumers think doctors don't do enough. They imagine that more tests and more treatments can only be good, and they clamor for instant access to new or experimental treatments for which there is only meager evidence of any value.

We suspect, in contrast, that for many well-insured patients, doctors are doing too much—creating risks and costs that are unnecessary. If this book simply encourages more conversations about whether we're doing too much in some areas of health care, we'll be happy. If consumers become even slightly more skeptical and more discerning about trying the "latest and greatest," we'd call it a success.

We'll propose avenues for change that seem consistent with the peculiar societal values of the United States. We'll argue that no single policy change or intervention will solve our problems with new medical treatments, and that changes will have to involve doctors' behavior, patients' behavior, corporate behavior, the media, and regulatory agencies.

As we wrote, we wanted to include some personal stories, but with two authors, we faced some ambiguity if we wrote in the first person singular. On the other hand, using the third person and referring to Rick and Donald or to RAD and DLP seemed stilted. So we've adopted the convention of saying I (Rick) or I (Donald) had such and such an experience, and just using the first person thereafter for the rest of a paragraph or story. We hope this makes sense and will be easy to follow. When we use "we," of course, we mean we.

In some cases, we've described some of my (Rick's) actual patients. We've taken liberties with names, ages, genders, details about the healthcare providers, and some medical details in order to obscure their identities, but the essential details of the stories are accurate.

We've chosen to focus on whether and how well new treatments work, and why useless or risky treatments sometimes become popular. We've deliberately avoided some contentious moral issues, such as those raised by contraception, abortion, cloning, or stem-cell research. Our perception of the proper role for these technologies depends heavily on our religious, ethical, and political values. For most medical treatments, though, the basic issues are these: Does it work? Is it safe? How well does it work? For whom and under what circumstances does it work? How much does it cost?

Our hope in writing was to take the high road with some grace and humor, and to avoid getting too arrogant or self-righteous. And to paraphrase Janine Abercrombie, a newsletter editor, we also hoped to demonstrate that, unlike "hospital food," "a fascinating book about health care" need not be an oxymoron.

ACKNOWLEDGMENTS

The Robert Wood Johnson Foundation funded the effort on this project through a Health Policy Research Investigator Award. We're extremely grateful for this opportunity. It has been a luxury rather than a burden to study and write about something that we find so interesting and important, but that is a bit of a departure from our daily work. David Mechanic and Lynn Rogut, in particular, were supportive and flexible in meeting our various requests. Alvin Tarlov gave us critical encouragement. The opinions and conclusions in this book are ours and not necessarily those of the Robert Wood Johnson Foundation.

We had a lot of help in writing this book. Many of the ideas presented here have been the topic of discussions with our colleagues, whose indirect influence on this book has been important. These folks are too numerous to give them all credit, and we'd forget some anyway. To many of our friends and colleagues at the University of Washington, Columbia, Dartmouth, UCSF, Harvard, and elsewhere, thanks for your inspiration.

We were extremely fortunate to conduct interviews with several people at universities, state and federal agencies, professional societies, and the media. Special thanks to Gunnar Andersson, Len Cobb, Terry Corbin, Cathy DeAngelis, Todd Edwards, Jack Elinson, Dave Flum, Gary Franklin, Bob Gagne, Lee Glass, Rod Hayward, Roger Herdman, Joel Howell, James Kahn, Larry Kessler, Eileen Koski, Bruce Psaty, Scott Ramsey, Drummond Rennie, Sanjay Saint, Roger Sergel, Ken Shine, Hal Sox, Orhan Sulieman, Sean Tunis, Jim Weinstein, and Norm Weissman.

Another bunch of wonderful colleagues gave us critical feedback on things we wrote. They not only sharpened our thinking but extended it, added material, and improved our writing. These stalwarts included Michael Barry, Laurie Burke, Wylie Burke, Tim Carey, Tom Koepsell, Mark Schoene, Greg Simon, Sean Sullivan, Gil Welch, Michael Wilkes,

Steve Woloshin, and Jim Willems. The help of these interviewees and reviewers shouldn't be contrued as endorsements. The views and opinions expressed here are ours. We assume the exclusive blame for anything that isn't so good or isn't accurate.

Researching and writing a book requires extended periods for thinking, reading, searching, following leads, and writing. Time without interruptions was a precious commodity. Access to the University of Washington's Helen Riaboff Whiteley Center at Friday Harbor greatly facilitated the search for such time. It's hard to imagine how this book could have been written without the quiet time and support provided by the Whiteley Center and its wonderful staff. Similarly, Rick had the extraordinary good fortune to spend a month at the Rockefeller Foundation's Bellagio Study and Conference Center in Bellagio, Italy. Thanks to the extraordinary staff and my fellow residents there, as well.

Adrienne Hickey, the editorial director at AMACOM Books, gave us encouragement and good advice. Her enthusiasm for our ideas was enormously helpful. Jerome Groopman and John Geyman gave us valuable encouragement as well. Gwyneth Moya, Kelley Chaddock, Kathryn Henne, and Pam Hillman provided valuable assistance in finding materials, obtaining permissions, and preparing the manuscript.

Another group of supporters and critical reviewers weren't professional colleagues, but family members who were willing to plow through drafts of chapter after chapter. These critics made us realize how hard we would need to work in order to avoid the deadly academic writing style and the ubiquitous jargon of medicine and health services research. To the extent that we succeeded, Lynda Betts, Jane Deyo, Janet Pugh, and Larrian Thompson deserve much of the credit. Lynda read every chapter (some of them twice) and became our best editor. Thanks to Lynda and Shirley, especially, for their patience, enthusiasm, encouragement, and love.

PART I

CAN THERE BE TOO MUCH OF A GOOD THING?

The Hazards of Uncritically Embracing Medical Advances

1

What's the Problem?

Don't We Need Lifesaving New Treatments?

Formerly, when religion was strong and science weak, men mistook magic for medicine; now, when science is strong and religion weak, men mistake medicine for magic. —Thomas Szasz, MD[1]

No one benefits from putting the cart (new treatments) before the horse (good science). —Jose A. Bufill, MD[2]

CONSIDER some recent medical "breakthroughs" reported in the media:

- In 2002, James Quinn died in a Philadelphia intensive care unit. He had lived nine months with a new AbioCor artificial heart. For seven of those months, he had been in the hospital, where he suffered two strokes and was on a ventilator much of the time. Before he died, Quinn said, "This is nothing like I thought it would be. If I had to do it over again, I wouldn't do it. No ma'am."[3]

- In 2001, Bayer removed its cholesterol-lowering drug Baycol from the market. Between 1997 and 2001, manufacturers pulled fourteen drugs off the market because of unexpected toxicity and related deaths. The makers had marketed these drugs aggressively; they were taken by millions of patients and collectively are suspected in over a thousand deaths.[4]

- In 2002, researchers reported that hormone replacement therapy for postmenopausal women may often cause more harm than benefit, although it's been used for decades.[5] The same week, we learned that a popular arthroscopic operation for knee arthritis doesn't work.[6]

- In 2001, twenty-five-year-old Jennifer Rufer of Seattle discovered that she *didn't* have cancer after all. Blood tests had repeatedly suggested a rare form of uterine cancer, and she had endured an unnecessary hysterectomy, removal of part of a lung, and months of chemotherapy.[7] Rufer had wanted a big family, but the false-positive tests destroyed that dream.

- In 2000, the *New England Journal of Medicine* reported that an aggressive new treatment for breast cancer was no better than standard care, although it was more toxic and cost twice as much.[8] Over 42,000 women had received the new treatment, at a total cost of $3.4 billion.[9]

- In 2002, researchers reported the largest clinical trial ever conducted for high blood pressure, involving 33,000 patients. An old-fashioned diuretic drug proved more effective than newer drugs in preventing the complications of high blood pressure.[10] But the use of diuretics had fallen steadily for years before the trial, thanks to aggressive marketing of newer and higher-priced medicines.[11]

What's going on here? Aren't the latest medical advances always the greatest? Don't doctors know what they're doing? Why are ineffective treatments used at all? Isn't the FDA or someone in Washington on top of this stuff?

Many medical advances offer real advantages over older tests and treatments. Others offer little, if any, advantage, and many have alarming side effects. Even the effective medical innovations are often oversold and overused. The United States spends more than any other country on health care, but has shorter longevity, worse public health statistics, and worse health-care inflation than most developed nations.

Economists and decision makers agree that new treatments are a major reason for ever-rising health-care costs. This in turn leads to rising health insurance premiums and a growing number of uninsured. But these new treatments are a double-edged sword. Some of them are good, some are bad, and most are only partly understood when they become widely used.

As doctors and manufacturers introduce medical advances, good money too often trumps good science. Vested interests, marketing, politics, and media hype often have more influence on how new medical advances get used than the best scientific evidence. We've painfully watched this many times during our careers in medicine and health services research.

New tests, devices, or drugs are routinely introduced as "breakthroughs"—when, in reality, many are marginally effective, useless, or even harmful. Many aren't even particularly new, but rather are "me too" products. This breathless approach is good for business, but not always for patients or the public. The best scientific evidence may get pushed to the background, suppressed, manipulated, or ignored. Good science sometimes wins in the end, but often only after avoidable illness, discomfort, costs, and delays. As a Yiddish proverb suggests, "The truth never dies, but it leads a wretched life."

In talking about medical technology, we mean to include drugs, surgical procedures, medical devices, diagnostic tests, assistive devices, and even lifestyle change strategies, not just electronic gadgets. However, we're not talking about information technologies, like electronic medical record systems, which are generally underused in medicine.

Many policy debates on rising health-care costs have largely ignored the necessity of introducing medical advances in a critical, carefully targeted fashion. This is in spite of economists' views that new treatments are a major driver of rising costs. Health-care analyst J. D. Kleinke argues that "All the energy expended in administrative, policy, and business spheres . . . [is] independent from and ignorant of actual medical practice."[12] Many policy makers simply assume that new drugs and new treatments can only be good. New health-care financing schemes rarely address the causes of rapid cost inflation, focusing instead on ways of shifting costs and tinkering with financial incentives.

On the other hand, some critical observers, like the ethicist Daniel Callahan, argue that we should dramatically slow technological progress in medicine, as it's largely unaffordable.[13] In a culture that is enamored of innovation and new technology, slowing medical advances may prove unacceptable. We'd be happy if all concerned simply stopped buying and marketing useless, harmful, or marginal treatments, which account for billions of dollars annually that could be put to better use.

Myths About Medical Advances

We suspect that there are some commonly held myths about medical advances that perpetuate the use of expensive but marginally useful treatments. Some of these myths, which we hope to dispel, are:

- "Experimental" and "standard" care are well defined.
- Doctors adopt medical advances only on the basis of good science.
- Newer is always better.
- More medical tests are always better; information can only be good.
- Action is always better than inaction.
- Doctors adopt new treatments only if those treatments offer good value for money.
- We can cure most medical conditions.

These beliefs are widely held among consumers and doctors alike. But they often lead to useless, harmful, or unnecessarily expensive care.

Furthermore, these myths contribute to a growing sense of anger and disappointment among consumers. Many people are outraged by the high cost of care, flip-flopping experts, conflicting medical opinions, loss of insurance, and fear of being undertreated or overtreated. As patients, they find that they don't know how to make good choices because they often have inadequate information. They often find expensive tests or treatments to be disappointing. On the one hand, they don't want major advances withheld because of their cost; on the other hand, they fear that doctors will make treatment decisions without considering their ability to pay.

Another source of frustration is that chronic diseases are now the main reasons for seeking medical care. In the past, most medical care was for acute conditions—broken bones, infections, appendicitis—for which we could offer a short course of treatment and expect a cure. Now, doctors most often are treating incurable conditions such as diabetes, high blood pressure, congestive heart failure, certain forms of cancer, and hardening of the arteries. These are chronic precisely because we don't have cures.

Many people may imagine that having a heart bypass cures heart disease, or that insulin cures diabetes. Nothing could be further from the truth. These conditions usually require lifelong medications and lifestyle changes in the form of new diets, physical activities, and smoking habits. Even with aggressive treatment, these patients don't have the same prognosis as people without the diseases. Organ transplants don't make people "as good as new." They can prolong survival, but they often require fussy ongoing treatments, intensive monitoring, lifestyle changes, and a quality of life that's far from normal. Despite their high-tech qualities, these treatments aren't like having a broken bone set and being "fixed."

The Dubious Need for Some Medical Services

Doctors sometimes make use of medical advances, at some risk and substantial cost, for the flimsiest of reasons. When I (Rick) was a medical student, I took a cardiology elective working with patients who had been referred for cardiac catheterization. This process involves threading a long tube through the aorta to the heart and injecting dye into the arteries that supply the heart. It's usually safe, but serious complications (like a heart attack) sometimes occur. In some cases, we found that a referred patient's medical history and examination findings weren't at all suggestive of significant coronary heart disease. The cardiology fellow acknowledged there was little reason to perform the procedure on these patients. But the patients had often traveled for some distance, and we were loathe to disappoint them or insult the referring physician. The fellow said philosophically, "You go to a barber, you get a haircut." But that couldn't disguise the fact that we were offering risk and cost without expecting any real benefit.

Recently, the financial and health stakes of dubious cardiac catheterization have become even greater. With the availability of balloon angioplasty, which opens narrowed arteries by inflating a tiny balloon inside the narrowed area, cardiac catheterization has become not just a diagnostic test, but also a treatment opportunity. And with the addition of coronary stents (small wire tubes that prop open narrowed arteries), the treatment opportunities and costs have expanded further.

Unfortunately, these treatments are increasingly being used for patients who don't even have chest pain or other symptoms—a situation in which the risks are clear, but the benefits are speculative. But like my cardiology fellow thirty years ago, a cardiologist in Dallas notes, "If Joe Smith, the local internist, is sending you patients, and if you tell them they don't need the procedure, pretty soon Joe Smith doesn't send patients anymore.

Sometimes you can talk yourself into doing it even though in your heart of hearts you don't think it's right."[14]

In some cases, the medical needs are more compelling, but using the latest treatments can still be hard to justify because the benefits are minuscule or nonexistent. An example would be aggressive treatment of an elderly patient who is near death from an incurable chronic disease. Most treatments have smaller benefits in this situation than in others, and the risks are usually greater.

One of my (Rick's) own patients may illustrate the point. John Gillespie was an eighty-two-year-old man with long-standing high blood pressure, diabetes, and rheumatoid arthritis. He had survived removal of a kidney for cancer and surgery for prostate cancer, as well as a recent removal of part of the colon for a ruptured diverticulum. His remaining kidney function was subpar. To top it off, he had severe narrowing of the aortic valve in his heart, a condition that had led to chest pain and mild enlargement of the heart.

John came to the emergency room one night complaining of shortness of breath. After careful evaluation of his heart condition and symptoms, the cardiologists and heart surgeons recommended that he have his aortic valve replaced. He and his family agreed. To make a long story short, he underwent the surgery, had a succession of serious complications, and lingered in the hospital for six weeks, mostly in intensive care. He never recovered the ability to communicate, and he was dependent on a breathing machine for the entire hospitalization.

We finally discharged John to a specialized nursing home that provided ventilator care, and he died a few weeks later. I found myself wondering if we'd done John any favors. He might not have lived any longer without the surgery, but he might have enjoyed a better quality of life for a few weeks.

Nonetheless, doctors, patients, and families may find it difficult to just stand by and provide comfort care. We often say, in effect, "Don't just stand there; do something." But this collective bias for action sometimes unintentionally violates the Hippocratic dictum: "First, do no harm." In some circumstances, the best advice—but the most difficult to follow—would be, "Don't just do something; stand there."

The pressure from the public and from industry to develop and disseminate new treatments is intense. In some cases, patients have no effective treatments for their diseases and are willing to pay—or at least have their insurance pay—for anything new that comes along. But most innovations aren't treatments for fatal diseases. Instead, they're aimed at discomforts and inconveniences, many of which already have effective treatments. And some new technologies ultimately prove ineffective or harmful, although this may become clear only after many patients have received them. Also, in most cases, "new" seems to be synonymous with "outrageously expensive."

The result is sometimes cost without benefit, and this is the situation that most concerns us. A closely related situation is one in which there is high cost and tiny benefit. This is a thornier problem, but one that we can't entirely ignore. Either situation means profit for someone, at the expense of patients' dollars and perhaps their health. Sometimes, "tried and true" proves better than "latest and greatest."

Most patients are insulated by insurance from the full costs of medical advances, so it seems to them that there is little reason for restraint. Of course, this reasoning presumes that there's never a risk. Doctors, hospitals, and manufacturers are only too happy to oblige most patient requests, because they stand to benefit. The insurance industry sometimes balks, but it can always raise premiums. The folks who are paying the lion's share of the bills—mainly our employers and the government—may seem like the only ones who care whether new advances are worth the cost.

But where do employers and the government get the money to provide health insurance? From all of us: consumers, taxpayers, and employees. Employees pay not only through direct premiums, but through lower wages as well. We pay for medical care in the price of goods and services. When you buy a new car, you pay more for health-care costs than for steel.

In the end, all parties share the blame for uncritically promoting useless or marginal innovations: patients, doctors, hospitals, the media, drug companies, device manufacturers, advocacy groups, politicians. The net result is that insured people get a richer and richer package of treatments, but fewer and fewer people can get insurance. And some of the treatments that the insured are buying are worthless.

When Do New Treatments Stop Being Experimental?

It may be surprising to learn that there are no standard definitions of *experimental* and *standard* care. There's no "Good Housekeeping Seal of Approval" that new operations, devices, tests, or drugs must receive before they become standard care. There's not even agreement about what evidence of effectiveness should be required if there were to be such a seal.

Many people imagine that FDA approval constitutes such a seal. It's true that for drugs there must be a reasonable demonstration of safety and efficacy, but the FDA makes no claims concerning value for money. The FDA doesn't require comparative studies to determine which of several competing drugs is most effective. As a result, products with trivial benefits often receive regulatory approval, regardless of their cost. An expensive new drug may offer no advantages over a cheap old one, but if it works at all, the FDA generally must approve it. For medical devices, the FDA's approval process is less rigorous than it is for drugs, and for new surgical procedures, there's no approval process at all. The FDA also gives little scrutiny to nutritional supplements—a multibillion-dollar industry.

There's no standard for judging when new medical advances are worth the cost, or when insurance should cover them. Attempts by researchers to establish such limits have never reached consensus. Every insurance plan or health-care organization makes this determination on its own, with wide variability in the process. Insurers often cover new treatments because others do, because effective marketing creates demand, or because lawsuits are threatened—not because of convincing evidence that the new treatments work.

Our thesis is that the evolution of clinical practices shares a great deal with the evolution of public policy—it's the result of competing interests, rather than a linear translation of scientific knowledge into practical application. Students of human behavior, economics, and political science may think it naïve to expect the development and diffusion of medical treatments to follow a rational process. But doctors are sometimes surprised when they see marketing or media hype triumph over scientific knowledge. Furthermore, we think that the public believes there is a linear scientific path.

We think most patients would be outraged to learn that, thanks to effective marketing, they may get an extremely expensive drug for high blood pressure rather than cheaper drugs that are more effective. We think they'd be outraged to learn that they are getting expensive surgical implants, even though a similar operation without the implants may be safer and just as effective. We think they'd be outraged at paying for diagnostic tests that are useless, or that increase anxiety and lead to unnecessary treatments. And we think they'd be outraged at buying treatments that turn out to be bad for their health rather than good. All these scenarios are daily events. No outrage materializes because most of the time, neither patients nor doctors even recognize them.

This is a greater problem in the United States than in most other countries, because we have no central financing of health care and no central capacity for technology assessment. In most developed nations, a central drug board decides when to cover the cost of new drugs, and it is able to negotiate lower prices than U.S. consumers face. Most countries have a professional agency that evaluates the evidence supporting new devices, tests, or procedures and makes consistent decisions about their use. These countries still face rising costs, but they are able to moderate the increases. In times of prosperity, concern about the adoption of new treatments may seem unimportant, as all things seem affordable. But in tight financial times, the problems of rising insurance premiums, growing Medicare taxes, and shrinking insurance coverage become more obvious.

Does High-Tech Medicine Crowd Out Low-Tech Benefits?

One problem is that the amount of money available for medical care is finite. We spend almost 15 percent of the gross national product for health care. This is a ton of money, but not an infinite supply. If we spend billions on high-tech services that reach only a few patients, this may prevent us from spending money on simpler services that could offer greater benefits to more people. Medicare literally spends billions, for example, on left ventricular assist devices that help the heart pump blood, implantable cardioverter-defibrillators to shock the heart if it enters a fatal rhythm, and lung volume reduction surgery in patients with end-stage emphysema. These services have big lobbies that include manufacturers, patients, and medical specialists.

But Medicare doesn't pay for things like better nursing staff ratios in hospitals, many forms of preventive care, or (until 2006) drugs. For many people, these are extremely valuable services, but Medicare can't afford them as long as high technology gets the first claim on health-care dollars.

Scientific Data and Social Values

Part of the challenge in approaching medical advances is to balance legitimate but conflicting social interests. We want to facilitate access to experimental technology in order to allow the earliest possible use of promising new treatments and to support high rates of innovation.[15] This is appealing to desperate patients, good for job growth, and politically popular. On the other hand, we may want to restrain access to new technology in order to ensure patient safety, produce valid information on benefits and risks, and constrain health-care costs. This may be better stewardship of societal resources. Our sense is that current incentives give too much weight to rapid introduction of new medical advances and not enough weight to careful evaluation. One result is that visions of cure and false urgency often drive out reflection in making health-care decisions.

We have no illusion that the adoption of medical advances can be based on scientific considerations alone. Decisions about whether to provide new treatments always incorporate the values of a society, and therefore must be political as well as scientific. Is a new treatment worth it? Should lifesaving technology for a few be valued over preventive treatment for many? Is a new treatment mainly for enhancing lifestyle or for treating disease? What do we define as disease? Who should pay for which kinds of treatment? As a society, we have to make these value judgments, and science can't make them for us.

On the other hand, we should make these judgments with good information regarding the benefits, risks, and costs of a new treatment. To the extent that this information gets suppressed or distorted by biased research, marketing and media hype, or wishful thinking on the part of doctors, it can lead to bad decisions. Our plea is to minimize the distortions and make the best information freely available to consumers, doctors, and policy makers. The process of adopting medical advances should be political, but scientific evidence should set the range of reasonable debate.

2

Medical Innovations and American Culture

The Call of the Sirens

We have met the enemy and he is us. —Pogo

You will come to the Sirens, who bewitch all men who come near. . . . "Come hither, Odysseus . . . stop your ship so you can hear our voices. No one has ever sailed his black ship past here without listening to the honeyed sound from our lips." —Homer, *The Odyssey,* Book 12

MEDICAL INNOVATIONS in America issue an almost irresistible call, like the Sirens in the Greek classic. In Homer's *Odyssey,* the Sirens were mythical creatures whose call to passing sailors from their island was so seductive that the sailors inevitably turned their ships to reach the Sirens, only to be shipwrecked in treacherous waters. When Odysseus passed on his voyage, he had his sailors put wax in their ears and bind him to the mast so that they wouldn't heed the Sirens' call and be swept to their deaths.

We're a "technoconsumptive" culture. We're pulled irresistibly to new technology, often without recognizing the risks. We seem to assume that high-tech medicine can only be better than low-tech medicine, that more medical care is better, that newer is better, and that more aggressive is better.

Yet sometimes this isn't so. In a study of more aggressive care versus more conservative care for certain patients with heart disease, the more aggressive strategy—with more cardiac catheterization and balloon angioplasty—was associated with a higher death rate.[1] The implication was that the more aggressive strategy is sometimes followed without a clear reason.

Two researchers from the University of Texas tried to explain why such procedures might sometimes be done without a clear indication. They concluded,

> In an era in which invasive cardiac procedures are manifestations of high-technology, resource-intensive medical care, many patients and their family members expect and insist on aggressive management. The term "conservative management" may project the impression (to physicians and patients alike) of obsolescence, inadequacy, and inferiority rather than of thoughtful reflection. . . . In the event of an adverse outcome, the patient and his or her family may be more understanding and forgiving if an aggressive approach was pursued (i.e., if "everything possible was done"), even if such an approach contributes to the adverse outcome.[2]

Similarly, experts reflecting on unnecessary surgery comment on the "aura of excitement" surrounding surgery, which doesn't usually accompany nonsurgical approaches.[3] Even diagnostic testing may be overrated in the public mind. In 1997, a controversy erupted about the value of mammography for women under age forty when an expert panel of doctors and researchers suggested that there was no proven benefit. Most women, however, were already convinced of the value of mammography in young women, and many who were surveyed thought screening should begin before age forty.[4] Asked why they thought the issue had become so controversial, most said that it was a matter of cost containment, not a question of effectiveness. These examples suggest that we're predisposed to assume that medical tests and treatments can only be good.

In fact, formal surveys suggest that Americans are more enamored of medical technology than consumers in other developed countries are. In the United States, 34 percent believe that modern medicine "can cure almost any illness for people who have access to the most advanced technology and treatment." In contrast, only 27 percent of Canadians and 11 percent of Germans believe this is true. Two-thirds of Americans report being "very interested" in news about medical discoveries, as opposed to 44 percent of Europeans. Among seniors, the differences were even greater, with 79 percent of Americans being "very interested" versus 42 percent of Europeans. Europeans were just as interested as Americans were in other inventions and discoveries outside of medicine, however.[5]

Advance after advance marches by, tempting us to seek it out for ourselves or for a loved one. Organ transplants, joint replacements, magnetic resonance imaging, chemotherapy, implantable defibrillators, microsurgery, drugs for almost every medical condition—the list is endless. In fact, the cultural activity of health care is indistinguishable from the use of new advances. Even if the right treatment doesn't exist at the moment, no one can blame seriously ill people for imagining that a breakthrough might be just around the corner. Or for thinking that if we only spent enough money, we could find a cure for nearly anything.

Why is medical technology so dramatically appealing in American culture? What are the social, political, and cultural forces behind it? Why does technology spread almost instantaneously from Manhattan to Mukilteo?

Technological Utopia in American Culture

In a pioneering book, historian Howard Segal showed how the age-old idea of America as a potential utopia was coupled, sometime during the nineteenth century, with a strong belief in technological progress.[6] Many of us live with an image of modern life as a steady march of progress in which we benefit from science at a faster and faster pace.

But medical progress isn't linear. There are fits and starts, trials and errors, blind alleys, two steps forward and one step back. Medical advances involve risks and benefits. In some cases, the risks outweigh the benefits, and new treatments can prove harmful.[7] Some treatments are only partially effective or are effective only in highly specific situations.

"Medicalizing" Common Problems

In between medical advances and the consumer stands the doctor, who controls access to prescribed treatments. Many of us today turn to the doctor to solve problems—physical, psychological, and social—that we might once have taken to a priest, bartender, or grandmother. Obesity, menopause, baldness, rowdiness, shyness, and even aging are now seen as medical problems that demand a medical solution.

Severe obesity, because of its impact, is clearly a medical problem. But being slightly overweight and thinking that this is unattractive is less straightforward. Aesthetics, culture, and body image shape our perceptions. Furthermore, obesity often has nonmedical and environmental roots: the growth of the "fast food nation," the marketing of highly processed foods, infatuation with TV, the loss of sidewalks and bike trails, and the ascendancy of the automobile, to name just a few.

Nonetheless, the technological imperative often drives us to doctors for solutions to all sorts of problems, medical and nonmedical. Our cultural preference seems to be for medical solutions (taking weight loss pills or undergoing weight loss surgery) rather than social or environmental solutions.

Individualism, the Group, and Expectations

Doctors are "imprinted" during medical training to provide the best possible care, which is generally interpreted as the newest and most technological care.[8] Medical students and residents are far more likely to be chastised by their faculty mentors for failing to order tests than for ordering too many. The admonition to "be complete" is pervasive in medical education.

In turn, Internet searches and consumer advertising often prime patients to arrive at the doctor's office with specific requests for the latest treatments. To patients searching the Internet, a preliminary report given at last month's scientific meeting seems as credible as findings that have been widely studied, published, and confirmed—maybe, because of its newness, even more credible. Some patients shop around to find a doctor who will give them what they want, even if it's ill advised. Examples include unnecessary testing or antibiotics for the common cold.

Both professional and patient autonomy build on the concept of a "free market," which has been applied to American health care for decades. Both doctors and patients want to use new treatments without someone second-guessing their decisions. But market forces can barely function when most costs are covered by insurance and full information is rarely available to consumers.

Another driving force is the expectation that doctors will act in the best interests of the individual, no matter what the cost and no matter how it affects society as a whole.[9] This is how doctors are trained to think. But policy makers have a different perspective; they ask, "How can I best promote the health of an entire population?"

Some in government, like former Colorado Governor Richard Lamm, argue that medical ethics, as commonly structured and interpreted, is bad public policy. If we spend staggering amounts of resources to extend one person's life by a week, we have less with which to provide prenatal care, cover the uninsured, or improve schools and police services. These things might offer more good to more people. Lamm argues that doctors refuse to consider diminishing returns when they look at the multitude of things we can do with modern medicine.[10]

American concepts of individualism and autonomy sometimes butt head to head with a desire for fairness. Should we provide basic services to everyone, or should we provide an increasingly expensive array of technology only to those who can afford insurance or who have deep pockets? This question underlies the current debates about health-care reform and universal insurance coverage.

Broader American social values also contribute to the use of new treatments. There's a strong belief that America is exceptional and can accomplish all things by the application of technology.[11] Richard Nixon, for example, declared war on cancer, anticipating that investment in this fight would find a cure. In his 1971 State of the Union address, Nixon made a special request for an additional $100 million for the National Cancer Institute. When he signed the National Cancer Act into law, he declared, "I hope in the years ahead we will look back on this action today as the most significant action taken during my Administration."

More than thirty years later, we've made only incremental progress in reducing mortality from cancer, and the disease and the treatments themselves still elicit fear. We may need to replace our expectations of "breakthroughs" with more realistic notions about the pace and nature of clinical advances.

Entitlement, Youth Culture, and Impatience

Many Americans have a sense of entitlement—they feel that the latest medical advances are "owed" to them. Expecting to live longer and better through medical procedures, often without paying for those procedures directly, is a common expectation. Most insured Americans expect "free" colonoscopies, cheap drugs, and immediate access to a physician. They expect MRI scans and blood tests on request. Even those who seek out "Volkswagen" insurance policies expect "Mercedes" care when the time comes.

Our youth-oriented culture and our continual search for the "fountain of youth" create demand for medical advances throughout the life span. For its preoccupation with health, beauty, and the perfection of youth, our culture has been described as narcissistic.[12] Medical technology is inextricably linked to the youth culture, not only through cosmetic surgery, but through an entire host of medications that help us do what we all want to do—remain active, youthful-appearing, and vital until the end. We take Viagra for erectile dysfunction, Propecia for hair loss, and Botox to erase wrinkles. We can even have surgery to make the voice sound younger, though at a relatively high risk.

Americans are also in a hurry for fixes. Most patients want diagnosis and treatment without delay, even for minor or chronic complaints. "Doc in the box" operations in shopping centers are popular for just this reason. Some of our colleagues have told us that if their doctors don't have e-mail, they'll change doctors, a view echoed by others.[13] Our attitudes toward the availability of new treatments often parallel our attitudes toward routine medical care. We're in too big a hurry to wait for careful evaluation of new drugs, devices, or operations.

Of course, there are forces that counter our belief that every medical problem can be solved, that the fountain of youth is around the corner, or that unrestricted access to expensive new treatments should be the norm. Insurance plans and managed-care organizations limit some uses of new treatments. Congress periodically takes up the cost of medical care. Some people are anxious about how viable Medicare will be by the time they retire. More reports like those that started Chapter 1 appear in the daily papers, giving a sobering picture of some new technologies. But public demand for new treatments often triumphs, and health-care plans cave in and provide the treatments. This can happen even without evidence that the treatments work.[14,15]

Rapid Spread of Medical Innovations

Many social and cultural forces feed the spread of innovations, foremost among them the belief that anything new is inherently good. A corollary is that everyone should have immediate access to all innovations. A frontier mentality fosters fascination with each "first," like the first artificial heart. This fuels demand for access to the latest and the best. Marketing creates demand through advertising, news, and word of mouth.

The vision of technomedicine fuels technoconsumption. Medical centers seek new treatments in order to appear up-to-date. Being the first on the block to have the latest treatment is an ideal for doctors, hospitals, and consumers. Those who build and sell medical treatments foster this ideal. Prestige accompanies the latest treatment. Who wants an older device or operation when a new one is available?

Sometimes, what seems new may not be. However, the perception of newness is often more important than the reality. Everett Rogers, guru of technological diffusion, notes, "If the idea seems new to the individual, it is an innovation."[16] This may partly explain the successful marketing of "me too" drugs that offer little advantage over older drugs. Manufacturers have sometimes simply renamed a product and called it new, as Eli Lilly did when it repackaged Prozac as Sarafem. Lilly then marketed Sarafem for "premenstrual dysphoric disorder" instead of depression, with a large new marketing campaign.

In a media age, innovations spread through mass marketing. The Internet also spreads news and creates demand through list serves, web sites, chat rooms, and spam. Health news is a common topic for magazine articles and cocktail party conversation. What used to be sequestered in grandma's medical book or in a medical library is now all around us: on paper, the radio, the Internet, and television.

Constant specialization in medicine and the ever-narrower scope of specialist practice facilitates the spread of new treatments. Patients often believe that a specialist has more advanced knowledge of treatments and can apply them more precisely than the generalist physician. Some patients visit complex and well-equipped institutions and get involved in an assembly line of tests, probes, evaluations, and consultations, all of which use the latest innovations. As we'll see, the more tests you have, the more likely it is that one result will be abnormal, leading to a cascade of further tests and treatments. These are always good for doctors and hospitals, but not always for patients.

End-of-Life Care: Is Death Optional?

Medical procedures are becoming more and more prevalent in care at the end of life. And this is an integral part of hope.[17] Yet more and more patients and their families have become aware of the potentially harmful power of the "technological imperative" in the care of terminally ill patients. Daniel Callahan, a medical ethicist, describes this as the "compulsive use of technology to maintain life when palliative care would be more appropriate." He notes that there often is an underlying assumption "that death is the principal evil of human life."[18]

Callahan notes that even when patients have advance directives against lifesaving technology, they aren't guaranteed the care they want. He says, "Death is still denied, evaded, and, in the case of many clinicians, fought to the end, regardless of the patient's wishes."[18]

Medical progress sometimes creates the illusion that death is avoidable. Our medical interventions sometimes create the impression that the death of a particular patient at a particular time is an accidental event, not an inevitable one. The chairman and CEO of Human Genome Sciences, a biotech company, has declared, "Death is a series of preventable diseases."[19]

A consequence of these attitudes and illusions is that there's often a wide gap between what we say we want and what actually happens at the end of life. Almost 80 percent of Americans hope to die at home, without pain, in the company of close family or friends, having put their affairs in

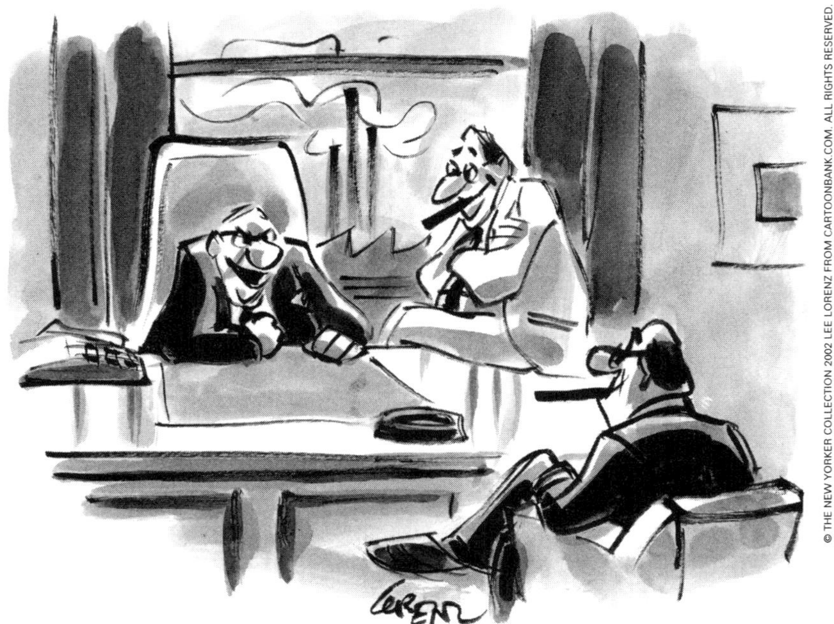

"Well, we've licked taxes—that just leaves death."

order. Most want to feel that their relationships are as complete, whole, and peaceful as possible. But 75 percent of Americans actually die in hospitals or nursing homes. Of those, a third die after ten days in an intensive care unit.[20]

The longer we use medical treatments at the end of life, the greater the cost can be, both human and economic. Giving up hope and giving up treatment aren't easy for either doctors or patients. But Callahan argues that death need not be seen as public enemy number one. Chronic illness and disability, he argues, may be what people fear most, and efforts at innovation might usefully be turned in that direction.[18]

Infatuation with Technology: The Example of the Artificial Heart

The artificial heart program in the United States illustrates our infatuation with medical technology and the ups and downs of medical progress.[21] The time line for the program extends from the 1950s to the present, as we approach FDA approval of the new AbioCor artificial heart. Patients and health professionals have dreamed of a totally implantable artificial heart for decades. A totally implantable device would mean no external machinery to tether the recipient.

Congress has generously funded research into the implantable devices, starting forty years ago at the National Institutes of Health. Doctors at that time assumed that developing an artificial heart was essentially an engineering problem and that hearts could be mass-produced, installed, maintained, and monitored, just like replacing parts in your aging car.

Experience proved otherwise, and interest waned until 1967, when the charismatic and handsome Christiaan Barnard performed the first human heart transplant. Barnard's much-heralded surgery spawned further development of the artificial heart program and culminated in a National Institutes of Health (NIH) report that outlined the obstacles as technical: biomaterials and power supply.

In December 1982, Seattle dentist Barney Clark received the first totally artificial heart as a permanent replacement—the Jarvik 7. The heart was not "totally implantable" because it had to be connected to a power source outside the body. On the thirteenth postoperative day, the implanted heart began to fail, and Clark developed an overwhelming infection. He died after 112 days.

But Barney Clark made the artificial heart program famous throughout the world. The media portrayed his surgery as a dramatic bionic event, rather than as a medical experiment. No other medical event had been covered so intensely in the media. Corporations began to talk of mass-producing the hearts, assuming that they would gain acceptance through wide use. As he left the operating room after assisting with the second implantation of an artificial heart, the developer of the heart, Robert Jarvik, commented to the press that the surgery had gone so smoothly that it seemed "routine."[22]

But the progress in the artificial heart, like most major technological advances, occurred at significant cost, both social and economic. Public expenditures on the artificial heart program were high, making some people uneasy about the possibility that the program might siphon off resources needed for other heart research or to provide wider access to basic medical services.

LANDMARKS IN THE DEVELOPMENT OF THE ARTIFICIAL HEART

1953 A heart-lung machine designed by Dr. John Gibbon is used in a successful open-heart surgery, demonstrating that an artificial device can temporarily mimic the functions of the heart.

1964 The National Heart, Lung, and Blood Institute sets a goal of designing a total artificial heart by 1970.

1966 Dr. Michael DeBakey of Houston successfully implants a partial artificial heart.

1967 Dr. Christiaan Barnard performs the first successful human heart transplant. The patient, fifty-three-year-old dentist Louis Washkansky, dies eighteen days after surgery in South Africa.

1969 A total artificial heart is implanted into a patient by Dr. Denton Cooley of the Texas Heart Institute. The patient gets a heart transplant three days later but then dies a day and a half afterward.

1982–1985 Dr. William DeVries carries out a series of five implants of the Jarvik total artificial heart. The first patient, Barney Clark, survives for 112 days. Only four others received the Jarvik as a permanent replacement heart; one, William Schroeder, lived 620 days, dying in August 1986 at the age of fifty-four. Other patients received the Jarvik as a temporary device while awaiting heart transplants.

1994 The Food and Drug Administration approves the left ventricular assist device, which helps failing hearts continue to function.

2001 Doctors at Jewish Hospital in Louisville, Kentucky, implant the first self-contained, mechanical heart replacement into a patient. The device, called the AbioCor, is battery-powered and the size of a softball.

2002 James Quinn dies in a Philadelphia intensive care unit after nine months with an AbioCor heart. Seven of those months were spent in the hospital, and he suffered two strokes

2004 Twelfth patient receives an AbioCor heart, survives eighty-five days. Abiomed, the maker, announces plans to apply for FDA approval by the end of the year, under a "Humanitarian Device Exemption." News reports indicate that up to 4,000 patients a year may be candidates.

Sources: Associated Press; http://www.cnn.com/interactive/health/0106/heart.chronology/frameset.exclude.html; *Boston Globe,* Feb. 23, 2004, p. D1; *Boston Herald,* May 18, 2004, p. 37.

In October 1988, the director of the National Heart, Lung, and Blood Institute at the National Institutes of Health asked the Institute of Medicine (IOM) to evaluate the artificial heart program.[23] The request was prompted in part by an NIH decision to cancel contracts for further development of a totally implantable artificial heart. I (Donald) was a member of that IOM committee, which investigated both the outcomes of end-stage heart disease and the potential impact of a totally implantable artificial heart.

The committee projected that the need for mechanical hearts would be between 35,000 and 70,000 per year through the end of the century. After 2010, the aging of the population would mean a large number of additional candidates. The committee recommended heart transplantation, rather than artificial hearts, as the treatment of choice. The committee concluded that the cost-effectiveness of a total artificial heart was significantly worse than that of other heart disease treatments.

Throughout its deliberations, the IOM committee noted the complex relationship between corporate culture and the artificial heart program. Creating and marketing the Jarvik heart was a business, as is production of the new AbioCor heart. Investors have provided large sums of capital, anticipating a substantial market and large profits. Without private investment, development would probably be impossible, and private-public partnership in building this technology is likely to continue.

Some people have defended the program by invoking national pride, arguing that if the United States didn't develop a total artificial heart, then Japan or Germany would. This raised the specter that the United States would be "left behind" technologically.

In 2001, Robert Tools received the world's first fully implantable artificial heart, saying that it was an easy decision to let surgeons swap his sick heart for a machine. Tools said, "There was no decision to make, really. I would have died without it." He died seven weeks later with it.

The promise of a better artificial heart remains attractive, and some believe that an artificial heart will become a realistic, permanent option for patients with heart failure. An inherent faith in technology, augmented by private business interests, promotes this idea, and suggests a not-too-distant scenario.

The NIH imagined that it would have an artificial heart in 1970. We suspect that the implicit assumptions were: "It's a mechanical problem. Build replacement parts. Technology can fix this. It's easier to invest in technological cures than in behavioral prevention. Death should be avoidable." Thirty-four years later, we're still waiting to see how successful an artificial heart can be, and whether it will siphon resources from other needs. It still offers both exciting promise and a sober reminder of the complexity of the human body.

Consequences of Technoconsumption

Medical advances aren't the major driving force behind improvements in the health of the population as a whole. Public policies regarding water quality, housing, transportation, food quality, education, and even speed limits are more powerful determinants of population health. These policies represent a different kind of technological diffusion, changing environments rather than individuals.

High-technology medicine is intended to help a relatively few people with a particular disease or problem. It contributes little to the well-being of the population as a whole. Nonetheless, medical advances sometimes provide us with the tools to extend the lives of loved ones and prevent disability. It's not easy to weigh the wants and needs of individuals against those of the population as a whole. We have a bias in favor of saving identified individual lives, as opposed to larger numbers of statistical, unidentified lives.

It's also not easy to understand—let alone alter—the social, cultural, and political forces that promote diagnostic and therapeutic technology over health-promotion strategies. Yet health-promotion strategies may produce greater gains in population health. These strategies might include creating environments that promote physical activity, healthier eating habits, and smoking cessation.

It's increasingly important to consider whether we're overusing medical treatment, exaggerating its benefits over its risks, and failing to keep a balance between social change and technological development.

3

Why More Isn't Always Better

Red Herrings, Side Effects, and Superbugs

I remembered an Irish woman who once said to me, "you know, if only you doctors could find a cure for these wretched antibiotics, you would be doing us all a good turn." —John Lister[1]

There were other tests, some of which seemed to me to be more an assertion of the clinical capability of the hospital than of concern for the well-being of the patient. —Norman Cousins[2]

AS WITH buying a house or eating ice cream, it seems that getting more of a good thing is always better. Most of us assume that more medical care can only be a good thing. Americans are convinced that American medicine is the best because we get the most, and that the more we spend for medical care, the better it is.

For many basic medical services, this holds true. Childhood vaccinations, antibiotics for life-threatening infections, and surgery for appendicitis or heart disease can be lifesaving. At a population level, better access to basic services makes a big difference.

But as a nation, we may be at a point of diminishing returns. Increasing our expenditures on health care beyond a certain point may not improve the health of the nation one whit. There could even be a point where spending more for tests, drugs, and surgery will make things worse, leading to irrelevant findings, avoidable side effects, and unnecessary surgery.

Whether, as a society, we've reached that point is a matter of dispute. Everyone in the health-care industry—drug and device makers, hospitals, nurses and doctors—benefits financially when people spend more on medical care. They're quick to agree that more is better. With almost 15 percent of the economy going into health care, a huge number of American jobs depend on this idea. So it's no surprise that any suggestion to the contrary meets stiff resistance.

Even if our society as a whole has reached a point of diminishing returns with regard to health-care costs, some individuals may not be at that point. Someone with no insurance or with limited access to care may be in a very different situation. If such a person were able to make additional expenditures on health care, those expenditures might buy significantly better health. But those who are well insured and face no barriers to care may often be at the point of diminishing returns, or even beyond. For these people, added expenditures are more likely to buy unnecessary tests or treatments, some of which have unintended consequences.

Even if buying more health care is expensive, it often seems that cost is no object. That's because insurance—meaning everyone else—is subsidizing the bills. But those who pay the lion's share of the bills, including major employers, Medicare, and Medicaid, may be more skeptical. Many are wondering if we've collectively reached a plateau of benefit for cost. A few heretics suspect that we've actually passed the point of diminishing returns and are at a point where more expenditures buy worse health, instead of better health, for the public at large.

In the 1970s, the RAND Corporation started a novel experiment, comparing the effects of free medical care to those of insurance that required patients to pay a fraction of the cost. They found that people who got free medical care used much more. For poor people, that was good. Better access to care resulted in better health. But for people with average incomes, the added expenditures didn't improve their health at all. In fact, their increased use of medical care paradoxically led to more worry, pain, and activity limitations.[3–5]

A more recent study was more narrowly focused, but also suggested that beyond a certain point, more access to medical technology doesn't help. This study focused on the highly specialized world of neonatal intensive care units. These units are rich in medical technology—full of heart monitors, breathing machines, and intravenous infusion devices. These units are where premature babies (sometimes unbelievably small) achieve seemingly miraculous survival. Are more neonatologists and more neonatal intensive care units always a good thing?

The study compared regions of the country with a large supply of these units to regions where there were fewer. As you might expect, babies were more likely to survive in regions where there was a moderate supply of these units than in regions where there were very few. But in areas that exceeded the moderate supply, having more specialists and neonatal intensive care beds didn't help. There simply was an oversupply, leading to use of intensive care units when they weren't needed. In other words, having some neonatal intensive care available is good, but there's a point beyond which adding more doesn't help. The researchers noted that intensive testing and treatment for infants who don't need it can lead to errors and complications, and can interfere with bonding between mother and baby.[6]

An editorial accompanying this study in the *New England Journal of Medicine* suggested that neonatal intensive care units and specialists were proliferating in part for financial reasons. The units are moneymakers for hospitals, and doctors are attracted to the specialty because they can earn more than general pediatricians. The editorialist argued that the situation was "emblematic of how a market-driven health care system with inadequate public planning produces too much of a good thing."[7] We'd argue that this narrow example is emblematic of what's happening in many areas of medicine. Technology is good up to a point, but beyond that point, it's just cost without benefit.

Some People Who Get Care Don't Need It

How could more care actually make things worse? One of my (Rick's) patients illustrated how things can go awry when people get too much care. This fellow's visit to the emergency room for a nonemergency problem set off a cascade of treatments and serious complications that proved unnecessary.

David Grohman was an elderly retiree who came to the emergency room complaining of difficulty seeing. David had been in the movie industry, and was perhaps prone to dramatizing his complaints. His actual words, he later told me, were, "I'm going blind." Because of David's age, the emergency room doctor was concerned that David might have temporal arteritis. This is a rare condition involving arteries in the head that can cause permanent visual loss. Even though a screening test for temporal arteritis was normal, the doctor was anxious and hedged his bets by starting high doses of prednisone. This potent anti-inflammatory drug is similar to cortisone. Over the next few days, David experienced a well-known complication of prednisone: the new onset of diabetes.

Shortly thereafter, he suffered a severe complication of diabetes: a condition called hyperosmolar coma. He also had psychiatric symptoms that are known to occur with high doses of prednisone. He was hospitalized twice and had a biopsy of his temporal artery. The pathologist read the biopsy as normal, but hedged his interpretation. Because of the prednisone treatment, he couldn't rule out partly treated temporal arteritis. So the hospital doctors continued the prednisone.

When I saw David in the outpatient clinic, I decided to taper the dose of prednisone, which David had now been taking for about two months. When we succeeded in stopping it entirely, David's diabetes and psychiatric symptoms promptly disappeared. He had no further vision complaints, and on detailed questioning, it appeared that the original visual problem was simply presbyopia. This is the common problem of older adults who have difficulty reading or focusing up close.

This seemed to be a story not so much of bad care as of excessive care, initiated by uncertainty and anxiety in the emergency room. Had the emergency room doctor gotten more details about the symptoms and been more comfortable with even slight ambiguity, he might have spared David the serious complications and expensive hospitalizations. Had David waited until the next day and seen a doctor in the regular clinic instead of going to the emergency room at night, different decisions might have been made. In spite of two hospitalizations for life-threatening complications, the hospital doctors didn't seriously question whether the original diagnosis was correct or whether David needed the prednisone. The bias for action overrode obvious signs that the treatment was causing harm and the possibility that the original treatment decision was based on anxiety more than need. David suffered from too much medical care.

Some forms of excessive care, like the overuse of antibiotics, are becoming familiar to the public. Nearly half of all antibiotic prescriptions are for colds and related symptoms, even though most of these conditions are viral infections that don't benefit from antibiotics. Many of these drugs cause occasional side effects, turning useless treatment into harmful treatment. This "prescriptive promiscuity," as one expert calls it,[8] increasingly involves broad-spectrum antibiotics, which kill a wide variety of bacteria. Excessive use of such drugs is a major contributor to the emergence of resistant bacteria: germs that can't be killed with antibiotics.

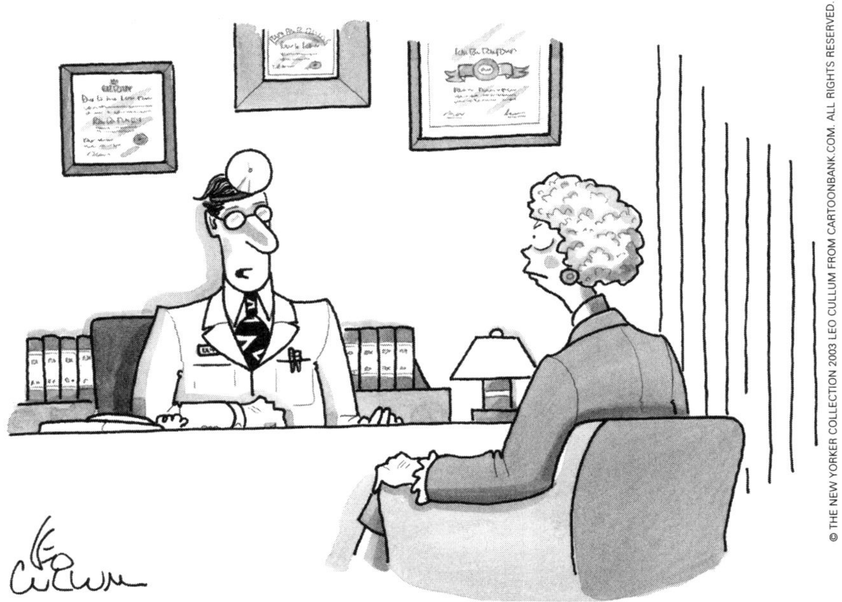

"You may believe you've been overcharged, but, remember, you're overmedicated."

These resistant bacteria are often called "superbugs." So giving antibiotics for colds generally falls into the category of useless therapy that sometimes turns harmful and can make things worse for all of us. Sometimes more isn't better.

It's increasingly apparent that expenditures for health care are only loosely associated with health itself. It's common knowledge that the United States spends more per capita on health care than any other country, yet our life expectancy and infant mortality are worse than those in most European countries and Japan.[9] This in itself may not be a symptom of too much medical care, but it does suggest that higher spending hasn't bought better health.

More surprising to many people is the enormous geographic variability in health-care use within the United States. For example, surgery rates for back pain literally vary all over the map. There's four times more back surgery per 1,000 people in Boise, Idaho, than in Manhattan.[10] Within Washington State, back surgery rates vary sevenfold among the largest counties. Some of the highest rates are in small communities, while the biggest city, Seattle, has a fairly low rate.[11]

Many experts suspect that this means that doctors in some areas do too much back surgery. The employers who pay the bills wonder why they should pay for services that seem to exceed the norm. But it may also be that too little surgery is done in some areas. This could result in unnecessary pain. What surgery rate is right?

To answer that question, we'd like to know what rate gives the best overall health results. However, this information is hard to come by. Like most things that bring us to the doctor, back pain isn't fatal, and the treatments are generally low risk. So we can't just look at death rates to decide what surgery rate is right. However, under the leadership of Dr. Bob Keller, a Maine orthopedist, we studied back surgery results in geographic regions with high, low, and medium rates of back surgery.

We did the study in Maine, where most orthopedic surgeons and neurosurgeons in the state were willing to participate. The results were surprisingly clear. We found the best surgery results, in terms of pain and disability, in the part of the state with the lowest surgery rate. We found the worst results in the area where surgery rates were the highest. The region with a middling surgery rate had middling results.

You may wonder whether surgeons in the low-rate area got better results just because their patients weren't as sick. In fact, this wasn't the case. Before surgery, patients in the low-rate area had equally severe pain and disability, and more abnormalities on spine-imaging tests.[12]

It seemed that the surgeons who were least likely to operate were best at determining which patients would benefit from surgery. They had a higher threshold for recommending surgery, and they got the best results. This in turn suggested that some of the surgery in the high-rate areas was unnecessary or even harmful. Again, sometimes more isn't better.

The possibility that some operations are unnecessary extends well beyond back surgery. International comparisons indicate that U.S. doctors perform surgery at a much higher rate than those in other developed countries.[13] That might be okay if all the operations were beneficial. But an early study of surgical second opinion programs found that almost 18 percent of recommendations for surgery weren't supported by the second evaluation, leading to questions about the need for them in the first place.[14]

A congressional subcommittee concluded that perhaps 2.4 million unnecessary operations are performed annually in the United States, at a cost of $3.9 billion and 11,900 deaths. Using expert criteria, studies have shown high rates of unnecessary heart bypass operations, hysterectomies, pacemaker insertions, and tonsillectomies. Dr. Lucian Leape, a surgeon at the Harvard School of Public Health, worries that the combination of risk and the promise of a dramatic cure gives surgery an aura of excitement. Doctors and patients alike may mentally minimize the risks when a "cure" seems within their grasp.[14]

National statistics confirm that some forms of medical care are inherently risky. In 2000, a national survey showed that a leading reason for hospitalization was complications from surgically implanted devices and grafts. These complications trailed only various forms of heart disease, pneumonia, and childbirth as a reason why people landed in the hospital. Adding complications from other types of medical treatment gave a staggering total. Treatment complications accounted for 914,000 hospitalizations, at a cost of $19 billion. Many of these complications were probably due not to errors, but to the inherent risks of medical treatment. This isn't a reason to avoid medical care, but it argues for caution.[15]

Some People Who Need Care Get Too Much

Like excessive antibiotic use, the complaint of overly aggressive care for terminally ill patients is becoming a familiar story. Some patients die with monitors, catheters, and intensive care that neither the patient nor the family wants. Such patients may be overtreated but under-cared for.

In a study of hospitalized patients over age eighty, researchers examined preferences for care and actual treatment in four hospitals scattered throughout the United States. Most of the patients who died in the hospital said that they didn't want aggressive care. Fully 70 percent wanted care that was focused on comfort rather than on prolonging life, suggesting that only 30 percent preferred life-sustaining treatments. Nonetheless, 63 percent received at least one life-sustaining treatment before they died, including admission to intensive care, mechanical breathing, surgery, and kidney dialysis.[16]

Only in retrospect may patients' families and doctors realize that they were drawn into aggressive care by frequent diagnostic tests, close monitoring, and conscientious efforts to identify "reversible" problems. Unfortunately, any benefit from making a new diagnosis or providing a perfect treatment for such patients may be minuscule. This is because they usually have multiple problems and are highly susceptible to complications.

A remarkable study of Medicare patients in their last six months of life seems to confirm that there's a problem. Dr. Elliott Fisher, with his colleagues at Dartmouth Medical School and the Maine Medical Center, found that doctors in some cities spend 60 percent more on care for these patients than do doctors in other cities. The high-cost cities included Los Angeles, New York, Miami, Chicago, Detroit, and Philadelphia, among others. The low-cost areas included San Francisco, Seattle, Minneapolis, Denver, and Rochester, New York.

Unfortunately, the quality of care was no better in the high-spending areas. Treatments that are known to be effective were used equally in the different areas. There was little difference in the use of major surgery or the quality of outpatient care. Instead, the extra $2,300 per person in the high-cost areas bought more doctor visits, more specialist visits, more tests and minor procedures, and more days in the hospital. Patients in the high-cost areas who were close to death were more likely to get feeding tubes, emergency kidney dialysis, and breathing machines. So for patients in the last six months of life, some areas of the country provide much more expensive care than others, without a clear advantage in quality of care.[17]

Fisher's analysis of Medicare data yielded some other startling findings. The researchers chose three common serious conditions—colon cancer, heart attacks, and hip fractures—to examine the costs and outcomes of treatment in detail. The likelihood of dying from one of these conditions was actually higher in regions with more expensive styles of care.

In yet another analysis, Fisher examined access to care and preventive services among all Medicare patients. He found that those in high-cost areas had no better access to care, and were actually less likely to get flu shots, mammograms, or Pap smears. Altogether, Fisher's study of Medicare patients showed that the higher cost of care in some areas didn't deliver longer life, better access to doctors, or better preventive care. It seemed to deliver cost without benefit. Sometimes more isn't better.[17,18]

Sometimes Patients Prefer More Care, Even When It Doesn't Help

Paradoxically, some studies suggest that patients may be more satisfied when more is done, even if what is done doesn't improve their health. Researchers at nine VA hospitals tested the benefit of more doctor visits and more frequent telephone follow-up for patients discharged from the hospital. They studied patients with chronic problems: heart failure, diabetes, or emphysema. Unexpectedly, patients who got closer follow-up were more likely to be rehospitalized and spent more days in the hospital than patients who just got their usual care. There were no differences in quality of life between the groups. Nonetheless, those with closer follow-up were more satisfied with their care.[19] This suggested that the added attention and care made patients happier but not healthier.

In a study of patients with persistent back pain, researchers assigned half to get back x-rays and the other half to receive no x-rays. Those who had x-rays were more likely to have pain at follow-up and had slightly worse daily functioning. Nonetheless, those in the x-ray group were more satisfied with their care than those who received no x-rays.[20] In this case, the added testing made patients happier, even though it may have made their health worse.

Yet another example comes from the treatment of men with early prostate cancer. Some doctors recommend a drug such as Lupron that stops production of male hormones. This treatment amounts to a medical castration. There's no definitive evidence that early treatment with these drugs alone can improve the length or quality of life in men with localized prostate cancer. The proven value of these drugs is only in reducing symptoms in men with more advanced cancer. A recent study showed that when doctors gave this treatment to men with early disease who had no symptoms, it led to more impotence, breast swelling, hot flashes, and discomfort than in men who weren't treated. However, despite having worse symptoms and quality of life, the men who got treatment, as opposed to watchful waiting, were more satisfied with their care.[21]

This finding—that patients sometimes like more care even if it doesn't improve their health—has important implications for the costs of medical care and what we as a society want to pay for. Many people with medical problems like more attention and having more things done. Maybe they feel that their problems are being taken more seriously, maybe they feel more reassured, maybe they feel more cared for, or maybe they prefer actively doing something to a "wait and see" approach.

For those with insurance, the response may be, "Who cares? It's relatively harmless, and people like it." Because insurance picks up the tab, it seems free. But the rising cost of insurance—in some cases, to pay for things that don't improve health—is exactly why more and more people can't afford insurance. And as we've seen, unnecessary care isn't always harmless. So an important question becomes, how much are you willing to increase your insurance premiums or Medicare taxes to accommodate care that satisfies but doesn't improve health?

Risks of Too Many Tests: Red Herrings and False Impressions

Newer diagnostic tests are aggravating the problem of excessive care. CT and MRI scans offer amazing inside pictures of the body. But they also reveal tiny abnormalities that would once have gone unnoticed. Intuition tells us that this must be good, but it turns out that many of these abnormalities are red herrings.

Again, the problem of back pain offers good examples. Experts have concluded that perhaps 85 percent of patients with back pain can't be given a definitive diagnosis, despite the best medical evaluation. In part, this is because so many structures in the spine can give rise to pain, including muscles, ligaments, bones, nerve roots, and parts of the discs between vertebrae. X-rays and MRI scans often can't distinguish which of these is the true source of an individual's pain.[22,23]

And we now know that bulging, degenerated, and even herniated discs in the spine are common among healthy people with no symptoms.[23] When doctors find such discs in people with back pain, the discs may be irrelevant, but they are likely to lead to more tests, patient anxiety, and perhaps even unnecessary surgery. In fact, back surgery rates are highest where MRI rates are the highest.[24] In a randomized trial, we found that doing an MRI instead of a plain x-ray led to more back surgery, but didn't improve the overall results of treatment.[25]

Because we see more things on these scans, certain medical problems seem to be becoming more common year after year. This is not because abnormalities are getting more common; it's only that we're more likely to discover them. But finding things makes doctors and patients more enthusiastic about doing the tests and seems to justify them. Many of these abnormalities are trivial, harmless, and irrelevant, so they've been dubbed "incidentalomas."

Nonetheless, these incidentalomas sometimes get treated. It's easy to be fooled into thinking that if the patient does fine, it's because we found an abnormality and treated it.[22] But with an incidentaloma, the patient was destined to get better anyway because the condition was a nondisease to begin with. However, patients are grateful for a good outcome and often attribute their success to finding the abnormality early on.

So excessive testing creates a dual illusion: Abnormalities seem ever more common, and our treatments for them seem ever more effective. These illusions reinforce the habit of doing tests, creating a vicious cycle.[26] This may partly account for the popularity of CT and MRI scans among consumers, some of whom are willing to pay out-of-pocket for screening with these tests.

In addition to unearthing irrelevant abnormalities, every diagnostic test is occasionally wrong. Just as every treatment has some risk of side effects, every test has some risk of inaccurate results. *False positive* refers to a positive test in someone who really has no disease. *False negative* refers to a negative test in someone who really does have the disease. These false-positive and false-negative test results can mislead both doctors and patients. Interpretation of test results is rarely straightforward. Statistically speaking, the more tests you have, the more likely it is that you will have an abnormal result. Although doctors often identify erroneous results through repeat testing or ancillary tests, false positives can result in unnecessary anxiety and unnecessary costs. And they can sometimes lead to disastrous mistakes in treatment.

The story of Jennifer Rufer is extreme, but it illustrates the point. Rufer was a twenty-two-year-old married Seattle woman who hoped to have lots of children. Then blood tests repeatedly suggested a rare form of cancer in her uterus. She underwent chemotherapy, but the test stayed positive, leading to a hysterectomy. Even after surgery, the test remained abnormal; it was repeated a total of forty-four times. Her doctor, fearful that the cancer had spread, ordered more chemotherapy and a full-body scan, which showed a suspicious spot on her lung. A portion of her lung was removed, but the test still remained abnormal. Rufer's husband, David, spent the first years of their marriage supporting Jennifer through her ordeal, watching her lose weight, and posing for what they thought would be their last Christmas picture together.

Eventually, a different test kit was used, and it gave a conflicting result. Rufer's blood samples were then reviewed by doctors at Yale University, who concluded that her tests had been false positives all along. The original test, made by Abbott Laboratories, had had other false positives reported. A lawsuit against both Rufer's doctor and Abbott Laboratories followed. In 2001, this resulted in a jury award of $15 million for pain and suffering; $452,000 more for economic damages, including lost wages and the cost of having children using a surrogate mother; and $750,000 to

David Rufer for pain and suffering. Newspapers reported that one juror nearly cried when talking about what happened to Rufer, saying, "Here's somebody who went to the doctor for medical help and got hurt for the rest of her life. I can't even talk about the tragedy involved in this case." [27–30]

Do Doctors and Hospitals Create Their Own Demand?

One problem is that having trained many doctors and specialists, we must let them make a living. Lots of medical care is in a gray zone, where there's no single correct course of action, so it's easy to imagine that doctors and hospitals might begin to lower the threshold for doing tests or giving treatments. This can help them to stay financially viable. In studying back surgery rates internationally, we found that surgery rates correlated fairly well with a country's per capita supply of orthopedic surgeons and neurosurgeons. Both the surgery rate and the number of surgeons were highest in the United States.[13] Thus, it may be that in some cases, doctors create a demand for their own services.

Other evidence for this possibility comes from studies of Medicare that have examined what happens when Medicare cuts reimbursement to doctors for a particular service. When the price of a specialized service drops, doctors tend to do more or order more, so that the higher volume compensates for the drop in price per service. Doctors see patients more often, order more tests, and perform more surgery.[31] Similarly, in areas where there are more hospital beds, more patients get admitted to the hospital. The axiom that "a hospital bed built is a hospital bed filled" was named "Roemer's law" in honor of the researcher who described the phenomenon.[32]

In his studies of Medicare spending, Dartmouth's Elliott Fisher found that having more hospital beds and doctors in a region didn't increase the use of effective treatments. Instead, a greater supply increased the use of more discretionary things, where any benefit was less clear. These included more office visits, tests, consultations, hospital admissions, days in the hospital, and treatments at the end of life. There are no clear-cut guidelines for these decisions, which Fisher labels "supply sensitive."[33,34]

Sociologist Henry Vandenburgh, in his book *Feeding Frenzy,* describes supplier-induced demand run amok. He reports the methods used by some for-profit Texas psychiatric hospitals to recruit patients in the early 1990s. These hospitals created "suction" intake departments, aiming to hospitalize at least 30 percent of callers who responded to advertisements. They used professional patient finders, who set up support groups for parents of rowdy teenagers. Some patient finders received the equivalent of $1,500 for each patient they brought into the hospital. Doctors were also sometimes paid for referrals to the hospitals. In some cases, counselors were posted at public schools, free of charge, to direct teens with "good" insurance to the hospital. Similarly, employees were posted with probation officers, with police officers, and in emergency rooms, where they competed for patients by offering free assessments. Once patients were admitted, doctors were manipulated by administrators into avoiding discharge until the patient's insurance payments were exhausted. Fortunately, these practices were eventually exposed, and the worst abuses were eliminated by a combination of managed-care incentives, new regulations, and certificate of need restrictions on hospital beds.[35]

The Sting

Employers, who pay most of the bills, are increasingly concerned about buying inefficient and ineffective medical care. The Midwest Business Group on Health recently estimated that $390 billion is spent each year on overuse or inefficient use of medical care. The figure amounted to a third of all health-care expenditures.[36]

It may be hard to believe that a third of all medical costs are wasted. But the RAND Corporation arrived independently at a similar estimate.[37] As examples of wasteful care, the Midwest Business Group cited overuse of surgery, tests, and medicines. It also cited the consequences of failing to provide effective preventive care. The report suggested that the problem wasn't the price of medical services. Instead, the Midwest Business Group was mainly concerned that some services were unnecessary or of poor quality. The American Hospital Association and the American Medical Association were quick to dismiss the group's findings.

If some services are overused and many complications are avoidable, why is there little public outcry? First, remember that many people are more satisfied when they get more care, even if that care doesn't improve their health. Also, most people who get unnecessary care don't know it. If your back operation was unnecessary, but you got better anyway, you're likely to feel that you had good care. The patient who takes unnecessary antibiotics has no way of knowing it. More likely, he'll be outraged if his insurance company refuses to pay for the care. Thus, there are rarely identifiable victims.

Those who remember the movie *The Sting* will recall that the good guys—Redford and Newman—wanted a ruse that would let them swindle a murderous Mafia boss out of staggering sums of money. The ruse had to be so good, though, that the vengeful bad guy would never even suspect that he'd been had.

Doctors and hospitals usually don't knowingly swindle patients, but huge amounts can be spent on useless tests or treatments. There aren't clear-cut good guys or bad guys here. But the sting is that most patients never recognize the waste or the unnecessary risk, and are usually grateful for their care. They assume that more is better. Medical professionals, hospitals, and medical manufacturers conveniently benefit from this assumption, and typically share it.

A friend in San Francisco, Dr. Seth Landefeld, introduced us to the Japanese word *muda. Muda* refers to wasted resources, lost opportunities, and unintended consequences. He noted that we can all point to medical miracles, or at least marvels, and be proud of them. But he went on to describe several patients whose well-meaning care resulted in complications, pain, or extended suffering. He concluded, "So many choices made by doctors and patients lead to *muda* rather than marvels, choices that may too often be influenced by unrealistic hopes for a miracle. . . . There is always room in medicine for hope, but not for biased or magical thinking."[38]

4

Why Newer Isn't Always Better

Unpleasant Surprises, Recalls, and Learning Curves

The scientists of the 1940's and 1950's were coming up with drugs that treated what was never before treatable . . . . It was a heady time. Arrogance came out of real accomplishment, not thin air. But along with accomplishment was this incredible shortsightedness. I don't know if the two can be divorced. —Dr. David Mock, whose mother received diethylstilbestrol[1]

"MY DOCTOR told me he had the magic bullet," according to Chris Vanselous, recounting her story to the *Washington Post*. She had miscarried six babies when her doctor prescribed diethylstilbestrol, or DES, which was then a new synthetic estrogen. Vanselous recalled, "He said I'd have a bigger, healthier, brighter child." She did have a baby this time, but her daughter, Jill, was born with abnormal reproductive organs that led to infertility.

In 1999, after growing up and marrying, Jill settled a lawsuit with drug maker Eli Lilly, once the largest distributor of DES; she hoped that funds from the settlement would help her in adopting a child.[2] In addition to causing infertility in some daughters of women who took DES, the drug, we now know, is associated with a rare form of vaginal cancer in the daughters. Recent studies suggest a higher risk of breast cancer, as well.[3,4]

A biochemist synthesized DES in 1938, and it became popular in 1947, when two Harvard University professors theorized that high doses could prevent miscarriages. In the 1950s, though, studies began to show that the drug didn't prevent miscarriages at all—one of many cases in which theory and reality diverge. The drug hadn't improved Chris Vanselous's chances of having a baby; she was just lucky the seventh time around.

Then, in the late 1960s, an association with vaginal cancer was observed among the daughters of women who had taken DES in pregnancy. In 1971, the FDA issued a bulletin warning doctors not to prescribe DES for pregnant women.[3,4]

Doctors, patients, and the media had initially hailed DES as a wonder drug. It was widely prescribed for pregnant women to prevent miscarriages, and was often prescribed "just in case" to assure strong babies. Doctors prescribed it for millions of pregnant women between 1938 and 1971. It also was widely used to suppress lactation after childbirth, as a morning-after contraceptive, to slow growth in tall teenage girls, and to treat acne. Farmers fed it to livestock as a growth stimulator, so it showed up in hamburger, veal, and chicken for consumption. It was a highly profitable drug, made by some two hundred drug companies and sold under three hundred names.[1,5]

But then the bad news about complications began rolling in. After thirty years, DES went from being a wonder drug to being "the time bomb drug" in the media.[1,5] When Chris Vanselous first took DES, she undoubtedly thought that the new drug was a major advance, and so did her doctor. Time proved them wrong.

Newer is better, we think, especially when medical technology is involved. It seems logical that anything new must have built on what we had learned from our previous experience with drugs, operations, or devices, and thus must be an improvement. Many people assume that the Food and Drug Administration (FDA) wouldn't approve anything that wasn't better than existing products. Direct-to-consumer marketing always implies that newer is better, and so does the marketing aimed at doctors.

In the aggregate, it's true that medical advances offer real benefits. But false starts like DES are surprisingly common. Take a step back and consider some recent "breakthroughs" that were widely used before they were debunked. Doctors and patients alike hailed high-dose chemotherapy with bone marrow transplantation for late-stage breast cancer as a breakthrough. Patients sued to get insurance coverage for the new procedure, and states passed laws requiring coverage. But in the end, the procedure proved no more effective than standard care, and was more toxic and more expensive.[6,7]

Less dramatic but equally important was the recent news that old-fashioned diuretic drugs (water pills) are more effective than newer and more expensive drugs for preventing the complications of high blood pressure. Despite their greater effectiveness, the diuretics had steadily lost ground to the newer drugs, which companies had been marketing heavily both to the public and to doctors.[8,9]

Maybe the most familiar and dramatic reminder that newer isn't necessarily better is the occasional recall of new drugs from the market. Recalls generally occur because unexpected complications are discovered after a new drug becomes widely used. The same process occurs with new medical devices. How is it that new medical treatments sometimes get disseminated while they're still only half-baked?

Recalls and Risks of New Drugs and Devices

Sometimes the "latest and greatest" advances are fraught with risks that haven't been discovered when these advances hit the market. In fact, there's some heightened risk every time a new operation, drug, or gadget enters the medical world. A familiar example was phen-fen (phentermine and fenfluramine), the diet pills that were pulled from the market in 1997 after some patients taking the drug developed heart valve problems. Altogether, fourteen drugs were withdrawn from the market between 1997 and 2001 because of serious side effects. Many of these were "me too" drugs that had no advantage over readily available alternatives. None of the drugs was for a life-threatening condition.[10]

The withdrawal of Baycol, a cholesterol-lowering drug, was typical in many ways and illustrates some of the problems. The Bayer Corporation marketed the drug in 1997 in a low-dose tablet. It was introduced even though there were already five similar drugs on the market. These made up a class of drugs called statins that are chemically similar and that all lower cholesterol by inhibiting the same enzyme. Though it did indeed lower cholesterol, Baycol was less effective than other drugs at its initial low dose and caused more serious side effects at higher doses.[11]

The FDA warned the company in 1999 that some of its sales materials were "false, lacking in fair balance or otherwise misleading," and that they minimized "the most important risk information."[12] Data on the risks were accumulating, and the FDA noticed an increase in adverse events after approving a higher dose.

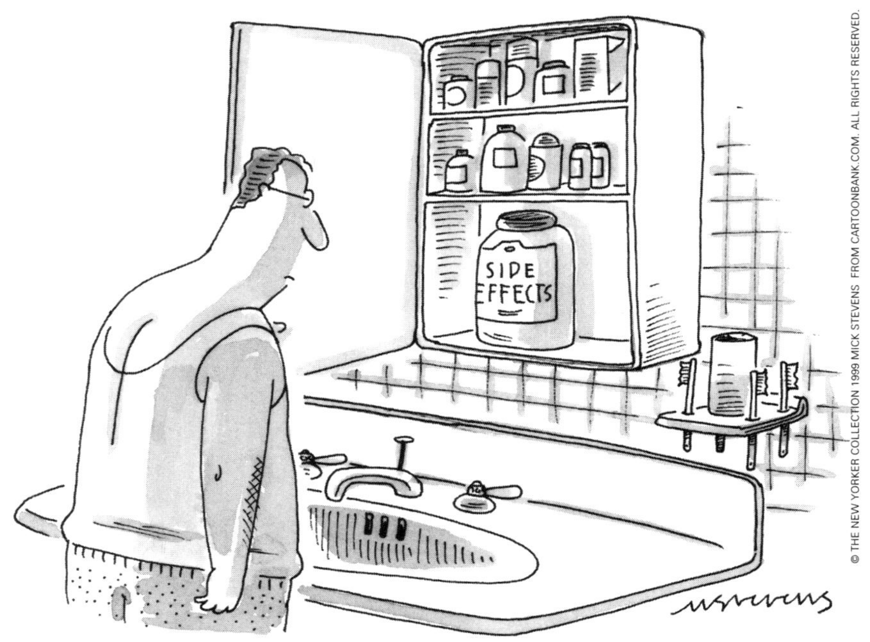

Despite these limitations, the company marketed the drug effectively, and some six million people took it. Sales in 2001 were expected to hit $600 million, and it was one of the company's fastest-growing products.[11]

In the meantime, though, reports had linked approximately one hundred deaths and sixteen hundred injuries to the drug. The drug was finally recalled in 2001. After reviewing the increase in complications, an FDA official said, "It took time and tragedy to understand it was different."[11]

Recalls of medical devices are also common. A recent analysis of FDA records showed that between 1990 and 2000, there were twenty-eight recalls of heart pacemakers, affecting over 300,000 devices.[13] The Bjork-Shiley convexo-concave artificial heart valve was a popular model, and surgeons implanted the valve in over 82,000 patients worldwide. But the valve was withdrawn from the market in 1986 because of an unexpectedly high failure rate.[14] Many patients still have them in place, and their doctors must now weigh risks and benefits in deciding whether to recommend repeat surgery to replace the defective valves.

Even seemingly simple products sometimes raise worrisome concerns. In 2003, sales of Gynecare Intergel, a gel used in gynecological surgery to reduce the formation of scar tissue, were suspended after seventy-two reports of adverse events, including three deaths and forty-eight injuries. Investigation is underway regarding reports of pain and repeat operations that might be linked to the gel. Roughly eighty thousand doses of the gel have been sold in the United States and other countries.[15,16]

These are examples from a long list of similar problems that might temper the rush to be first in line to try new medical treatments. Some critics argue that the FDA is too quick to approve new drugs and devices, thanks to pressure from industry, political posturing, and public demand. Other critics argue that the agency is too slow.

One problem is that manufacturers conduct pre-market testing on relatively small numbers of patients, with relatively short periods of follow-up. If they did otherwise, new products would be even slower to come to market. Testing is often restricted to relatively healthy patients without multiple medical problems or medications. These limitations on testing mean that unusual side effects—even serious ones—often remain undiscovered when new products reach the market. These harmful effects become apparent only after widespread use of the new products.[17–19]

A recent report suggested that the cost of complications and mortality from prescription drugs in the United States is more than $177 billion a year. This exceeds the expenditures for the drugs themselves. This is a crude estimate that depends in part on expert opinion and includes the costs of failing to take medication as prescribed. On the other hand, it doesn't include the costs of work absenteeism or decreased productivity related to side effects.[20,21] Even if the real costs are only half as much, drug complications add a huge sum to the national medical bill.

Exaggerating Benefits

Even when treatments prove effective, doctors tend to overestimate their benefits and underestimate their risks. Consider the story of Tom Nesi, a former director of public affairs at the drug company Bristol-Myers Squibb. In a *New York Times* article, Nesi described his wife, Susan, who was fifty-two when she was found to have a highly malignant brain cancer. They were told that the average survival with this condition was about eleven months, but they hoped for more.

They sought care from a prestigious medical center that offered several innovative treatments. One, called a Gliadel wafer, is a dime-sized wafer that is implanted in the brain when the tumor is surgically removed. The goal is to deliver chemotherapy directly to the tumor site. The Nesis were told that this would extend Susan's life, on average, about two months. In the ensuing months, Susan underwent three brain operations and six hospitalizations. After the third operation, she was almost totally paralyzed and unable to speak or eat. In her final months, she required two weeks in a critical care center, a full-time home health aide, a feeding tube and electronic monitor, home hospital equipment, occupational therapists, social workers, and medication. Her costs of care were around $200,000.

Susan lived three months longer than average, so many doctors would describe the innovative treatment as a success. After the disastrous third operation, her surgeon told Tom: "We have saved your wife's life . . . we have given you the ability to spend more quality time with your loved one." Two weeks later, sustained by the feeding tube, Susan wrote on a notepad, "Depressed . . . no more . . . please."

Tom then faced a decision as to whether to stop the feeding tube and withhold liquids. He concluded his story by noting, "I think we need to ask ourselves whether offering terminal patients limited hope of a few more months is really beneficial. The question is not whether days are extended, but in what condition the patient lives and at what emotional and financial cost."[22]

This is a story of well-meaning doctors and a desperate patient. The presumption of both parties must have been that new technology could only help. As usual, the bias was to do something, to be aggressive. In the end, the treatment may have been worse than the disease. In many such cases, doctors tend to see only the good side of their interventions. They sometimes dismiss, discount, or are wholly unaware of the downsides, which often diminish quality of life. And although new treatments often claim great benefits, we need to critically ask what the benefits are, and what we are giving up in order to have them.

Bad News Is Sometimes Uncovered Only Slowly

Sometimes treatments are widely used for years before problems are discovered. The story of DES is an example of the delay that sometimes happens in uncovering the risks of new medical treatments. It took decades for the worst complications to become known, and new research is still discovering problems among the children and grandchildren of women who took DES.

The history of hormone replacement therapy for menopausal women has followed a similar time course. This treatment has been popular for decades, and women still use it for symptoms like hot flashes. But many doctors and many women thought that it also reduced the risk of heart disease, making long-term use desirable. Only in the last three years have rigorous studies shown that these hormones offer no protection from heart disease; in fact, they increase the risks of blood clots, breast cancer, and other side effects. In 2002, researchers stopped the most definitive study early when it appeared that the risk of long-term use outweighed the benefit.[23,24]

Similarly, high-dose oxygen therapy for premature infants was widely used for more than a decade (1942–1954) before researchers linked it to rentrolental fibroplasia, a condition that blinded about ten thousand children. The condition, renamed retinopathy of prematurity in recent years, was a key factor in the blindness of popular musician Stevie Wonder, born in 1950. The doctor-caused epidemic was a result of conviction about the value of treatment, failure to suspect medical therapy as a cause, and a series of shortsighted or badly designed research studies that failed to uncover the risks.[25,26] Such dramatic examples come in a slow but steady stream, and further recommend caution in seeking new treatments.

Risks of New Surgical Procedures

Like new drugs and devices, new operations or surgical techniques sometimes become widely used before anyone realizes that they're flops. Dr. David Flum, a general surgeon at the University of Washington, cites a now obsolete operation for severe obesity that involved connecting the first part of the intestine directly to the last part (jejuno-ileal bypass), bypassing most of the small intestine. "This procedure was being widely used in the 70's and 80's, until we realized that people were developing malnutrition, not absorbing key nutrients, and even sometimes dying," he says. "It's an operation that was embraced because it was a novel idea, but it wasn't really given the appropriate level of testing, which became evident only after the procedure was done for several years." Doctors now use other types of obesity surgery that offer greater safety, although some experts worry that even the new procedures are riskier than doctors and patients realize.[27]

In 2002, researchers found that a popular type of knee surgery for arthritis doesn't work. The operation involves inserting a fiber-optic scope into the knee, flushing out any debris, and shaving rough areas of cartilage. (This is different from operations to repair torn ligaments or cartilage resulting from injuries, which are effective.) Although it took seven years to get the study funded by the federal government, researchers found that the operation for arthritis was no more effective than a sham operation, where a small incision was made in the skin, but nothing else was done.[28] Such eye-openers are another reason not to be first in line for a new operation.

In Surgery, Practice Makes Perfect—But Do You Really Want to Be Practiced On?

Even when new surgical techniques prove successful, there's a long and sometimes difficult shakedown period associated with their adoption. The introduction of the fiber-optic laparoscope for "minimally invasive" abdominal surgery offers an example. Consider the experience of a friend, Jim Hudson.

On a sunny June day in 1991, Jim reported to the hospital to have his gallbladder removed, expecting to eliminate the belly pain that had plagued him for three months. The fact that he was to have laparoscopic surgery calmed some of his anxieties. This was a brand new technique that used a fiber-optic scope and required only tiny incisions, instead of a gaping eight-inch incision. Scarring would be minimal. He'd be in and out of the hospital the same day, and visiting his horses at the farm the next. Instead, he nearly bought the farm.

Immediately after surgery, things didn't seem right. Jim was sweating heavily and passed out in the recovery room, so he was transferred to a hospital bed. After his wife insisted that something was drastically wrong, his nurse found that his blood pressure was barely measurable, so the surgeon whisked Jim back to the operating room for suspected bleeding. He was slit from breastbone to pubic bone so that his intestines could be pulled aside. There his surgeon found a nicked artery that "pumped blood half way across the room," as Jim was later told. Seven days and many pints of blood later (he lost one-third of his blood), Jim went home to a slow recovery. He took as souvenirs a fourteen-inch incision, concerns about his transfusions, and protracted squabbles with his insurance company over the long hospital stay. He was lucky he survived.

But is luck really what you want to depend on? Unwittingly, Jim was part of the learning curve for laparoscopic surgery, which was brand new in 1991. Doctors, nurses, and other staff were still learning the details. Complications still happen, and there's no guarantee that the same events wouldn't occur today. But the risk was higher ten years ago precisely because this was a new technique, and everyone was still learning it. The more experience a surgical team has with any type of operation, the lower the complication rate.

Don't get us wrong. Laparoscopic surgery for removing the gallbladder is a good thing. It's now the standard method. It's shortened recovery times and even reduced operative mortality (deaths per 1,000 operations) for most people who need their gallbladders out.

But Dr. Flum, the University of Washington surgeon, has studied the most common complications from laparoscopic gallbladder surgery. He

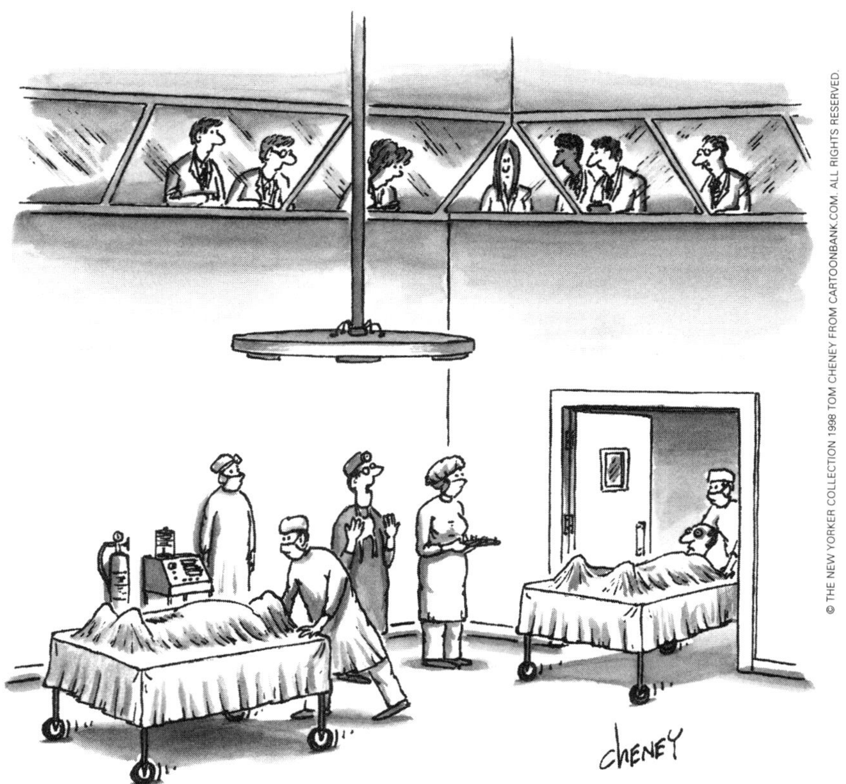

"Next, an example of the very same procedure when done correctly."

discovered that complication rates fell by 10 percent each year from 1991 through 1998.[29] According to Flum, the drop occurred because "everyone was gaining experience. Surgeons perfected the technique, and shared their experiences. Operating room nurses learned the routines. Everyone learned the pitfalls and how to avoid them. Not only does experience improve an operation, it improves our skill at figuring out who's most likely to benefit."

Surgery for heartburn (to reduce the reflux of stomach acid into the esophagus) is another example that illustrates the learning curve. The most common technique, called the Nissen fundoplication, is increasingly popular. In this operation, part of the stomach is folded up around the lower end of the esophagus to make a tighter entrance into the stomach. Like gallbladder surgery, this operation once required an extensive incision, but it's now done with the fiber-optic scope.

As with gallbladder surgery, Flum found that complications with the laparoscopic approach fell steadily after its introduction. One complication is accidentally nicking the spleen, which nestles close to the stomach. Because of bleeding, this usually requires removing the spleen. Unlike the heart or the liver, the spleen isn't critical for survival, but it does have a valuable role in fighting infection, so it's nice to keep it. Flum found that the rate of spleen removal as a complication fell by more than half during the five years after the operation was introduced.[30]

So complication rates for a new operation generally improve over time, but they're also closely related to how many of the operations an individual surgeon has done. For example, Flum finds that surgeons who have done less than twenty gallbladder operations with the laparoscope have twice as many complications as more experienced surgeons. Unfortunately, when an operation is brand new—as laparoscopic gallbladder surgery was in 1991—all surgeons are relatively inexperienced. And while twenty cases improve performance substantially, Flum thinks that surgeons just keep getting better with even more experience. "It's probably after about 150 operations that the complication rate gets as low as it can get," he says. "And I personally think that inexperience is linked to most everything bad that can happen."

Of course, surgeons have to learn somehow. In medical school and residency training, they gain experience under close supervision. But new operations come along in a steady stream after surgeons' training is complete, and they somehow have to gain experience with these, too. We should all be grateful to the first few patients who undergo a new operation. But unless your hand is forced, you may not want to be one of them.

A corollary of the learning curve is that doctors who do larger numbers of a particular operation or procedure will be more proficient and have better results. The same applies to hospitals. But a surprising number of operations are done by doctors who do only a few operations of that type a year. A recent report by the Center for Medical Consumers in New York highlighted the problem. For many delicate medical procedures, such as cardiac catheterization, placement of coronary artery stents, hysterectomies, and lung biopsies, almost half of the doctors who performed the procedure at all did only one or two a year.[31]

In the previous chapter, we saw that more isn't always better. Here we've argued that newer isn't always better. Sometimes it is, but don't assume that this is automatically true. Even when a newer approach is better, there's often a shakedown period during which risks are unusually high. These conclusions run contrary to some deeply held cultural beliefs in American society.

Both doctors and patients are often eager to try new things. But the notion that more and newer is always better is one that we've got to get over if we want medical care to get safer and more affordable. The popular notion sometimes holds, but not always. FDA regulations aren't designed to guarantee that it's true, doctors tend to underestimate risks, and marketing can result in rapid adoption of products that ultimately prove inferior or unsafe. Sometimes "tried and true" proves better than "latest and greatest."

5

Social Hazards

What We Lose by Uncritical Use of New Treatments

We're eating pancakes some nights as it is. I said to my husband, "what are we going to do, sell the house so we can pay health insurance?" —Trish Patafio, homemaker[1]

THE MEDICAL world adopts new treatments with blinding speed. This is especially true if doctors perceive the new treatments as "cutting edge" and if the reimbursements are good. In 1981, doctors performed 26 liver transplants in the United States. Just six years later, 1,182 were performed. By 2001, over 5,000 liver transplants were being done each year.[2,3] In most years, about 10 percent of the two hundred top-selling drugs are new.[2] When a new operation for patients with emphysema was described at a medical meeting in 1994, it set off a frenzy to provide the new operation. An article based on the presentation appeared in January 1995. By October 1995, the operation had been performed on over a thousand Medicare patients and was being offered in at least thirty-seven states.[4]

But as we've seen, some medical advances get adopted before we know enough about them. In many cases, this is related to successful marketing, professional enthusiasm, and public demand. In contrast to the traditional lament, "How do we get people to use new approaches?" we think today's challenge is how to slow down and critically evaluate the consequences before using new approaches too widely.

Health-care analysts agree that new technology is a major reason for rising health-care costs, if not the most important reason. Harvard economist Joe Newhouse examined several factors that increase costs. These included wasteful administrative costs, a possible physician surplus, defensive medicine, expensive care for the terminally ill, and other such factors. He concluded that each contributes a small amount to rising costs, but the main driver is new technology.[5]

"It's not increased waste, it's not fraud, it's not increased lawsuits, it's not that people on average are older," agrees economist Michael Chernew of the University of Michigan. Acknowledging that some of these contribute to rising health-care costs, he says that the "predominant factor" is the enormous number of new medical techniques.[6] Coupled with our obsession with new technology, this is a recipe for spiraling costs.

Discussing Medicare cost increases in the 1990s, yet another economist said:

> It was not because physician fees for specific interventions were growing rapidly; they were not. It was not because hospital admission rates were increasing or patients were staying in the hospital longer; they were not . . . . In a survey of fifty leading health economists . . . 81% agreed with the statement, "The primary reason for the increase in the health sector's share of Gross Domestic Product over the past 30 years is technological change in medicine."[7]

Many people think of managed care—in HMOs, for example—as creating a barrier to new technology. But it has had only modest effects.[6] This is in part because new technology is irresistible to consumers, who have sued or moved their care elsewhere in order to gain access to it. In addition, doctors are quick to insist that hospitals or health plans acquire the latest drugs and devices. Most hospitals are happy to buy anything that will help fill the beds.

Some economists argue that because medical services get better as they get more expensive, Americans will be willing to pay the additional costs. This is the rosy view. Right now, though, facing rapidly rising insurance premiums, fewer employers are willing to bear the costs. There's little public appetite for tax increases that would sustain greater Medicare spending. Consumers are complaining about more out-of-pocket costs.

Rising Costs, Falling Insurance

Rapidly increasing health-care costs may not be as benign as the rosy view would suggest. Consider some recent news items:

- Being uninsured isn't just for the poor anymore: 1.4 million Americans, more than half of whom had incomes over $75,000, lost their health coverage in 2001.[8]
- Almost 44 million Americans have no health insurance, and the number of people with sporadic coverage is even greater. In a two-year span, 80 million Americans under age 65 lacked coverage for at least a month.[9]
- Even among people with employer-sponsored insurance, more than 11 percent of those with a chronic health problem failed to fill a needed prescription because of cost.[10]
- Even during the period of low health-care inflation and record national prosperity in the late 1990s, health coverage for retirees declined; some large corporations have dropped retiree benefits altogether; and many indicators point to greater drops in retiree coverage.[11]

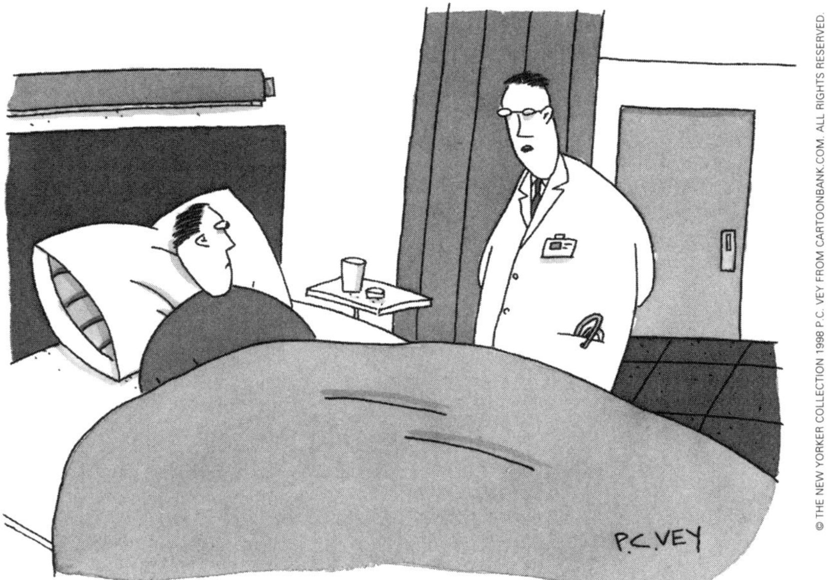

"In the future, everybody will have fifteen minutes of health-care coverage."

- Some 18 percent of California seniors don't fill a prescription or take less than the prescribed doses of a treatment to "make their medications last longer."[12]
- The rising cost of health insurance is driving some healthy people and their families to opt out of employer-sponsored health insurance.[13]
- Deductibles (the amount you pay before your insurance kicks in) and copayments (the fraction you have to pay even after your insurance kicks in) continue to rise.

As new technology drives up the cost of care, insurance becomes less affordable and available, and this is a social problem of steadily growing

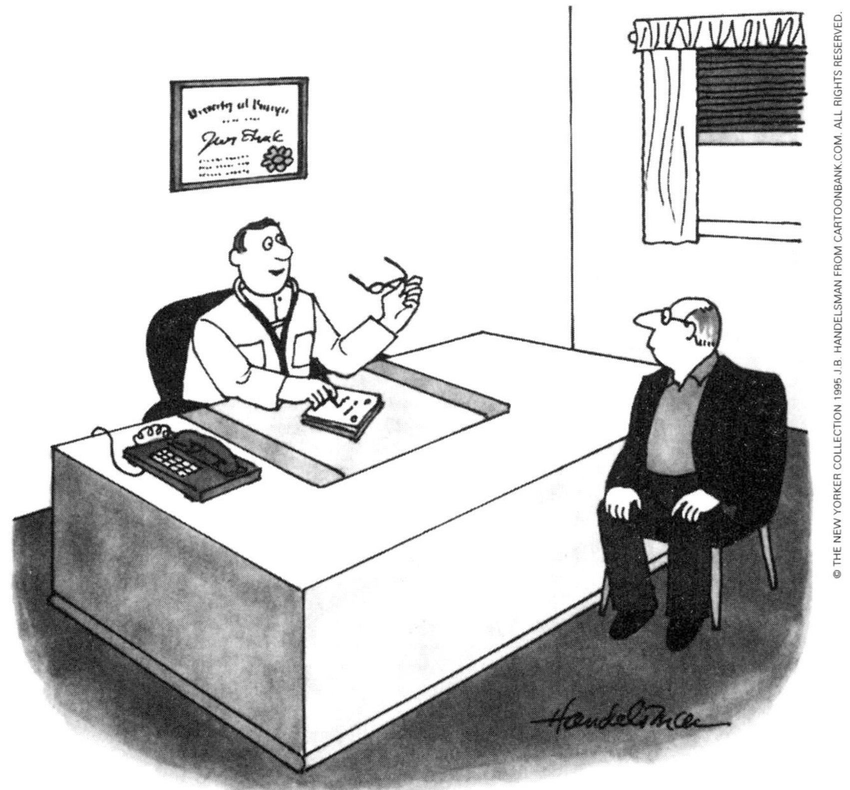

"You're in luck, in a way. Now is the time to be sick—while Medicare still has some money."

proportions. Most experts forecast continuing rapid increases in health-care costs. Most insurance plans will offer less coverage, and consumers will pay more out of pocket.[14]

It's likely that the number of uninsured will continue to rise. In fact, survey data indicate that the rapid rise in health-care costs from 1979 to 1995—much faster than personal income—accounted for almost all the decline in health insurance coverage.[15] These trends suggest to us that, contrary to the rosy view, Americans really aren't convinced that rising health-care costs are worth it.

With rising costs, falling taxes, and the upcoming addition of drug coverage to Medicare, even this mainstay of health insurance coverage is looking shaky. In 2004, the Medicare trustees moved their estimate of the program's bankruptcy forward by seven years from earlier estimates. The trustees now estimate that Medicare hospital coverage will be insolvent by 2019.[16] Although such dire predictions have a way of never coming true, they emphasize the need for new revenues, cost cutting, or both.

Other Consequences of Our Obsession with Medical Advances

Another cost of adopting technology too quickly is a reduced ability to evaluate it critically. When treatments are already in common use, patients are often unwilling to participate in the research that would establish the treatments' real effectiveness. For example, the wide availability of autologous bone marrow transplantation for breast cancer (a result of advocacy and legal and political action) slowed enrollment in the definitive clinical trials, jeopardizing their completion. When the trials were finally completed, they showed bone marrow transplantation to be no more effective, and perhaps more toxic, than conventional chemotherapy. And it sure cost more. By one estimate, we spent $3.4 billion on this treatment over ten years, when standard chemotherapy would have been less than half the price.[17]

Rapidly rising health-care costs also contribute to state budget deficits, reduced business profits, and painful consumer choices. As health care consumes more and more of the gross national product (14.9 percent in 2002, projected to rise to 18.4 percent by 2013[18]), fewer resources are available for other critical needs: infrastructure, education, environmental protection, and defense, to name a few. For some of us, it also means less for beer, home remodeling, Sonics basketball tickets, or visits to the family in California—things that also improve our personal quality of life.

Improvements in education and the environment might have bigger dividends for population health than more spending on medical care. Unfortunately, we can't point to individuals who have lived longer because of cleaner air, cleaner water, or better health habits. But most of us can point to individuals—including members of our own family—who have benefited from specific medical advances. And when it's a member of our family, of course, we want nothing but the best. But knowing what's best is often difficult, and, as we discussed in the preceding chapter, the "latest and greatest" treatments often prove disappointing but expensive.

We've argued that using too much medical care and embracing new treatments before they've been fully evaluated can waste resources and may sometimes be bad for your health. Part of the problem is that the process by which advances are disseminated is highly variable. Profit motives, political concerns, media, marketing, and the cultural allure of medical advances often drive dissemination as much as scientific evidence does. Unproven, ineffective, and marginally useful treatments are often introduced and reimbursed right along with those that have a solid evidence base.

Why Don't New Medical Treatments Lower Costs?

Intuitively, it might seem that new treatments would attack the fundamental causes of disease and lower costs. In the computer industry, technological progress means that computers get faster and cheaper year after year. Of course, that doesn't mean that expenditures for computers are falling. Instead, they continue to rise, as more and more people and businesses buy them and upgrade them. Similarly, the likely scenario for the foreseeable future is a continued increase in medical costs related to new treatments.

This occurs in part because new treatments may convert rapidly fatal diseases into chronic diseases, with heavy ongoing burdens. The newer drugs for AIDS and insulin for childhood diabetes are examples. Such treatments are often extremely valuable, yet they add to the cost of care rather than reducing it. Expensive new treatments "chip away" at diseases more often than they provide dramatic cures.[19] As imaging and surgical techniques become safer, doctors extend them to more patients, increasing the volume of services. Treatments for lifestyle concerns, such as impotence, baldness, and social anxiety, appeal to a large fraction of the population, greatly expanding the market for new products. Although many drugs give value for money, some increase costs with no benefit over cheaper alternatives.

Lewis Thomas, a well-known physician-researcher and writer, described three levels of medical technology. He used *nontechnology* to describe care for patients with advanced diseases—like incurable cancer or advanced cirrhosis—for which there may be palliation, but there is no hope of changing the course of the disease. He described *halfway technology* as noncurative, but able to delay death or improve quality of life. Organ transplants, kidney dialysis, cancer chemotherapy, and coronary angioplasty are examples.[20] He reserved *high technology* to refer to truly curative treatments or effective prevention techniques. Polio vaccine is a good example.

While many wouldn't consider polio vaccine to be high-tech, it reflects a deep understanding of the cause of the disease, the body's response, and how to effectively alter that response. Rather than offering expensive amelioration, it prevents the disease entirely. Before polio vaccine, the "high-tech" solution to severe polio was the iron lung. Unfortunately, most of what we consider high-tech is really halfway technology that offers no cures.

Bandwagons and Competing Agendas

As we noted earlier, we use the term technology to refer not simply to electronic gadgets, but to new medical treatments, diagnostic tests, surgical procedures, and drugs. We pointed out that there are no defined criteria for designating these technologies as experimental or as standard, nor is there an orderly process for the transition from one category to the other. We're often enthusiastic about treatments that have little scientific support, but careless in supporting treatments with strong support. The transition of new treatments from experimental to standard care is susceptible to a "bandwagon effect" in which doctors, the public, media, advocacy groups, and marketing help to sustain unproven ideas.[21] Even when new technology works, there may be less expensive ways to achieve similar or better outcomes.

Many doctors and consumers alike imagine that the development of new treatments follows a neat linear path, something like this:

> Basic Biological Research (scientists) → Development of New Products and Strategies (industry) → Testing New Approaches in Actual Practice (medical researchers) → Approval by Regulatory

Agencies (FDA) ⟶ Consideration of Value for Money (by somebody, we hope) ⟶ Widespread Use

Instead, we think the process is messy, complex, and affected by a host of competing agendas; it may look more like Figure 5-1.[22] In part because of this unruly process, ineffective medical "advances" sometimes gain wide acceptance before they're proven useless. Each can result in substantial costs and side effects.

For example, stomach freezing for peptic ulcer disease was based on the observation that cooling reduced stomach acid. There followed the sale of some 2,500 gastric freezing machines and growing controversy over the procedure's efficacy. Four properly randomized trials led to the demise

FIGURE 5-1. Influences on the Use of New Medical Technology.
Reproduced with permission from R. A. Deyo, Annual Review of Public Health, 2002, *no. 23, p. 36.*

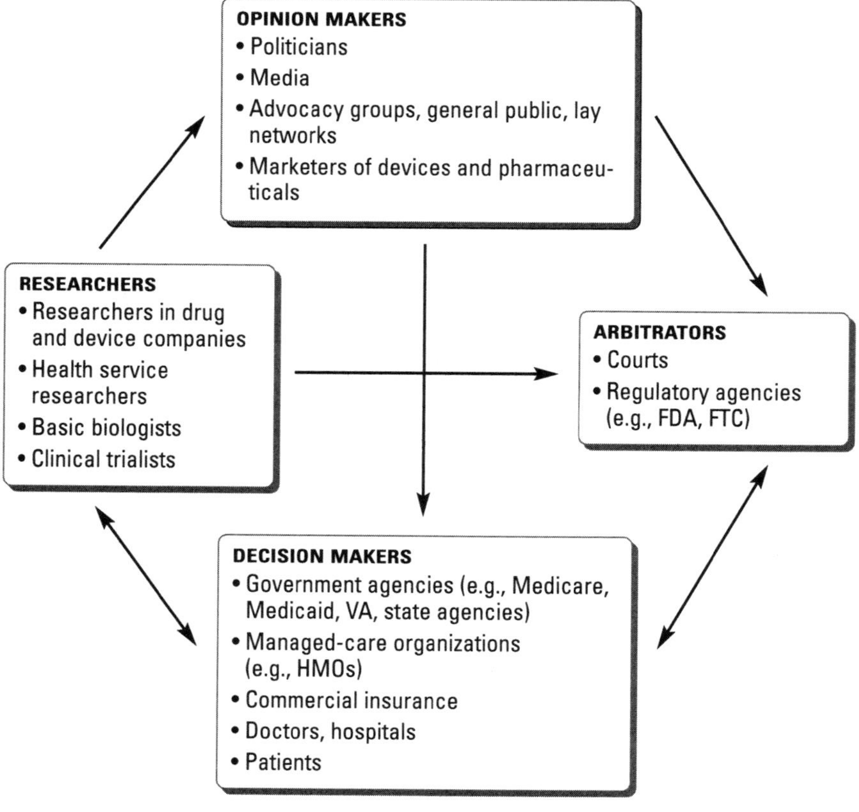

of the technique, but only after 15,000 patients were treated, with some untimely deaths as a result. [23]

More recently, the drugs encainide and flecainide were introduced for treating abnormal heart rhythms. They effectively suppressed abnormal heartbeats among patients who had had a recent heart attack, but when tested in a clinical trial, they caused more deaths than placebo therapy.[24] Electronic fetal monitoring remains in routine use, despite well-designed clinical trials demonstrating little benefit to the baby, but an increased likelihood of Cesarean section or forceps delivery.[25] The previous chapter described the use of diethylstilbestrol (DES) for premature labor, high-dose oxygen for premature infants, and several other examples. In each case, multiple factors played a role in the adoption of the technology, and ineffective treatment became standard care through complex social, political, and economic processes.

Everett Rogers, who wrote the definitive book on diffusion of innovations, suggests that scientific evidence affects the adoption of new technologies only moderately. Other factors that influence local opinion makers and consumers often overwhelm scientific considerations.

Rogers says that a shortcoming of research on dissemination is its pro-innovation bias. Advocates often give little attention to the consequences of new technology, assuming that it will have only beneficial results. However, the undesirable, indirect, and unanticipated consequences of an innovation usually go together, as do the desirable, direct, and anticipated consequences. Rogers also suggested that overadoption of new technology is an understudied aspect of its diffusion.[26]

In adapting diffusion theory to health care, others note that doctors often adopt medical strategies before the relevant technologies have been adequately tested. The contribution of the new strategies to patient care may be unclear and sometimes dangerous, and their one certain contribution is an increase in health-care costs.[27]

But new technology itself isn't the villain. Rather, the villain is the process by which advocates, the media, and health-care providers adopt new technology. As with nonmedical technology, social rather than scientific forces may play a central role in its diffusion. At each step in the evolution of medical strategies, characteristic errors in both reasoning and research may occur. Better research methods and more critical use of published studies may not help unless the social forces are taken into account.[27]

Are Current Cost-Containment Efforts Doomed to Failure?

Dr. William Schwartz, a distinguished kidney expert, argued in 1987 that all current medical cost-containment strategies will inevitably fail. He believed that gradually eliminating useless care could save billions but would offer only a temporary reprieve from rising costs. He predicted that eliminating unnecessary hospital days would save money, and this may account for some of the temporary blunting of cost increases by managed care. But he also correctly predicted that the underlying rate of cost increases would resume after unnecessary hospital days were eliminated, because of ongoing innovation.[28]

A recent analysis by the Henry J. Kaiser Family Foundation seems to bolster Schwartz's argument. In a review of increases in health-care costs from 1961 to 2000, the report concluded that none of the cost-control efforts of the last thirty-five years has had a lasting impact. These included the introduction of Medicare and Medicaid regulations, wage and price controls, "voluntary efforts" under the Carter administration, and, most recently, managed care. The apparent failure of all approaches may reflect "the American people's uncontainable desire for the latest and best health care."[29]

Different insurance schemes and financing mechanisms may help, but they won't entirely prevent rising costs. Altering financial incentives may help, but it doesn't address the underlying problem. Rapidly rising medical costs are a problem everywhere in the world, under every type of insurance system, not just in the United States. Deciding whether and when to adopt new treatments is an ongoing challenge under every health-financing scheme.

Some new treatments provide cost without benefit; more often, they provide big cost with small benefit. As Dr. David Eddy, an independent health-care analyst, suggests, "As a society, sooner or later we will have to determine whether there are some benefits that are just too small to justify the cost."[1] No one wants to deny the possibility of big breakthroughs, regardless of costs. But most of the time, deciding whether the bang is worth the buck will have to be considered, and the process needs to be consistent if we want to constrain costs without forgoing major innovations.

PART II

HOW THINGS REALLY WORK

Opinion Makers and Regulators of Medical Advances

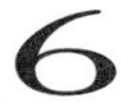

What Will You Swallow?

How Drug Companies Get You to Buy More Expensive Drugs Than You May Need

A desire to take medicine is, perhaps, the great feature which distinguishes man from animals. —Sir William Osler, 1891[1]

Pharmaceutical companies will soon rule the world if we keep letting them believe we are a happy, functional society so long as all the women are on Prozac, all children on Ritalin, and all men on Viagra. —Author unknown[2]

ON A RECENT Saturday morning, I (Rick) got a page at home from Ethel, an elderly patient. Because of a new rash, she'd consulted a colleague in our university clinic the previous afternoon. Her diagnosis was shingles, a painful eruption caused by a virus, and the clinic doctor had given her a prescription for the antiviral drug famciclovir. But Ethel had been to her local pharmacy and had discovered that it would cost $170 for a seven-day supply. Being a low-income Medicare patient with no insurance coverage for drugs, she couldn't afford the medicine, and she wondered if a less expensive drug could be prescribed. I changed her prescription to an older and less expensive drug, acyclovir. After several phone calls, I found a pharmacy where Ethel could fill her prescription for just $25.

In changing the prescription, I considered that famciclovir and acyclovir have roughly similar effectiveness, although famciclovir can be taken three times a day, rather than the five times a day needed for acyclovir. Experts suggest there is little to recommend one drug over the other for this particular problem.[3] Both drugs are generally safe, but occasionally cause unpleasant side effects, including nausea, vomiting, headache, and itching.

Any benefit from either drug was uncertain, however, in this particular patient with shingles. Such medication is most effective for this condition when it is started within three days of symptom onset. It now was five days from the start of Ethel's symptoms.

So this elderly woman had initially received a seven-day prescription that would cost $170, was unlikely to help, and would expose her to at least a modest risk of side effects. My prescription was also of dubious value, although it was less costly. I wasn't inclined to dissuade Ethel from taking medication because I hadn't evaluated her myself, and she was now persuaded that medicine would help stop her pain.

These events began with effective promotion of a new drug and a doctor who was probably not aware of costs, because most patients have insurance and cost seems irrelevant. A patient who was in pain wanted something done, faced an unaffordable drug price, and contacted me as her primary doctor. Considering Ethel's request, the timing, and the need to help, I acquiesced and gave her a prescription that was unlikely to help her much, but would meet her expectations. Stories like this are routine, and they surely increase your insurance premiums and Medicare taxes. But they represent cost with little benefit, outside of providing reassurance and support.

An Overview of the Drug Industry

How did we get into this situation? Doctors, patients, and insurance incentives certainly share the blame. But we'll focus here on the role of manufacturers in promoting drugs, creating demand, and keeping prices up. We're quick to acknowledge that the drug industry does some good things. Some new drugs are valuable innovations, critical in the successful management of disease. Industry research is essential to bringing new products to market. In some cases, better drug treatments have reduced other treatment costs, resulting in overall savings.[4,5]

But many drugs are "me too" products with little to distinguish them from others already on the market. "Me too" drugs increase costs and are sometimes promoted to the point of excessive use. Most of them are effective, but some ultimately prove less effective or less safe than cheaper alternatives.

What are "me too" drugs? Think of all the anti-inflammatory drugs on the market. Most people are familiar with ibuprofen and naproxen (now available over the counter), and with another dozen or so drugs that still require prescriptions—Daypro, Feldene, Voltaren, Tolectin, Clinoril, Celebrex, Vioxx, and others. These all work in basically the same way, and there's no evidence that one is more effective than another, although they vary in safety. Similarly, there are several statin drugs for lowering cholesterol, nonsedating antihistamines, proton-pump inhibitors such as Prilosec for ulcer disease, SSRIs for depression, and drugs in several categories for high blood pressure. These are called *classes of drugs,* and the first drug in a class—the innovator—is often a real advance. The rest are generally "me too" drugs that differ slightly chemically, work the same way, and may offer little advantage, but are hailed as breakthroughs in marketing campaigns.

In some cases, having several drug choices is advantageous. A patient may have better results or fewer side effects with one drug than with others, or may prefer taking fewer pills. However, having more than three or four drugs in a class is usually redundant, with the additional entries having

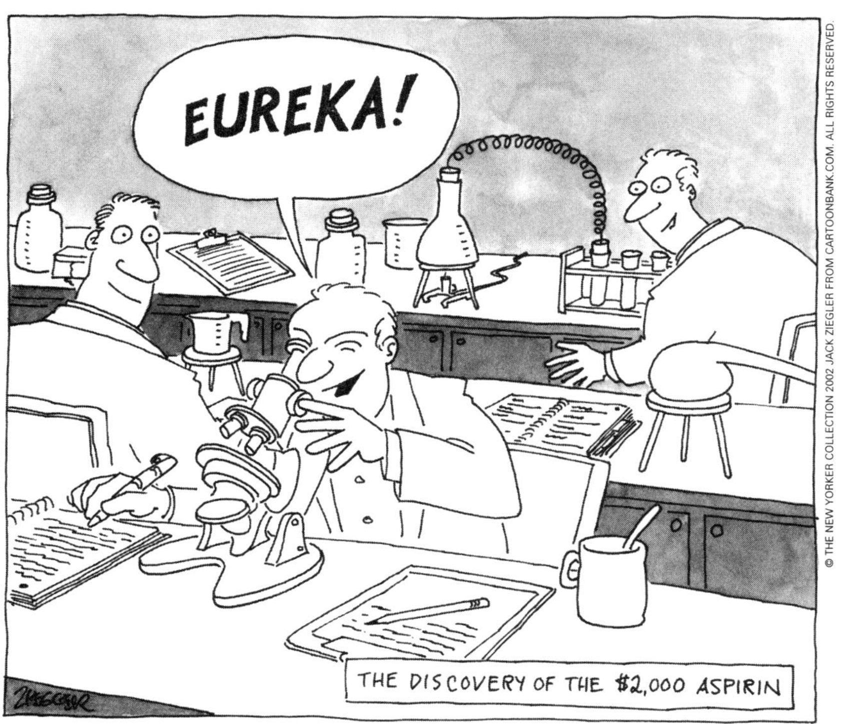

little clear advantage. Multiple entries in a class account for most competition among products, although market forces have only a little to do with pricing. New entrants to a class may be given a lower price than the innovator drug in order to compete, but only slightly lower—a form of "shadow" pricing.

Nearly everyone complains about the high price of medicines. From the drug company's perspective, though, its first obligation is not to patients, but to shareholders—to maximize profits. And the high cost of drugs might be palatable if manufacturers were simply charging what the market will bear. But it's less palatable when the market is manipulated, with drugs promoted to patients who don't need them, expensive drugs promoted over equally effective but inexpensive drugs, competition suppressed, and research manipulated to exaggerate a drug's effectiveness.

Market forces for buying drugs are unlike the market forces for buying cars because consumers are less able to determine by themselves whether they need a drug, which one they need, and what alternatives are available. They rarely have enough information to decide whether a more expensive drug is "worth it" compared to a less expensive one. Insurance that insulates many patients from the full cost of drugs further distorts any semblance of a free market. Insurance reduces any incentive to weigh the cost versus the benefit of a particular drug.

Some analysts argue that even with their high costs, new and highly effective drugs are cost-effective. This means that they offer good value for money, not necessarily that they save money. Such analyses often focus on the innovator drugs that are first in their class, and ignore the new drugs that prove no more effective than their predecessors. They also tend to focus away from drugs for chronic conditions like back pain or diabetes. Even if we accept the argument, economists point out that we can easily go broke paying for expensive but "cost-effective" treatments.

Americans have the dubious privilege of paying higher drug prices than consumers in other countries, comparing drug for drug. A month's supply of the cholesterol-lowering drug Zocor (80 mg), for example, recently cost $71 on a Canadian pharmacy web site, compared to $124 on a U.S. pharmacy web site. A hundred tablets of the arthritis drug Vioxx were $131 on the Canadian web site, versus $248 in the United States.[6]

Boston University researchers have found that prices in Canada and Europe are just half to two-thirds of U.S. prices. Dr. Alan Sager, a BU professor, estimates that Americans would save $38 billion a year if we paid

MATT DAVIES THE JOURNAL NEWS
©2008.
10/8
SOMETIMES I CUT MY PRESCRIPTION PILLS IN HALF TO SAVE MONEY...
DRUG-CO.S
SOMETIMES I GO WITHOUT HEAT IN THE WINTER & I SKIP MEALS SO I CAN PAY YOUR PRICES...
& SOMETIMES I HOP A BUS TO CANADA TO FILL MY PRESCRIPTION FOR 75% LESS...
GASP!!
BUYING DRUGS IN CANADA IS MEDICALLY UNSAFE...

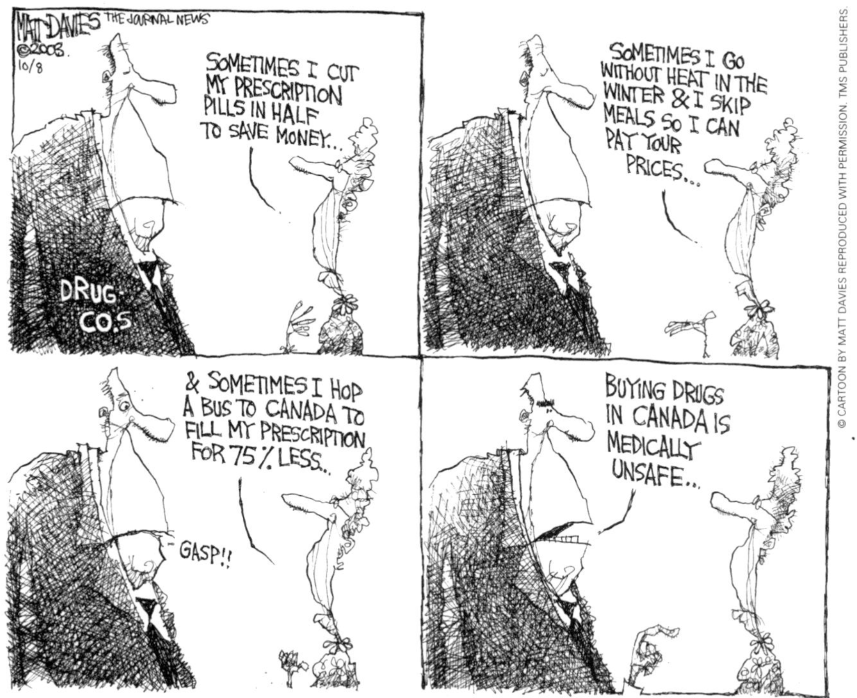

Canadian prices for the same brand-name prescription drugs.[7] This is why many of my (Rick's) elderly patients, without insurance coverage for drugs, drive from Seattle to Canada to fill their prescriptions.

The drug industry is colossal. In the United States, we spent $154 billion on drugs in 2001, more than triple the amount spent in 1990.[8] A government estimate for 2003 is $184 billion just in retail sales. That's more than the gross national product of Thailand. At least until 2003, drug manufacturers were the most profitable industry in the United States, ahead of commercial banks in second place. The median net profit (after taxes) for the drug industry in 2000 was 18.6 percent, compared to just 4.5 percent for all *Fortune* 500 firms.[9]

Drug Company Research

The drug industry argues that its high prices are justified by research costs and the risks involved in new product development. There are hundreds of false starts for every successful new drug that's brought to market; testing and evaluation is lengthy and expensive. So the cost of developing a marketable drug is hundreds of millions of dollars.

However, research costs for the top ten drug manufacturers averaged 14 percent of revenues in 2000. This was less than the 18.6 percent that the companies kept as profit after paying for research.[10] The profits don't pay for research. Profits are what the companies keep *after* they pay for research and all their other expenses.[11]

Research costs were apparently greater than promotional costs, although it's unclear whether some market research is included in the research figure.[9,12] Furthermore, promotional spending has increased much faster than research spending. From 1997 to 2001, research spending rose 59 percent, but spending on advertising rose 145 percent.[12]

Employment data also suggest that marketing actually gets a higher priority than research. Using the industry's own employment data, Alan Sager found that in 2000, the brand-name drug manufacturers employed almost 88,000 people in marketing, but only 49,000 in research. He also found that research employment fell 2 percent from 1995 to 2000, while the number of people employed in marketing rose 59 percent.[11]

Today, much of the innovation in the industry is going on in small biotech firms with relatively small budgets, rather than in the big drug companies. Larger companies then buy up these biotech firms or enter into manufacturing and marketing agreements with them.

Much of the research by the biggest companies is directed toward developing "me too" products or making small (sometimes trivial) changes to existing products. A report by the nonprofit National Institute for Health Care Management examined 1,035 drugs approved by the FDA over twelve years, starting in 1989. Only a third of the drugs were actually new chemicals; two-thirds had active ingredients that were already available in previously approved drugs. And only 15 percent were new chemical compounds judged by the FDA to offer significant improvement over existing medicines. In comparing the second six years of the period with the first six years, the institute found that "incrementally modified drugs" increased by 81 percent and new chemical entities increased by only 10 percent.[13] Thus, much of the industry's vaunted research was simply recycling old drugs, not developing new ones.

As a result, by 2002, despite astronomical drug prices, new drugs were coming into the market at the slowest rate in a decade.[14] Thus, the pipeline for truly remarkable new drugs is relatively small. The allocation of resources within these companies seems to belie the industry's mantra that research costs justify high prices.

What about the high risks that the industry supposedly takes? Economists point out that in truly risky industries, profit margins are highly variable, with wide swings from high to low in different years. In contrast, drug industry profits are consistent from year to year, suggesting that the risks are exaggerated. As an editor of the *New England Journal of Medicine* noted, an industry whose profits routinely exceed those of every other industry, as well as its own research costs, can't be considered very risky.[9] Others suggest that if you regularly went to Las Vegas and came home 18.6 percent richer year after year, you could hardly be accused of gambling the family's wealth.

Further mitigating the risk is the drug companies' substantial government subsidy. The National Institutes of Health actually fund much of the basic biological research that leads to new drugs, using your tax dollars.[15] Also, the industry's research and marketing costs are tax-deductible. Thus, according to news accounts, the average tax rate for the drug industry from 1993 to 1996 was 16 percent, compared to 27 percent for other major U.S. industries.[9] Finally, the government grants patents for new drugs for twenty years, providing the legal monopoly that allows pricing in the ionosphere. So we find it hard to justify the high price of drugs by pointing to extraordinary research efforts or high risks.

Direct-to-Consumer Advertising

Increasing drug prices and growing use of more expensive drugs are fueled by good marketing. In 2000, companies spent $15.7 billion on drug promotion—a figure that's hard to fathom. For context, consider a single medication: the new anti-arthritis drug Vioxx. In 2000, the manufacturer spent $160 million just on direct-to-consumer ads. This was more than Pepsi spent to advertise its premier product (Pepsi), more than Anheuser-Busch spent on Bud, and very close to spending on the most heavily advertised car, which was Saturn.[16]

When you watch the evening news on the major TV networks, you see these dollars in action. These programs typically draw an older viewing audience—exactly the consumers with the greatest drug use. The drug companies are major sponsors of these programs, paying millions for prime-time spots. Direct-to-consumer marketing is only one of several ways in which drug companies maintain high demand and high prices, but it's very effective.[12]

Everyone has seen ads for prescription drugs in newspapers or magazines, or on television. Probably most can hum the "celebrate" song used to advertise Celebrex. Those of us who are past fifty—exactly the target demographic for Celebrex—remember when "Celebrate" was just a top-forty song by Three Dog Night.

If it seems to you that you've seen more drug ads in recent years, you're right. Until 1985, drug makers marketed almost exclusively to doctors, who did the prescribing, after all. But in 1985, in response to drug industry requests, the FDA interpreted its rules in a way that clearly allowed print ads for the public. Not satisfied, the drug industry argued for rules that would allow briefer messages, with less detail on side effects. And in 1997, the FDA relaxed the level of detail required, clearing the way for television and radio ads that would last only a few seconds.[17] In fact, the industry is still lobbying for further loosening of advertising restrictions.

The United States and New Zealand are the only countries that allow direct-to-consumer advertising. And New Zealand is in the process of changing its mind.[18] Other countries, including Britain and Canada, have considered and rejected the practice (although most Canadians get U.S. television stations). In Europe, consumer groups recently argued that information for consumers should come from independent sources rather than from drug companies. They wanted information "to help establish informed choice for patients instead of just more brand awareness."[19]

In response to the new opportunity for direct-to-consumer ads, the drug industry has increased such promotion ninefold since 1994, to almost $2.5 billion in 2000. Most of this growth was in television advertising.[20] In a 2001 survey, nearly a third of adults indicated that they had talked to a doctor about a drug they had seen advertised, and of those, 44 percent had received a prescription for the drug they asked about. In other words, one in eight Americans have gotten a specific prescription in response to a drug ad.[21]

The rosy view of drug advertising is that it educates consumers, makes them more aware of diseases and treatment options, encourages them to seek more information, and empowers them to obtain more appropriate treatment.[22,23] In some cases, these benefits are real. In general, public attitudes toward these ads are also favorable, perhaps because they create a sense of empowerment.

A more complete view acknowledges that advertising is advertising.[24] It's intended to expand the market, increase market share, and sell a product. The information in the ad is slanted to promote a product over its competition. An ad for a Ford dramatizes the Ford's attractive features. It doesn't tell you that Toyota has a better frequency-of-repair record.

Similarly, drug ads aren't likely to tell you about alternative treatments that may be equally effective, less expensive, or even better for your health. They aren't required to. And it's not breakthrough drugs that are most heavily advertised to the public. As a former *New England Journal of Medicine* editor points out, "The less important the drug, the more marketing it takes to sell it. Important new drugs do not need much promotion. Me-too drugs do."[9]

A major shortfall of drug ads is that they generally don't indicate success rates or the magnitude of any benefits.[25,26] They rely on phrases like "proven effective" rather than indicating just how effective the drugs are. To study whether actual research results would affect consumer perceptions, a group of doctors at Dartmouth presented consumers with actual results from clinical trials corresponding to drug ads. When they saw the study results—in an easily digested format—most of the consumers were underwhelmed. Most preferred the actual data to the presentations in drug ads, and their perceptions of drug effectiveness plummeted.[27]

Consider the antihistamine Claritin as an example. *The New York Times Magazine* indicated that the manufacturer, Schering-Plough, put $322 million into direct-to-consumer advertising during 1998 and 1999—perfect timing to take advantage of the newly relaxed rules for television advertising.[28] Yet a clinical trial showed that patients taking Claritin have on the average a 46 percent improvement in symptoms, compared to a 35 percent improvement from a placebo (sugar pill).[29] Can anyone imagine an ad touting Claritin as being 11 percent better than a sugar pill?

Many allergy specialists argue that nasally administered cortisone-type drugs—such as Nasacort, Beconase, and Flonase—provide better relief than Claritin for nasal allergies. Head-to-head comparisons consistently indicate that this is true.[30–32] Don't expect to find that in a Claritin ad, either.

Other alternatives—while Claritin was still on patent—were inexpensive over-the-counter antihistamines. Newer antihistamines like Claritin are no more effective than older ones like Chlortrimeton (and possibly less so). The only advantage of Claritin is less sedation, but about half of us tolerate the old drugs without drowsiness, making them a cheaper

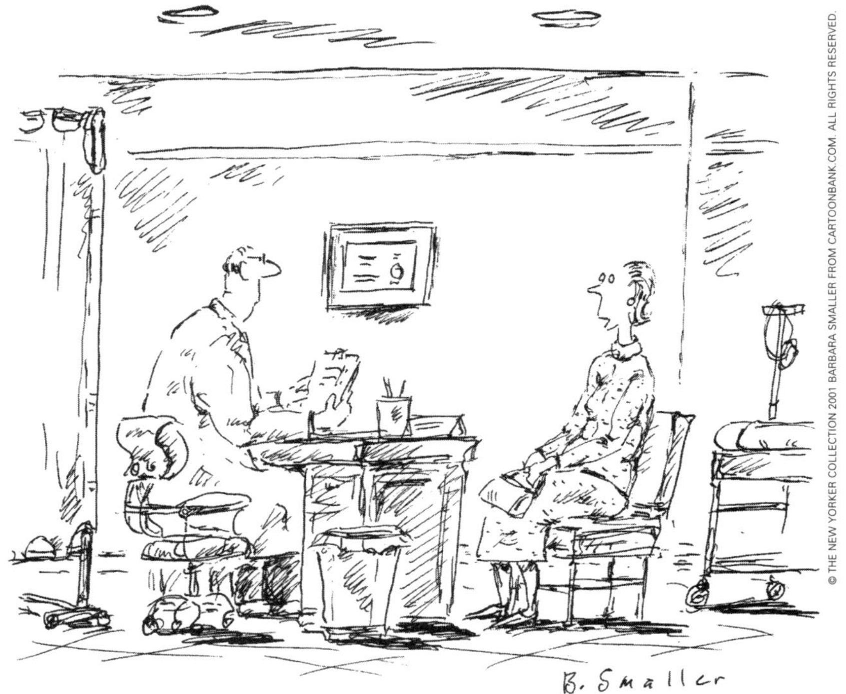

"I think the dosage needs adjusting. I'm not nearly as happy as the people in the ads."

alternative. That's not information you'll find in a Claritin ad. These omissions shouldn't surprise us—this is *advertising,* after all.

Did the big investment pay off for Claritin? Modest as the drug's benefits may be, data from the National Center for Health Statistics show that Claritin was the single most frequently prescribed drug at office visits in 1999.[33] It quickly captured 56 percent of the $1.8 billion market for nonsedating antihistamines.[34]

A University of California study confirmed the lack of important information in many drug ads. Researchers found that most direct-to-consumer ads provided no information on success rates, how a drug works, how long it must be taken, alternative treatments, or lifestyle changes that might reduce the need for medication.[26] And the FDA, which is charged with overseeing direct-to-consumer ads, has frequently complained about lack of balance, incomplete information, or misleading claims.[35]

Consumers may mistakenly think that drug ads have to be approved by the FDA before they appear. But in fact, the FDA generally doesn't have the authority to preapprove ads before they go public. The review comes when the ads are printed or aired, and there's often a significant delay in sending regulatory warning letters.[12,35]

From 1997 through 2000, the FDA issued about ten letters a month to drug makers for warnings or violations of advertising rules.[36] *The Wall Street Journal* reports that the agency has repeatedly contacted several companies, including Pfizer, Schering-Plough, Bristol-Meyers Squibb, and Glaxo Wellcome, about violations. These include "improper claims" and "minimizing" drug risks.[37]

However, the FDA can't levy fines, and its letters often come only after ads have achieved wide exposure. Furthermore, several drug companies have simply replaced one misleading ad with another after being cited for violations, according to a 2002 report by the congressional General Accounting Office.[12,35]

Surveys demonstrate a host of other common misconceptions regarding these ads. In a California survey, half the respondents thought that the FDA had to approve drug ads before they appeared, 43 percent believed that only "completely safe" drugs could be advertised directly to consumers, 22 percent thought that drugs with serious side effects couldn't be advertised, and 21 percent believed that only "extremely effective" drugs could be marketed directly to consumers. The study also showed that ignorance is bliss. Those who had the most misconceptions about the rigor of government regulation held the most positive attitudes toward drug advertising.[38]

Many doctors dislike direct-to-consumer advertising.[39] At first blush, this might seem to be a knee-jerk response to erosion of their paternalistic authority over patients. That may be part of the problem, but many of their concerns are more substantial.

In some cases, direct-to-consumer ads encourage patients to switch from their well-studied treatments to newer drugs whose safety and efficacy are less well known. Drug experts note that half the drugs approved by the FDA prove to have serious adverse effects that are unknown prior to approval.[40] A recent study in the *Journal of the American Medical Association* estimated that one out of five new drugs will eventually be withdrawn from the market or receive a so-called black box warning of serious potential side effects—risks that were unknown when the drug was first marketed.[41]

As a well-informed, critically thinking health-care researcher, I (Donald) waited many years for rigorous evidence on statin drug treatment for cholesterol, and then tried statins in order of their effectiveness and price. Like millions of Americans, my doctor and I settled on Lipitor, which was highly effective for me. Several years ago, after seeing a persuasive ad for Baycol, I asked my physician about it and then made the switch because Baycol was supposed to be equally effective and less costly than Lipitor. Luckily, Baycol wasn't as effective for me, and I switched back to Lipitor before Baycol was recalled because of serious side effects. In this case, direct-to-consumer advertising prompted a useless change that might have been risky.

Another concern is that patients with minor symptoms may be persuaded that they have a serious disease and seek expensive but unnecessary treatment. Some advertising makes physicians feel pressured to provide a "pill for every ill" when changes in lifestyle or eating habits, exercise, weight loss, or changes in the home environment may be more effective in improving health.

Requests for a specific drug may sometimes divert a doctor's attention from appropriate diagnostic evaluation. Dr. Michael Wilkes and his colleagues cite a hypothetical but plausible example: A patient sees an ad for an antidepressant, recognizes her symptoms as suggesting major depression, and seeks a specific drug in response to the ad. An alert physician conducts a careful medical history and examination, considers the possibility of hypothyroidism, performs the appropriate tests, and discovers that what she really needs is thyroid replacement therapy.[17] But the path of least resistance in a hurried doctor's office would simply be to acknowledge that depression is common and provide the prescription the patient requests.

Such concerns aren't purely hypothetical. Direct-to-consumer advertising clearly creates patient expectations and demands, perhaps for inappropriate therapy. In a survey of 78 doctors and 1,431 patient visits, researchers found that when a specific drug was requested, doctors prescribed it about 74 percent of the time. However, they were ambivalent about their decisions in 50 percent of cases when a patient requested an advertised drug, versus 12 percent of the time when drugs were not requested by the patient. The authors concluded, "If physicians prescribe requested drugs despite personal reservations, sales may increase but appropriateness of prescribing may suffer."[42,43]

Another study identified doctors who prescribed any of three targeted drugs "at a rate far greater than that warranted by scientific evidence of their effectiveness." Patient demand was the most commonly cited reason for prescribing the three drugs.[44] Patient expectations also prove to be a major reason for prescribing antibiotics for colds, an ineffective practice that may cause side effects and promote bacterial resistance to drugs.

Do ads really create a conviction on the part of consumers that they need a particular medicine? Surveys indicate that up to 15 percent of patients who ask for a particular drug would change doctors if they were not given the drug they requested.[45] These consumers, at least, seem convinced that their ad-informed decisions are better than their doctors'. Doctors often face a tough choice: spend a minute to write the prescription and send the patient home happy, or spend half an hour explaining why the latest and greatest drug promoted on TV is unnecessary and risk having a dissatisfied patient.

Direct-to-consumer advertising of prescription drugs poses a paradox. On the one hand, it assumes that patients can recognize when they might benefit from a product and seek it out. On the other hand, obtaining prescription drugs requires a physician, who has special training in diagnosis and treatment, to actually provide the medication. Drug companies have traditionally been protected from liability claims because a "learned intermediary" (the doctor) has to provide the prescription. The ad generates demand, but the doctor takes responsibility. With the drug industry marketing directly to consumers, this defense may become more questionable and open to court challenges.[46]

Finally, be aware that you may be getting pitched about drugs without even realizing it. An increasingly popular marketing ploy is the celebrity "educational campaign," designed to raise public awareness of certain medical conditions. These are conditions for which new products are available. As an example, actor Rob Lowe (formerly of *West Wing*) was retained by Amgen Inc. to appear on *Entertainment Tonight* and the *Rosie O'Donnell Show* to discuss fever in patients undergoing cancer chemotherapy. Amgen's new drug Neulasta is designed to help treat this problem, which Lowe's father had experienced. Unless a product is mentioned by name, these appearances need not conform to FDA advertising regulations. *The Wall Street Journal* reported that Lowe would probably receive more than $1 million for the campaign.[47]

Similarly, Lauren Bacall appeared on NBC's *Today Show*, describing a friend with blindness from macular degeneration and mentioning the drug Visudyne. The maker of Visudyne, Novartis, acknowledged paying Bacall for the appearance, but this was never mentioned by Bacall or the network, according to *The New York Times*. A Novartis representative said that the company chose Bacall for the marketing campaign because she would appeal to viewers over age fifty—the target population for the drug.[48]

Advertising to Doctors

Though consumer advertising is faster growing, it's dwarfed by promotions to doctors. After all, these folks write the prescriptions. In 2000, drug companies spent $13.2 billion on promotions to doctors and hospitals, and on free drug samples. So direct-to-consumer advertising was only 16 percent of the total advertising budget.[20]

How do doctors get pitched? Through gifts, one-on-one sales calls by drug company "detailers," ads in medical journals, company-sponsored continuing education programs, and free drug samples.

Consider this informal, incomplete list of freebies compiled by Thomas Moore at George Washington University, augmented with others reported in press accounts:

> Hundred-dollar bills, lip gloss, beach bags, coffee mugs, fruit baskets, pizza, audio cassettes, soap, personal computers, videocassette recorders, television sets, ice cream, coasters, tote bags, books, gourmet dinners, magnifying glasses, padlocks, custom videos, eyeglass holders, sunscreen, rulers, chocolates, wall posters, refrigerator magnets, calculators, videodisc players, coffeemakers, cameras, doorknob signs, stickpins, shopping bags, leather attaché cases, Swiss army knives, sweatshirts, submarine sandwiches, infant formula, stuffed animals, photo cubes, rock candy, free long-distance telephone calls, flowers, CDs, manicures, pedicures, car washes, bottles of wine, tanks of gas, Christmas trees
>
> Baseball caps, golf towels, golf umbrellas, golf outings, golf balls, tennis balls, tennis towels, ski scarves, ski caps, gym bags, photos with sports legends Jerry Rice, Dick Butkus or Ozzie Smith

Caribbean weekends, ocean cruises, ski weekends, trips to the Canadian Rockies, frequent-flyer miles, luggage tags, monogrammed luggage

Super Bowl tickets, airline tickets, tennis match tickets, baseball tickets, theater tickets, boxing tickets, tickets for a reception with Dallas Cowboy cheerleaders, symphony tickets, basketball tickets

Cholesterol tests, patient sign-in forms, paperweights, ballpoint pens, anatomical models, diagnostic equipment, document cases, file cards, magnetic paper clip holders, pencils, wall calendars, Post-its, clocks, penlights, cellophane tape, laser light pointers, letter openers, three-ring binders, desk calendars, instructional slides, pocket pen holders, EKG calipers, tape measures, felt-tip pens, pillboxes, stethoscopes, medical bags, notepads, clipboards, patient record forms, drug dose calculators, textbooks, medical journal subscriptions, prescription pads[49–51]

The list speaks for itself. Closer scrutiny of some items is also instructive. The "gourmet dinners" are often in fine restaurants, with an "educational lecture" supported by a drug company. I (Rick) kept the promotional flyers I received in my clinic mailbox during a recent year. These included invitations to dinner at the Palisade Waterfront Restaurant, Fullers, Kasper's, Top of the Town, Ruth's Chris Steak House, the Columbia Tower Club, the Hilton Seattle, The Four Seasons Olympic Hotel, and The Ruins. These are some of Seattle's finest and trendiest restaurants. As if the food weren't enough, incentives to attend dinners sometimes include $100 to $500 honoraria to provide opinions about products or to complete brief questionnaires on prescribing habits.[50,52,53]

A collective sense of outrage may rein in some of the most egregious gift giving. In 2002, the drug industry trade group implemented a voluntary code of commercial practices, recommending only modest meals and gifts of minimal value. Under this code, gifts should be associated with a physician's practice and be intended to benefit patients. However, fine dinners and "consulting fees" have continued. Furthermore, social scientists point out that even small gifts have the desired effect of unconsciously influencing decisions. Drug companies know that gifts influence doctors, which may explain why many companies restrict their own employees from accepting even small gifts.[54]

Another typical invitation (I get about two per year) was to participate in an "advisory board" sponsored by Ortho-McNeil, maker of the pain medicine Ultram. I had no prior contact with this company, but I was invited to a three-day meeting at the Rihga Royal Hotel in Manhattan, with an honorarium, hotel accommodations, meals, and round-trip airfare. Spouses were "warmly welcomed," and all accommodations except airfare were extended to them, as well. "Token consulting" with generous benefits is discouraged by the AMA, but is not defined, leaving lots of gray areas. Like most doctors, I'm absolutely, positively certain that such activities wouldn't sway me one whit from objective, optimal, evidence-based prescribing—no way, no how.

In 2000, there were 314,022 company-sponsored meetings and events at restaurants and hotels. Physicians accepted almost half of all event invitations that year, and 46 percent said that honoraria were important in their decision to attend, according to the Scott-Levin consulting firm.[55] The cost of these gifts, events, and honoraria, of course, is passed along to you in the price of your medicine.

Doctors have a collective delusion that these freebies have no influence on their prescribing habits. In fact, the more gifts a doctor receives from drug representatives, the more certain that doctor is that the gifts have no impact on prescribing behavior.[56] But patients have a hunch that such gifts might influence their doctors. When researchers asked patients to consider ten drug company gifts their doctors might receive, patients rated the gifts as more influential than did their doctors.[57]

These gifts are just part of the practice known as *drug detailing*. This refers to the use of salespeople—or "drug reps"—to make one-on-one calls to physicians, "educating" them about a company's products. Scott-Levin, the consulting firm, estimated that in just eleven months, U.S. drug companies spent $5.3 billion on sales calls to doctors and hospitals. The sales force grew from 35,000 drug reps in 1994 to 56,000 in 1998, equivalent to one drug rep and $100,000 for every eleven doctors.[58] But the proliferation hasn't stopped. By 2002, there were some 88,000 drug reps.[15] AstraZeneca added 1,300 reps just to promote its latest "me too" drug, Nexium. This is nearly identical to the company's Prilosec, which had just lost its patent.

Incidentally, Schering-Plough has just introduced Clarinex to replace Claritin, also a nearly identical drug that's lost its patent. Nexium, Clarinex: Apparently these drugs are supposed to be the "nex" thing you buy, rather than the cheaper versions that are losing their patents. According to the

Medical Letter, an authoritative source that accepts no advertising, Clarinex "will probably prove to be effective and safe, but there is no evidence that it offers any advantage over other second-generation H1-receptor blockers, including loratidine" (Claritin).[59]

You may wonder whether doctors really spend their precious time with these drug reps. A Scott-Levin survey of six thousand specialists found that almost all of them saw about ten reps a month.[60] A survey of internal medicine doctors found that 83 percent had met with drug reps during the previous year.[61]

How good is the information that doctors get from these door-to-door salespeople? A study in San Diego audiotaped presentations by drug reps and identified specific statements about drugs. Eleven percent of the statements were frankly inaccurate, judged by readily available reference information. You may not be surprised to learn that all the inaccurate statements were favorable toward the drugs being promoted.[62] Unfortunately, this is how many doctors get most of their drug information.

You may then wonder whether this promotion actually affects prescribing patterns. A few years ago, I (Rick) was the attending physician for a senior citizen with a severe kidney infection who required hospitalization and intravenous antibiotics. I consulted an infectious disease specialist to assist in treatment decisions, and I started a new, expensive antibiotic. After several days of continued fever and little improvement in the patient's condition, we changed antibiotics and saw a gradual recovery. Later, the specialist confided that he'd had little experience with the new drug and had been influenced by promotional material. He'd recommended switching drugs only after a senior colleague pointed out that older drugs were much more effective against the bacteria we'd identified. Obviously, doctors and drug promotions share the blame for errors like this. Such stories are worrisome, because happy endings aren't inevitable.

The pattern of using heavily promoted new drugs rather than older ones appears to be common. Recently, researchers examined prescriptions for routine urinary tract infections in locations all over the country. Despite guidelines from the Infectious Disease Society of America recommending Bactrim as the first line of treatment (at $1.79 for ten days), only 24 percent of prescriptions were for this drug. Instead, Cipro (at $71 for ten days) and Macrodantin (at $20) accounted for two-thirds of the prescriptions.[63] One of the study's authors, Dr. Elbert Huang of the

University of Chicago, told reporters, "If every drug can work and one drug is promoted more heavily, doctors tend to prescribe the one they've heard more about."[64]

To examine the direct effects of drug promotion, researchers at the Cleveland Clinic studied the use of two intravenous drugs in the hospital before and after doctors attended company-sponsored Sunbelt symposia on the drugs. Usage increased threefold for each of the drugs, creating a pattern significantly different from national usage. Yet a majority of the doctors attending the symposia said that such enticements wouldn't influence their prescribing.[65]

Ads in medical journals are another important way for drug companies to reach doctors. The budget for these is far less than that for one-on-one promotions, though, and even less than the budget for direct-to-consumer ads. Still, it added up to $484 million in 2000.[20]

How good is the information in drug ads that appear in medical journals? In a widely publicized study, Dr. Michael Wilkes and his colleagues sent 109 ads to a group of experts and asked them to judge whether the ads met FDA guidelines. They felt that 92 percent of the ads failed to meet at least one standard, and 15 percent failed to meet eight or more standards.[66] Predictably, the industry howled, saying that only 8 percent of the ads had actually been cited for violations. Wilkes pointed out that the FDA was understaffed for this work and may well have lacked the necessary in-house specialty expertise.

Of course, misleading ads can be useful for marketing, even if they prompt warnings from the FDA. According to Thomas Moore of Georgetown University, Warner-Lambert succeeded in gaining market share for its cholesterol-lowering drug Lopid based in part on advertising for uses other than its approved use, which was for a rare type of cholesterol disorder. The company was required to acknowledge its error and place corrective ads, but only after Lopid had become the second-best-selling cholesterol drug.[67]

Free Drug Samples

Finally, doctors and patients are influenced by drug samples—$7.9 billion worth in 2000. This was more than expenditures on direct-to-consumer ads, gifts, detailing, and medical journal ads combined.[20] Free samples sound pretty altruistic. Why do manufacturers spend so much on them?

There's nothing like free samples to get a doctor to use a drug, to gain firsthand experience with it, and to become comfortable prescribing it. And there's nothing like getting started on a drug to increase the likelihood that a patient will continue it.

To be fair, there are potential benefits of free samples. They may allow doctors to provide medicine more quickly, to assess its effectiveness before writing a full prescription, to evaluate side effects, or to determine a best dose. They may help reduce costs for indigent patients, and they could help to teach patients about appropriate use. Patients love free samples.

On the other hand, free samples have some disadvantages. They may promote products that are less effective or more expensive than alternatives, encourage patients to seek drugs that aren't covered by their insurance or health plan, and bypass the counseling that pharmacists provide regarding drug use and interactions with other drugs.

It also turns out that many samples end up being used by the doctors, their families, and the office staff. In one family medicine clinic, all the doctors, resident physicians, nurses, and staff were surveyed about their personal use of samples. Of fifty-three respondents, all but two had used drug samples, ranging from a single dose to a month's supply. The employees used 230 samples over a year, with a retail value of $10,000.[68] In essence, these samples were another free gift.

But the biggest concern is that samples may promote suboptimal treatment. In a study using case scenarios, the perceived benefits of drug samples led many doctors to report that they would use drugs other than their preferred first choice. For example, in a scenario involving high blood pressure, 27 percent of doctors said that with drug samples available, they'd give a sample that wasn't recommended as first-line therapy by the Joint National Committee on Detection, Evaluation, and Treatment of High Blood Pressure.[69] The first-line drugs are generally more effective, less expensive, or both.

Furthermore, 69 percent of those who would give a sample for high blood pressure indicated that they would write a prescription for the same medicine when it ran out—despite its being neither their own first choice nor a recommended first-line drug. Since most patients take blood pressure medicines for a lifetime, this must be music to the ears of a drug marketer. Resident physicians (those in training) indicated that they'd use samples even more than staff doctors, raising a concern about suboptimal prescribing patterns in the long run.[69]

Perhaps the best summary of marketing to physicians comes from the drug industry itself. In a recent debate at the University of Pennsylvania, Dr. Robert Freeman, an executive at AstraZeneca, told the audience, "We do marketing directly to physicians because we know it works. We all try to differentiate ourselves. And we do that by advertisement. We do that by marketing. We do that by promotion. And again I would point out, it's very effective."[52]

Though their comments may be self-serving, spokespersons for the advertising industry seem to have it right. "Creating consumer demand for prescription pharmaceuticals is now an attainable marketing objective," said one advertising executive. And a consultant predicted, "The winners in the prescription drug category are not going to be the ones with the best patents or products, but those that are the best marketers."[70] In other words, the use of new drugs—and their costs—will have only a little to do with scientific evidence of benefit, but a lot to do with effective marketing.

7

Making Friends, Playing Monopoly, and Dirty Tricks

Other Industry Strategies

With all due respect, this committee and this Congress jump when the drug industry says "jump"; it rushes to pass legislation when the drug industry wants it to pass legislation. —Representative Sherrod Brown (D-Ohio)[1]

PhRMA, this lobby, has a death grip on Congress. —Senator Richard J. Durbin (D-Illinois)[2]

DOCTORS may prescribe, but politicians write the laws that regulate the drug and device industries, tax incentives, Medicare and other federal health-care programs, the use of patents, and medical care in general. For drug and device manufacturers, members of congress are especially important friends. Campaign contributions and lobbying costs are among the expenses for making them friends.

Making Friends

In the 2000 presidential election year cycle, including 1999 and 2000, the pharmaceutical and health product industry contributed almost $27 million to political candidates, according to the Center for Responsive Politics. The top recipients were George W. Bush, Orrin Hatch, Bob Franks, and Rick Lazio—the Republican presidential candidate and three Republican Senate candidates. However, Democratic candidates shared the largesse, with Bill Bradley, Joseph Lieberman, and Al Gore also scoring in the top ten. Each of the top ten received over $100,000.[3] The industry sponsored lavish events at both national political conventions. Overall, though, the industry favored Republicans, with about two-thirds of the dollars going to the GOP.

The issue that was of greatest concern to the industry was a Medicare prescription benefit. While more government spending for Medicare drugs might seem good for manufacturers, the industry was opposed to the Democrats' plan, which included a component of price control.[3] For example, Democratic representative Thomas Allen from Maine had proposed to let pharmacies buy drugs for Medicare patients at the same price paid by the VA, Medicaid, and big HMOs. This would have cut costs to Medicare patients almost in half.[4]

But there were other important issues at stake. Some companies were lobbying for patent extensions on their top moneymaking drugs. When Schering-Plough was seeking a five-year patent extension for Claritin, then Senator John Ashcroft signed on to legislation that would help. The same month, Schering-Plough dropped $50,000 into a joint soft money account set up by Ashcroft and the National Republican Senatorial Committee, according to press accounts.[5]

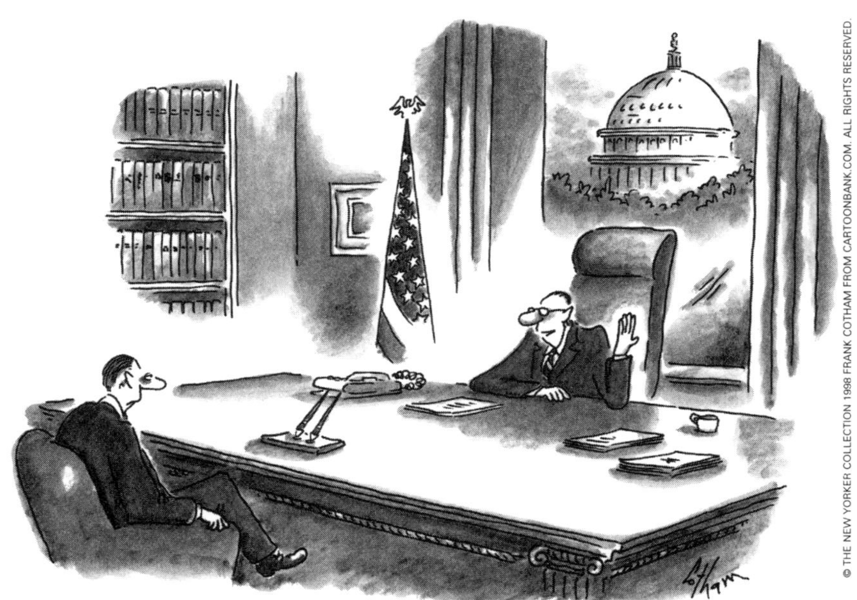

"I keep my core beliefs written on my palm for easy reference."

Similarly, during the 2000 election campaign, Senator Orrin Hatch of Utah received over $169,000 in drug industry contributions. This included use of a company airplane from Schering-Plough. Leaving no stone unturned, Schering-Plough also donated $50,000 to the Democratic Senatorial Campaign Committee. Senator Robert Toricelli of New Jersey, home state of Schering-Plough, accepted the donation. Though Toricelli wasn't up for reelection, he was sponsoring a patent extension bill.[6]

Contributions didn't go only to congressional representatives, of course. In 1999, former Surgeon General C. Everett Koop, "America's family doctor," supported a bill that would extend patent protection for Claritin. According to press reports, the Koop Foundation had just received a $1 million grant from Schering-Plough, the maker of Claritin. When critics suggested that the gift might be influencing his position, Koop responded: "I have never been bought, I cannot be bought. I am an icon, and I have a reputation for honesty and integrity, and let the chips fall where they may. . . . It is true that there are people in my situation who could not receive a million-dollar grant and stay objective. But I do."[7]

According to *The Wall Street Journal,* the investment in campaign contributions generated some important returns. Those returns on investment included Republican opposition to Medicare drug coverage proposals that included price controls. They also included delays in implementing patient privacy rules opposed by the industry.

Furthermore, the drug industry's support of Republican candidates earned it some important positions in the administration. The CEO of Merck and top officials at PhRMA (the Pharmaceutical Research and Manufacturers Association) became advisers to the Bush transition team. An executive from Lilly became director of the White House Office of Management and Budget.[8]

Generous as the drug industry's campaign contributions were, lobbying expenses dwarfed them. In the 2000 election cycle, these totaled $177 million, along with $65 million on issue ads. These ads try to shape public opinion on issues that are important to the drug companies. In 2002, the industry hired 675 lobbyists, well over one for every member of Congress, according to lobbying disclosure documents compiled by the watchdog group Public Citizen. The list included 26 former members of Congress and another 342 who had worked in Congress or other federal government positions. The major issues targeted by lobbyists? Again, Medicare drug benefit plans, patents, and drug pricing.[9]

Who were these lobbyists? You may be surprised at how many of their names you recognize. Many of them were former politicians who are influential and well connected in the halls of Congress. They include former Senators Connie Mack (R-Florida) and Birch Bayh (D-Indiana). PhRMA employed former Democratic Representative Vic Fazio of California. Pfizer hired former Democratic Senator Dennis DiConcini of Arizona and former Republican Representative Norman Lent of New York, as well as Orrin Hatch's son Scott. Merck has employed former Democratic Representative Tom Downey of New York. The list of former aides, advisers, and relatives of members of Congress is long and distinguished.[9]

One of the most potent weapons against a Medicare drug benefit that would reduce prices, though, wasn't the hired gun in Washington. It was an innocent-sounding, ersatz grassroots organization called Citizens for Better Medicare. It's best known for an aggressive TV and newspaper campaign against adding drug benefits to Medicare that featured "Flo," who warned against letting "big government" into her medicine cabinet. The group could raise and spend unlimited sums, without disclosure, as long as it didn't directly intervene in an election—such as by endorsing a candidate.[10–13]

The group was founded by Tim Ryan, former marketing director of PhRMA, the industry trade group for drug manufacturers. According to *The Wall Street Journal,* he did so at the "behest and expense" of major drug companies.[14] Other founders were from the Healthcare Leadership Council, which is made up of fifty drug companies, health-care providers, and hospitals. According to the Center for Responsive Politics, the biggest donors—Bristol-Myers Squibb and Pfizer—each contributed over a million dollars to political campaigns through the group. Altogether, the group's members contributed $9.9 million in soft money, contributions to political action committees, and individual contributions to federal candidates in the 2000 election cycle.[13] Although this group has little to do with pushing any particular drug, it has a lot to do with maintaining high drug prices overall.

Other organizations with support from PhRMA helped with television ads supporting Republican proposals for a Medicare drug benefit. The United Seniors Association, self-described as a "conservative seniors' organization," ran a $3 million ad campaign in about a dozen cities during May of 2002. The organization's president, Charles Jarvis, denied that PhRMA funded the ads, claiming that they were a grassroots effort. But a PhRMA spokesperson indicated that her organization had recently given United Seniors an "unrestricted educational grant" of an undisclosed amount. Jarvis acknowledged to *The Wall Street Journal* that most of the costs associated with the effort, including an additional $4 million Internet and direct mail campaign, were supported by a "general educational grant" from PhRMA. These funds supported House candidates who favored Republican Medicare proposals backed by the industry.[15]

As for lobbying to obtain patent extensions, an important strategy has been to work the desired language into critical legislation dealing with other issues. In 1996, Searle used a stealth approach to get a two-year extension on its patent for Daypro, an anti-inflammatory drug. How? By successfully getting a clause into the omnibus budget bill. This was legislation that Congress had to pass to prevent a government shutdown.[16]

For the 2003–2004 election year cycle, PhRMA budgeted $150 million to influence Congress, states, foreign governments, and public opinion. This figure, reported from confidential documents obtained by *The New York Times,* included the following items:

- $73 million for advocacy at the federal level, mainly with Congress
- $5 million to lobby the FDA
- $49 million for advocacy at the state level
- $18 million to fight price controls and protect patent rights in foreign countries

Specific items listed in the plan included $16 million to fight a get-out-the-vote initiative in Ohio that would lower drug prices for those without insurance coverage for drugs. Another was $9 million for PR, including op-eds and articles by third parties. And $2 million was allocated "to build intellectual capital and generate a higher volume of messages from credible sources" sympathetic to the industry.[2]

Playing Monopoly

Companies that develop new drugs get to patent them for twenty years. The industry is actively trying to increase the duration of these patents. This means that there can't be generic drug competition during that time, although other companies may develop similar drugs that compete. Some of the time under patent is often spent in the testing and development phases, but Stephen Hall of *The New York Times* estimates that the exclusive run in the marketplace averages about sixteen years.[17]

These patents are important for allowing companies to recoup the costs of drug development, which are high. The high profits that accrue during the life of the patent are a reward for innovation and an incentive to continue innovating. They also keep drug prices high. When patents expire, the price of a drug typically falls dramatically as generic competitors are introduced. So drug companies have every incentive to extend their patents as long as possible.

By various estimates, developing a new drug typically costs somewhere between $100 million and $800 million.[18,19] The higher figure comes from industry-funded estimates, the lower one from consumer advocates. These costs include lots of false starts for every drug that actually proves to be safe and effective, and the process typically requires seven years per marketable drug. Once a drug is marketed, the costs of manufacturing a pill are small, so development costs are the largest part of the investment.

Although these figures are daunting, the returns usually more than cover the bills. Consider the global sales of some top-ten drugs for a single year, 2003. Lipitor, for lowering cholesterol, earned $10.3 billion. Zocor, another cholesterol-lowering drug, was second at $6.1 billion. In tenth place was Zoloft, an antidepressant, at a mere $3.4 billion.[20] These drugs are admittedly best-sellers, but the point is that even a single year of sales can recoup development costs many times over. Extending a patent for even a few months can mean billions of dollars for the manufacturer. We shouldn't be surprised, then, when companies go to extraordinary lengths to extend those patents.

The New York Times quoted a former FDA official, who preferred not to be named, as saying, "It's always cheaper to litigate [to extend patents] than to lose market share. If you can keep a generic off the market for one day, three days, five days, two months, or two years, that's a lot of revenue." The *Times* estimated the cost of a lawsuit at $5 million, pointing out that it's less risky than new drug research, and that the return can be excellent.[17]

In 1984, Congress tried to simultaneously expedite the availability of less expensive generic drugs and reward the brand-name companies for developing new drugs. The Hatch-Waxman Act allowed the FDA to approve generic drugs without having generic manufacturers repeat the research to prove the drugs' safety and efficacy. At the same time, the brand-name drug companies were given an automatic patent extension of five years. This was intended to make up for time lost on patents while products were going through the FDA's approval process. The approval process can be lengthy, shrinking the duration of the patent after the drug hits the market.

Unfortunately, the law left loopholes that drug manufacturers zealously exploited. Drugs don't simply come "off patent" anymore, because the makers can patent not only the chemical compounds, but also the manufacturing process; other ingredients that may stabilize the active drug; the color, size, and shape of a pill; and the breakdown products of the drug after it's metabolized in the body.

The result, as described in *The New York Times,* is a series of strategically staggered patents, known as "layering," that can delay the emergence of generic drugs and lead to complicated litigation. For the companies that develop new drugs, the law also provided a powerful incentive for litigation: an automatic thirty-month patent extension if they sue generic drug makers for alleged patent infringement. Link this with the layered patents, and companies have the opportunity to pursue sequential suits and sequential patent extensions.[17]

In one example, Bristol-Myers Squibb submitted a new patent on BuSpar to the FDA just hours before BuSpar, its anti-anxiety drug, was to lose its patent. The company had already had exclusive sale of the drug for fifteen years and had made over $600 million from BuSpar in 2000 alone. The new patent was for a metabolite of the drug, and it forced a generic competitor, Mylan, to stop shipment of 46 million pills of its generic version. Mylan won a suit in federal court, but Bristol-Myers Squibb earned about $253 million in the meantime, according to *Consumer Reports.*[16,21,22]

Bristol-Myers Squibb appealed the court decision on Mylan's suit. But it then faced lawsuits from eighty insurance companies and twenty-nine states alleging that it had paid another generic drug company $72 million to keep a generic version of the drug off the market. Finally, consumer groups and three generic drug makers also filed lawsuits.[23,24,25]

GlaxoSmithKline played a similar card for its antidepressant drug Paxil. In 1998, a generic drug maker filed an application with the FDA to market a generic version of Paxil, but SmithKline Beecham (as the company was then called) alleged patent infringement, triggering the thirty-month extension. Since then, the company has filed suits regarding an additional four patents related to Paxil, starting the thirty-month clock anew. Altogether, GlaxoSmithKline extended its exclusive rights by five years.[26,27]

Drug companies also use other strategies to extend lucrative patents. A 1997 law promoted more testing of drug safety and efficacy for children by granting six-month patent extensions to companies that conduct formal studies in children. The law has led to more data about drugs for children, including information about dosing, safety, and formulation of several drugs. This is good.

However, drug companies are sometimes using the law to test drugs with infrequent application to children, such as those for high blood pressure, adult-onset diabetes, and high cholesterol. Companies gain an extra six months of monopoly, often worth millions of dollars, while the testing in children typically costs from $200,000 to $3 million, according to *The Wall Street Journal*.[28]

Consider the example of Pepcid, a drug for heartburn that had already been tested and found safe in children, but had never been approved by the FDA for children. Mothers were offered incentives to enroll their children in a new study. Mary Robinson, a Philadelphia x-ray technologist, got $300 plus a $50 gift certificate to Toys R Us for enrolling her seven-year-old daughter. The manufacturer, Merck, in turn made an estimated $290 million from the six-month patent extension it won.[28]

In another example of this strategy, Merck won a patent extension for its cholesterol drug Mevacor in 2001 based on pediatric testing. Merck's stock price immediately jumped almost 5 percent.[29] The FDA estimated that the law will raise the cost of prescription drugs by about $13.9 billion over twenty years and result in $29.6 billion in additional revenue for brand-name drug makers.[30]

Big employers, who pay most of our health insurance premiums, and state governments, who fund Medicaid, are among those most concerned about drug costs. It's no surprise that a coalition of ten governors, several labor leaders, and eleven major corporations—including General Motors, Wal-Mart, and Verizon Communications—has asked Congress to close some of the loopholes in the Hatch-Waxman Act that are used to extend patents. The coalition believes that reforms could save $600 million over three years for seventeen brand-name drugs alone—drugs whose patents are due to expire soon.[31]

It's also no surprise that PhRMA is vigorously opposed to the coalition and has made concerted efforts to stop companies from joining it. PhRMA has succeeded in pressuring some companies to quit the coalition or reduce their role. The drug industry's position is that reforms in the patent laws would stifle innovation and research by reducing revenues.[31]

Given the enormous incentive to delay competition, brand-name drug makers have used another strategy to delay the emergence of generic drugs. They simply pay generic companies not to produce a competing version. For example, in 1998, Geneva Pharmaceuticals won FDA approval to market a generic version of Hytrin, a drug used to treat enlargement of the prostate gland. Instead of launching the drug, though, Geneva entered into an agreement with Abbott Laboratories, which had developed the drug. According to the Federal Trade Commission (FTC), Abbott paid Geneva $4.5 million per month not to market the generic version—more than Geneva was likely to make from sales of the drug.[16]

Other generic companies couldn't jump in because of yet another provision of the Hatch-Waxman Act: one that gives the first approved generic manufacturer a six-month exclusive head start before other generics can compete. Both companies denied any illegal activity, but agreed to a settlement with the FTC.[16] During a suit filed by several states against Abbott and Geneva, Colorado Attorney General Ken Salazar said that state agencies paid $137 for 100 tablets of Hytrin, while the Geneva version was priced at about $18.[32]

Other examples abound. When Barr Laboratories, a generic drug maker, challenged Bayer's patent on the antibiotic Cipro, Bayer reportedly agreed to pay Barr $28 million a year until the planned expiration of the patent.[33] The FTC alleges that Schering-Plough paid a division of American Home Products $30 million and Upsher-Smith Laboratories $60 million to delay marketing generic versions of K-Dur, a potassium supplement often prescribed to patients taking diuretics. Similarly, the FTC complained that Hoechst Marion Roussel entered into an agreement with Andrx Corporation, paying millions of dollars to delay marketing a generic alternative to Cardizem CD, a drug used to treat angina.[34]

Yet another strategy for winning at Monopoly is to cut off the supply of ingredients to your competitors. The FTC charged that Mylan Laboratories conspired with three chemical suppliers to deny other generic drug makers access to the ingredients necessary for making two anti-anxiety drugs, clorazepate and lorazepam. After blocking the supply of ingredients to its competitors, Mylan raised the wholesale price of both drugs more than twenty-five-fold. The increases cost consumers an estimated $120 million, according to the FTC. Though it denied wrongdoing, Mylan agreed to pay $147 million to compensate patients, insurers, managed-care organizations, and state agencies and to pay attorney's fees, according to *Consumer Reports*.[16]

Dirty Tricks

PAYING HEALTH-CARE PROVIDERS TO USE DRUGS

Dr. David Franklin went to work for the drug company Warner-Lambert in 1996, and resigned later the same year. He concluded that he'd become a crucial component in an apparent plan to illegally market the epilepsy drug Neurontin. He proceeded to file a whistle-blower suit alleging that Parke-Davis (a subsidiary of Warner-Lambert, in turn now owned by Pfizer) illegally influenced and paid kickbacks to doctors who prescribed the epilepsy drug Neurontin for purposes never approved by the FDA.[35,36]

It appears that some companies go a step beyond marketing drugs, effectively paying doctors, pharmacies, or health plans to use them. Neurontin may be a prime example. Sadly, this may be more common than anyone wants to believe. According to *The New York Times,* 37 percent of Maryland doctors report that they've accepted some kind of compensation from drug companies.[37]

Neurontin is approved for use as an adjunct, or second drug, for treating seizures, and also for treating pain due to shingles. However, the drug is widely used for treating other chronic pain problems and certain psychiatric conditions, even though it's not approved for such uses. Doctors can legally prescribe a drug for such "off-label" uses, but drug companies aren't allowed to advertise these unapproved uses.

Several state attorneys general and the U.S. attorney's office in Boston have been investigating the marketing practices for this drug, which now has sales of over $2 billion a year.[38,39] The *Boston Globe* reported that court documents included a memo to Parke-Davis sales reps instructing them to "target neurologists with the greatest potential" by offering an all-expenses-paid weekend at a Florida resort, including a $250 honorarium for every doctor. A transcribed voicemail message from a manager told representatives, "When we get [to doctors], we want to kick some ass. We want to sell Neurontin on pain. All right?"[40]

The federal suit alleged that the company paid doctors to allow sales reps to watch as they examined patients. This allowed the reps to make

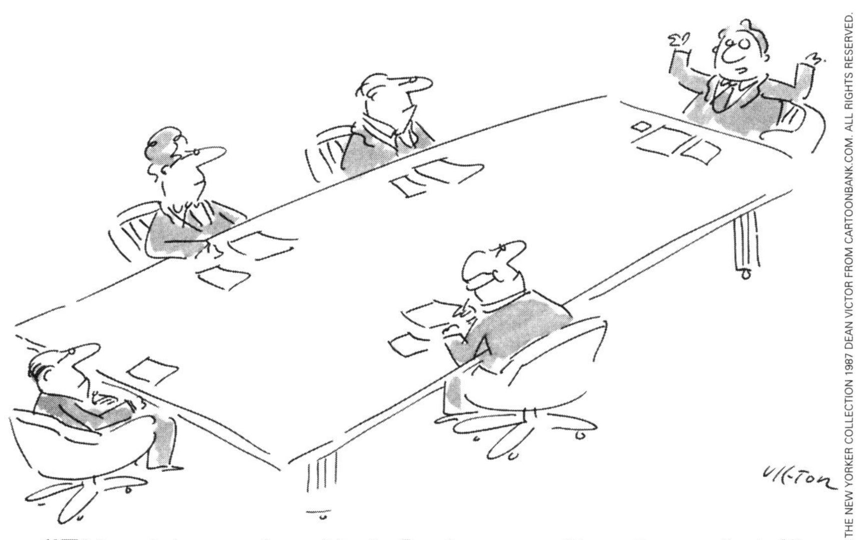

"This might not be ethical. Is that a problem for anybody?"

suggestions as to which patients might benefit from Neurontin. The payments were reportedly $350 for each day of access. It also claimed that the company paid some key doctors $1,000 each to sign their names to at least twenty ghostwritten articles for medical journals. The articles concerned off-label uses of Neurontin, and would serve the purpose of promoting such uses. The suit also alleged that the company urged prescribing higher doses than those approved by the FDA. Yet another claim was that the company paid doctors to promote Neurontin to their colleagues at dinners and weekend retreats at destinations like Aspen, Colorado.

According to court documents, the top speaker for Neurontin was Dr. B. J. Wilder, a former professor at the University of Florida. Wilder apparently received more than $300,000 for lectures over a three-year period. Other court documents suggest that Warner-Lambert hired an accredited continuing education company with the goal of increasing Neurontin prescriptions for pain, one of the unapproved uses. The company recommended creating courses for doctors that would have the desired effect, according to the *Boston Globe.*[35,37,39,40]

The suit further claimed that these marketing practices cost Medicaid programs alone tens of millions of dollars. Legal or not, the marketing campaign appeared to be successful. *The New York Times* reports that off-label uses account for almost 90 percent of Neurontin sales.[41] It also reported 2003 sales of Neurontin as $2.7 billion.

The New York Times reported that Dr. Franklin was most troubled by the company's insistence that he encourage doctors to prescribe higher-than-approved doses. Franklin said, "It was untried ground. . . . I recognized that my actions may be putting people in harm's way." Franklin said that marketing executives had told him that Neurontin appeared to be safe in high doses, so it was reasonable to encourage doctors to try it for almost any neurological condition "just to see what happens." He also reported that he was trained to exaggerate research results and hide reports of side effects.[36,37]

Franklin said he "was terrified" to file the suit, but his career has survived, and he now works for a medical device company.[36,37] Pfizer, which now owns Warner-Lambert, said that it did not promote Neurontin for off-label uses and was unaware of credible evidence that the Parke-Davis subsidiary made false claims.[35] Nonetheless, in May 2004, Pfizer pleaded guilty to civil and criminal charges and agreed to pay a $430 million settlement.[41]

For drugs that must be administered in doctors' offices—including some cancer chemotherapy, certain AIDS drugs, and new arthritis drugs like Remicade—doctors may not be paid directly, but they can profit handsomely. Doctors buy these drugs at deeply discounted prices and administer them to patients in their offices, usually intravenously. The doctors are then reimbursed by Medicare and other payers at close to the "average wholesale price"—a much higher figure set by the drug maker. The difference between what the doctor pays and the average wholesale price often amounts to hundreds of dollars per dose, a profit to the prescribing doctor. The higher the drug price, the more the doctor usually keeps, so manufacturers sometimes perversely compete to price their drugs *higher,* hoping to attract more doctors' business.

An example is alleged in a lawsuit filed by a group of unions, health benefits funds, and consumer organizations. They argued that Johnson & Johnson's subsidiary Centocor boosted demand for Remicade (used in treating rheumatoid arthritis) by "bribing" doctors to prescribe it and to seek "inflated reimbursement" from Medicare. The suit also claimed "unspecified illegal bribes and kickbacks" to doctors for prescribing Remicade.[42]

Remicade can cost more than $20,000 a year. *The New York Times* quoted Dr. Paul April, a rheumatologist in Tulsa, Oklahoma, as saying that the rheumatology field was "abuzz" with discussion of the money to be made, and that doctors were choosing Remicade over Enbrel (a similar new drug) because of the extra money they could make. He said, "Remicade is a good drug, but it is being overused because there is money to be made by using it."[43]

The *Times* indicated that until a reporter asked about it, Centocor had a web site that stated that one "benefit" of prescribing Remicade was the "financial impact" on the physician's practice. It included a worksheet to calculate "estimated revenue per patient," pointing out that the revenue was primarily the difference between what Medicare pays doctors and the lower amount doctors pay for the drug.[43] Though the outcome of the suit remains unclear, similar allegations are being brought by federal investigators against the makers of several cancer drugs.

For example, in 2001, TAP Pharmaceuticals reached a criminal and civil settlement over charges that it had defrauded Medicare and Medicaid by exaggerating wholesale prices for Lupron, its prostate cancer drug. Federal prosecutors alleged that TAP had artificially inflated the drug's wholesale price to increase sales, selling the drug to doctors for $100 to $150 less and encouraging them to bill at the higher wholesale price.[43] One remarkable part of the settlement included the company's admission that members of its sales force had helped doctors charge the government for free samples of Lupron, a violation of federal law. TAP ended up agreeing to an $875 million fine.[44,45]

The TAP case also began with a whistle-blower, Douglas Durand. Like David Franklin at Warner-Lambert, Durand had just taken a new job with TAP and was astonished at some of the company's sales tactics. In *Business Week,* he indicated that TAP had developed a plan to give a 2 percent "administration fee" up front to any doctor who agreed to prescribe Lupron. In addition, the company had offered every urologist in the country—about ten thousand doctors—a big-screen TV, as well as computers, fax machines, and golf vacations. According to Durand, some doctors made so much by prescribing Lupron that "They'd brag, 'Oh, there's my Lupron boat, my Lupron summer house.'"[45] Clearly, physicians share the blame for some marketing excesses.

Of course, Lupron's main competitor, Zoladex, was also aggressively marketed by its maker, AstraZeneca. In one example, a New Jersey urologist, Dr. Saad Antoun, pleaded guilty to billing insurers for free samples of Zoladex and pocketing between $30,000 and $70,000 as a result. News accounts indicated that Antoun switched from prescribing Lupron to Zoladex after a company representative explained how he could make just as much money by using Zoladex.[46]

Then in 2003, AstraZeneca pleaded guilty to violating the Prescription Drug Marketing Act and agreed to pay $355 million to settle civil and criminal charges for marketing schemes similar to those used by TAP for Lupron. Douglas Durand commented, "It was egregious, the behaviors of both companies, in terms of fraud against consumers." He claimed that the companies knew of each other's illegal sales methods and kept a "peaceful coexistence."[47]

Sometimes, drug company largesse has benefited health-care organizations rather than individual doctors. Another story involving Parke-Davis featured yet another whistle-blower, John David Foster. Foster alleged to prosecutors that the company gave the Ochsner Health Plan in Louisiana a $250,000 "educational grant" to encourage placing the cholesterol-lowering drug Lipitor on the organization's preferred drug list. Federal prosecutors maintained that the grant was a "disguised rebate" that helped keep Lipitor prices artificially high. This, in turn, cost the Medicaid program $20 million more than necessary, according to the government. Without admitting any wrongdoing, Pfizer, which subsequently bought the company, agreed in 2002 to pay $49 million to settle the allegations with the federal government and forty states.[48] Altogether, six drug companies paid $1.6 billion to settle whistle-blower suits between 2001 and 2003.[49]

USING PHARMACIES FOR PROMOTION

A different strategy raises concern about patient confidentiality. Some companies have used pharmacy records to target patients for inducements to change drugs. In 2002, the Florida attorney general's office began investigating whether Eli Lilly and Co. had sent free samples of the antidepressant Prozac to patients who were taking other antidepressants. A Florida woman who received a sample brought suit against Lilly, Walgreen Co., and her doctors, alleging that Walgreen allowed access to her records and provided Lilly with a list of antidepressant users. Lilly subsequently disciplined three sales managers and five reps over the incident, saying that the actions were inconsistent with company policy.[50,51]

In 1998, a pharmacy-based program had created a similar stir. Two drug chains in Washington, D.C., sent prescription records to a database marketing firm. The marketing firm, in turn, mailed reminders for refills or information about new drugs. One mailing targeted patients using nicotine treatments, telling them about the new drug Zyban, for smoking cessation. It was signed "Your CVS pharmacists," but the fine print noted that the mailing was supported by Glaxo Wellcome Inc., the maker of Zyban. Some mailings concerned other drugs, and the marketing company had sent about 200,000 mailings on behalf of one drug chain alone. Drug makers paid the pharmacy chains and the marketing firm for the mailings, and patients didn't know that their medical information was being used in this way.[52,53]

The president of the marketing firm thought, "This is good medical and good entrepreneurial practice, which is the nice thing about it."[54] Patients thought differently, and the pharmacy chains canceled the program after news stories elicited outrage. One spokesperson said, "The customer response was extremely negative, and because of privacy concerns we decided to discontinue. . . . Our phones rang off the hook."[54]

In some cases, these efforts touted more expensive versions of the patient's current medications. In others, the campaign targeted drugs whose patents were about to expire, hoping to maximize sales before prices dropped. In spring of 2002, Senator Charles Schumer of New York asked the FTC to investigate these practices, arguing, "These letters preempt the patient-doctor relationship, predisposing patients to a more costly course of treatment."

The National Association of Chain Drug Stores argued that this was simply a way of better informing patients, and PhRMA responded that competition among drug companies must be a good thing.[55] But in 2002, the Bush administration enacted new rules to prevent this marketing strategy, which had been steadily growing, citing concerns about patient privacy.

WRITING GUIDELINES

Because the medical research literature is so large, complex, and fast-growing, it's common for professional societies and health-care organizations to write clinical guidelines to help doctors with common treatment decisions. These guidelines aim to incorporate data from the best research, often combined with expert opinion, to recommend the most effective treatment approaches. These guidelines are intended to influence large numbers of physicians. We might hope that the panels that write these guidelines are free of commercial interests.

But in 2002, a group of researchers surveyed one hundred authors who were involved with thirty-seven guidelines endorsed by North American or European medical societies. Among these authors, 87 percent had some financial interaction with the drug industry. Some 58 percent had received financial support for research, and 38 percent had been employees or consultants for drug companies. In most cases, the companies made drugs that were considered in the guidelines. Only one guideline disclosed that some authors had personal financial interactions with the drug industry.[56]

An example of such conflicts of interest occurred with a guideline for treating strokes prepared by the American Heart Association (AHA). In August 2000, the AHA upgraded its recommendation for clot-busting drug therapy for acute strokes from "optional" to "definitely recommended." The drug it recommended was alteplase, a new biotech product made by Genentech. But the AHA subsequently faced intense criticism. According to an article in the *British Medical Journal,* Genentech had donated $2.5 million to the AHA to build its new headquarters in Dallas. Furthermore, Genentech had contributed $11 million to the AHA over a decade.[57]

Journalist Jeanne Lenzer conducted an independent investigation and learned that six of the nine panelists responsible for the guidelines had ties to Genentech. The AHA hadn't published this information with the guidelines. Though the AHA had required the panelists to file conflict of interest statements, it would not release the statements for public review. Two of the panelists acknowledged their ties only after being presented with other evidence of their connections to Genentech.

The one panelist who didn't support the recommendation, Dr. Jerome Hoffman, had no company ties. He was asked to write a dissenting commentary, but this was never published or mentioned in the guidelines. At his request, his name was removed from the list of guideline authors. But—for unexplained reasons—it was also removed from the list of panelists. This left the appearance of no dissent to the final guideline.[57]

In the meantime, the AHA had been conducting a campaign to refer to a stroke as a "brain attack," similar to "heart attack," to give the same sense of urgency about treatment. That campaign indicated that alteplase could "save lives," although none of the trials had shown a reduction in mortality from its use in stroke.

What was the evidence supporting alteplase for stroke? Randomized trials were fairly consistent in showing an advantage for alteplase in reducing disability, but not reducing mortality. Furthermore, it was only effective if it was given within three hours of stroke onset.[57,58] Experience in actual practice (outside the tightly managed research setting) has sometimes been discouraging, with some reports of increased, rather than decreased, mortality.[59,60]

Using the stringent entry criteria of the U.S. trials, including the requirement for treatment within three hours of stroke onset, few patients actually stand to benefit. By one expert estimate, the treatment will benefit less than 1 percent of stroke patients. Even if every patient sought care within three hours (an unlikely scenario), only 4 percent of patients would benefit.[61] The most generous estimate concluded that about 8 percent of stroke patients stand to benefit.[62] The American Heart Association recently withdrew statements that alteplase for stroke, at $2,500 per dose, "saves lives."[58]

Other professional societies have been more cautious about the evidence for alteplase. The American Academy of Emergency Medicine and the Society for Academic Emergency Medicine have concluded that the evidence does not yet warrant making it the standard of care for stroke.[57,63] Dr. Robert McNamara, president of the American Academy of Emergency Medicine, was quoted as saying, "We're being hoodwinked. The whole thing is fueled by drug company money. It leaves a bad taste in your mouth."[64]

European groups have also been more cautious, and European research studies are continuing.[65] A recent review concluded that alteplase may reduce disability from stroke despite a short-term increase in death. The risk-benifit tradeoff is complex, and the reviewers concluded that the treatment was "promising," but that the data "do not support the widespread use of thrombolytic therapy in routine clinical practice at this time."[66] Whatever the final place of alteplase in stroke management may be, many experts now seem to agree that guideline authors should provide full written disclosure of any conflicts of interest, and that these disclosures should be made available to readers.

All of these strategies—making influential friends, playing Monopoly, and dirty tricks—have an important effect on how new drug technology gets used and how much it costs. In some cases, the drugs involved have unique or valuable properties. However, political influence and dubious marketing strategies have often determined how they're used, more than scientific evidence or free competition in an open market.

8

Stacking the Deck?

How to Get the "Right" Answer in Clinical Research

There are three kinds of lies: lies, damn lies, and statistics. —variously attributed to Disraeli and Mark Twain

IF YOU HAVE arthritis, an injection of "oil" to "lubricate" your joints sounds very alluring. Some of my (Rick's) patients have used just such a metaphor in requesting injections of hyaluronic acid, recently marketed for treating osteoarthritis (the common "wear and tear" kind of arthritis). Hyaluronic acid is the component of joint fluid that gives it lubricating qualities, and it's low in arthritic joints. "Adding a quart of oil" is an almost irresistible approach, and preparations of hyaluronic acid made it seem possible.

The results of a clinical trial published in 2002 seemed to support the notion. Researchers randomly assigned 120 patients with osteoarthritis of the knee to get injections of hyaluronic acid; an oral anti-inflammatory drug; both; or neither. Placebos were used to assure that neither doctors nor patients knew who was getting active treatments. After several weeks of treatment, pain and walking ability were measured. The analysis and conclusions of the authors indicated that the hyaluronic acid injections were effective. The study was supported by the manufacturer, Bioniche Life Sciences, Inc., and one of the authors was a company employee.[1] So far, so good.

Unfortunately, the researchers used a statistical analysis that was suboptimal for comparing treatment effects among groups, and failed to use the maximum amount of information from all subjects. (For aficionados of research design, the published analysis showed a pre- to posttreatment analysis within each of the four treatment groups rather than a comparison of change among groups, and failed to analyze the data as a factorial experiment, as it was designed.)

When two Boston University researchers reanalyzed the data correctly, they found that the injections were no better than placebo. And the improvement from the oral anti-inflammatory drug was many times greater than that seen with the hyaluronic acid injections. They also identified three other studies, even larger in size, all of which showed no benefit of hyaluronic acid injections compared to placebo injections.[2]

Other reviewers concluded that this treatment, marketed under the names Synvisc, Provisc, and Suplasy, "should be shelved under the heading 'Good idea—doesn't work.'"[3] In a more recent synthesis of all the literature, researchers concluded, "Our findings suggest the controversy surrounding the efficacy of intra-articular hyaluronic acid is justified and that the best available data does not support its efficacy."[4]

Many drug trials are conducted with impeccable methods and data analysis, often by independent researchers. But it's become clear that when research is sponsored by industry, it's more likely to get results that are favorable to the company's product than when the research is independently sponsored.[5–8] The flawed data analysis in the hyaluronic acid study illustrated one reason, although the statistical issues are a bit arcane. Some other explanations for favorable results in company-sponsored trials are easier to grasp.

Withholding Data

In a celebrated example, the makers of Celebrex sponsored a study published in the prominent *Journal of the American Medical Association*. The results of the six-month study indicated that Celebrex caused less stomach problems than older, competing anti-inflammatory drugs like ibuprofen.[9] What the company didn't share was that it also had data from one-year follow-up, which showed similar rates of stomach ulcers for Celebrex and its competitors.[10,11] The editor of *JAMA* was not amused.[12]

Withholding data from publication was an issue at *JAMA*, in particular, because of a previous incident.[13] In that case, the manufacturer of a thyroid hormone replacement blocked publication of an unfavorable study—one that it had sponsored—for seven years.[14] That delay helped the company retain its majority share of the market, and kept its value high for a merger that occurred before eventual publication.[15]

In another case, a researcher found that a drug he was studying caused side effects and sent his manuscript to the sponsoring company for review. In response, the company proceeded to publish a competing article with little mention of side effects and warned the researcher that it would never again support his work. Similar stories are common, though no one knows the real prevalence of this sort of activity.[16]

These and similar incidents gave impetus to a joint statement by twelve journals declaring they would not publish studies "that allow the sponsor to have sole control of the data or to withhold publication."[17] Sadly, it appears that even academic institutions are failing to adhere to the guidelines regarding trial design, access to data, and publication rights.[18]

Even if publication is not withheld altogether, results are sometimes delayed. Harvard researchers surveyed 2,100 life science faculty to determine how common delay of publication might be. There were 410 who indicated a delay of over six months in publishing research results. Of these, 28 percent indicated that the reason was "to slow dissemination of undesired results." Although this represented only 5 percent of all researchers surveyed, the impact on clinical practice may be important.[19]

Furthermore, a study from Carnegie-Mellon University reported that in a sample of university-industry research centers, 35 percent of signed agreements allowed sponsors to delete information from publications, 53 percent allowed publications to be delayed, and 30 percent allowed both.[14]

In some cases, studies are designed with multiple outcome measures, and only those that favor the new drug are included in the published version. Even if unfavorable results aren't completely blocked, one researcher says, "When results are disappointing, there is commonly an effort to spin, downplay, or change findings."[16]

For example, Dr. Curt Furberg, a professor of public health sciences at Wake Forest University, described a research study on high blood pressure. He ran a study comparing a new drug, called a calcium-channel blocker, with an older diuretic drug that was also used for high blood pressure. When he found that the diuretic seemed more effective than the new drug, the company, Sandoz (now Novartis), disagreed with his analysis of the data, and writing up the results became contentious. Furberg told *U.S. News & World Report,* "We went through the draft and presented our version of the results to the company. But the company kept changing it back to an older version that we didn't agree with." After ten drafts, Furberg and four other authors gave up and took their names off the paper, despite five years of effort.[20]

Even aside from intentional suppression of bad news, positive studies (those showing a benefit for a drug) are more likely to get published than negative studies.[21–23] The reasons for this phenomenon are multiple. In some cases, researchers lose their enthusiasm when results are disappointing, and simply don't pursue the project through to publication. In some cases, negative results run counter to conventional wisdom or prevailing theories, leading researchers to suspect the results must be wrong or to shy away from challenging authority—even though it may be the theory that's wrong and in need of correction.[24] Whatever the reason, the effect is to create a research literature that may overrepresent good results and underrepresent bad results, giving doctors and patients an erroneous view of treatment efficacy and safety.

Repeated Publication of the Same Data

Perhaps the opposite of withholding negative results is publishing positive results over and over. When the same study is published repetitively, sometimes with different authors and different titles, it creates the impression in the medical literature that there is more evidence, based on more patients, than really exists. It gives "an artificial impression of wide support for the efficacy of an intervention," in the words of two researchers who sought to review and summarize the literature on risperidone, a relatively new drug for treating schizophrenia. After a "vexing," "bewildering," and "intolerably time-consuming" effort, they discovered that twenty articles and several unpublished reports on the drug actually represented only seven small studies and two large ones. One of the larger studies had been reported in six publications, often without reference to the others, and with different authorship for each.[25]

Redundant reports have also been documented for the antinausea drug ondansetron (Zofran),[26] the antifungal drug Diflucan,[27] and nonsteroidal anti-inflammatory drugs.[28] In the case of ondansetron, reviewers of the articles found that when all studies were combined, it appeared that 11,980 patients had been studied, but when duplicate reports were identified, the number fell to 8,645. Furthermore, including the duplicate data inflated the apparent efficacy of the drug by 23 percent. The redundant publications weren't easy to uncover: Expert authors of eight other articles, reviews, and book chapters hadn't noticed.[26]

Repeated publication of the same data is theoretically prohibited by most major medical journals—including all the journals in which duplicate studies of ondansetron appeared.[26,28] Why would authors bother? In some cases, university-based researchers face a "publish or perish" academic environment. They want to increase their publication numbers even if there's no commercial value, because it enhances the prospects for promotion, prestige, or salary increases. But for company-sponsored trials, other motivations may be at play. It may bias information in favor of a new drug, create the appearance of stronger evidence than really exists, and even increase stock values.

Unfair Comparisons

Another unfortunate strategy is to compare optimal doses of a new drug with suboptimal doses of a comparison drug. A new drug might also be compared with an incorrectly administered comparison drug (e.g., oral instead of intravenous), or with a drug known to be ineffective for the purpose at hand. Comparison with a placebo is sometimes necessary if there's no other effective treatment available, or if it's required for FDA approval. But in many cases, effective alternatives are well known.

A clever example of misleading comparisons occurred in studies of Diflucan, an antifungal drug, among cancer patients at high risk for fungal infections. The three largest studies all had three treatment arms: Diflucan, the new drug; nystatin, an older drug known from the start to be ineffective for this use; and amphotericin B, an older drug that must be given intravenously because it's poorly absorbed orally. In each study, the data analysis combined the nystatin and amphotericin groups, ostensibly because of chemical similarities. However, because nystatin was ineffective, this analysis had the effect of diluting any apparent benefit of amphotericin. Furthermore, most of the amphotericin patients were given oral rather than intravenous doses.

Not surprisingly, Diflucan looked better. But other researchers teased out data from these and additional trials. Once they separated the results for nystatin from those for amphotericin, they found that, as expected, nystatin was no better than a placebo. But they also found that Diflucan was no better than amphotericin. The three large studies were all sponsored by the manufacturer (Pfizer); two included Pfizer employees among the authors, and the authorship was overlapping. In fact, the independent researchers couldn't be certain that they were completely separate studies.[27,28]

Studies often use patients for whom the drugs are most likely to be safe and effective, even though their widest use may be in very different kinds of patients. New arthritis drugs, for example, are often tested in middle-aged adults with no medical problems besides their arthritis. In actual practice, though, these drugs are most likely to be used by older adults, many of whom have multiple medical problems, and who often are taking other drugs at the same time. The data on drug doses and drug safety observed in younger, healthier adults are misleading when applied to older patients, for whom the risks are greater and appropriate doses must often be smaller. Many doctors and patients learn this only through difficult trial and error.

Pharmacologist Lisa Bero and physician journal editor Drummond Rennie at the University of California, San Francisco, have cataloged a lengthy list of errors and misleading features of study design and analysis in published drug trials. The list is far more extensive than the problems described here, and the biases are sometimes more subtle. Others—such as fabricated data or methods—aren't so subtle. Bero and Rennie concluded that published studies are sometimes defective because drug company funding has affected their content and quality. Among other recommendations, they and others suggest that funders shouldn't be involved in presenting the data, that the researchers rather than industry-supported writers should be the authors, that sponsors shouldn't have sole control of the data, and that sponsors shouldn't be allowed to block publication.[29]

Asking the Wrong Questions

Sometimes it pays to step back from these details of research design and reporting and simply examine what questions are being studied. Doctors and their patients would most like studies that compare a new drug with the best available alternatives, addressing effectiveness, safety, convenience, and cost. The FDA requires evidence of efficacy and safety, but it doesn't necessarily require comparison with the best available alternative. Nor does it require the evidence (such as complication rates) to be published in medical journals. Convenience and cost aren't part of the agency's mandate at all. As editorialists have pointed out:

> Manufacturers would not benefit from studies to determine whether inexpensive, off-patent drugs or nonpharmaceutical interventions could replace profitable, single-source products, or from studies to determine the rates of adverse drug reactions.[30]

Thus, the information that doctors want most when prescribing is often unavailable. Drug manufacturers might subscribe to the comment of Thomas Pynchon in *Gravity's Rainbow:* "If they can get you asking the wrong questions, they don't have to worry about answers."[31]

This may explain why some effective treatments don't get used as often as they should. My (Rick's) father experienced a heart attack some fifteen years ago. It was already clear then that a class of drugs called beta-blockers (propranolol, metoprolol, atenolol, and the like) could substantially reduce deaths after a heart attack. But a new class of drugs called calcium-channel blockers was hitting the market and being heavily promoted (brand names like Procardia, Adalat, and others). These drugs were for treating angina and high blood pressure, although there was a sense that they must be good for heart problems more generally.

Dad had neither angina nor high blood pressure, but after the heart attack his doctor prescribed calcium-channel drugs, nonetheless—in a situation in which any benefit from these drugs was speculative. He wasn't started on beta-blockers, which had a proven benefit in terms of survival. But most beta-blockers were off-patent then, had no corporate marketing machine behind them, and were underused for patients with heart attacks. Studies comparing beta-blockers and calcium-channel blockers for patients like him had never been done. A decade later, it seems that beta-blockers, but not calcium-channel blockers, confer the survival benefit in this situation.

While many useful studies go undone, many studies are done more for marketing than to establish scientific facts. Some postmarketing studies are simply intended to promote a particular drug. By recruiting many practicing doctors to participate, drug makers hope to undo those doctors' habit of prescribing a competitor's drug, or to promote unapproved uses of the drug. These thinly veiled efforts to entice doctors to prescribe a new drug are often referred to as "seeding trials."[32]

Contract Research

Although drug companies often collaborate with university researchers to conduct clinical trials, companies have become increasingly dissatisfied with this arrangement. University committees are slow to review and approve studies, and faculty members divide their attention among the research, teaching responsibilities, and patient care.

Companies are therefore turning to for-profit contract research organizations to conduct clinical trials. These companies employ scientists, pharmacists, statisticians, and managers, and may conduct all or parts of the studies. In the words of Tom Bodenheimer, a San Francisco internist and policy analyst, the trials performed by the contract organizations may be "heavily tipped toward industry interests."[16] Because the contract research organizations must compete for business from the drug companies, they may be more reluctant than university researchers to offend their sponsors.

In a tongue-in-cheek article, a group of distinguished researchers suggested how truly blunt patient consent forms might read for a contract research project:

> **Commercial Randomized Controlled Trial for Multicenter Fun and Profit Consent**
>
> We would like you to participate in a treatment trial of a new drug. We really don't know much about it because we didn't write the protocol and the trial is being run by a for-profit contract research organization (since their future business depends on achieving favorable results for their sponsors, we're confident that this trial will turn out the way they want it to). We've joined the study because we will receive a bounty of several thousand dollars for recruiting you into it, plus a big bonus if we can talk a dozen of you into it by the end of the month. The drug we are testing is a trivial (but patentable) modification of a generic drug from the same class. We don't really expect it to perform any better but we're pulling for "non-inferiority" and a tiny but statistically significant difference in unimportant side effects. We'll be able to use that result in a series of direct to consumer television ads, so that future unsuspecting patients will demand this exorbitantly priced, me-too drug from their physicians. Of course, if the results do not favor the new drug, we will bury them without a trace.[33]

Growth in Industry Sponsorship

Even aside from contract research organizations, conflicts of interest are common. Commercial sponsorship of medical research, which often leads to conflicts of interest, is growing rapidly. In 1980, industry sponsored about 32 percent of clinical research, but by 2000, the figure was 62 percent. The federal government's share of research was falling during these two decades.[34] Entanglements among universities, drug and device companies, doctors, and other researchers have become almost ubiquitous.

A recent review article from Yale illustrates just how pervasive conflicts of interest in medical research may be. In an evaluation of 1,140 original research studies, a fourth of the biomedical researchers had industry affiliations. A third of the articles in major medical journals had lead authors with personal financial interests in their research. Furthermore, the Yale study found that two-thirds of the universities engaged in biomedical research held equity in start-up companies that funded research in the same universities.[34]

This review found that these ties appeared to influence research results. Industry-sponsored studies were three times more likely to yield pro-industry conclusions than research that was not sponsored by industry. In addition, industry sponsorship was related to restrictions on publication and on sharing data with other researchers. Industry-sponsored faculty were more likely than other faculty to report delays in publication of their research, often to slow the release of unfavorable results. In many cases, companies withheld accumulated results from researchers.

Sadly, most universities have developed only weak safeguards against major conflicts of interest. A survey of ten research-oriented medical schools found that only one prohibited researchers from having equity, consulting agreements, or decision-making positions in the companies sponsoring their research. In another survey, only 19 percent of schools had limits on their faculties' research-related financial interests.[34]

Guest Authors and Ghostwriters

Consider also the problem of guest authors and ghostwriters. It's increasingly common for research reports, editorials, and review articles to be penned by a professional writer hired by a drug company, contract research organization, or communications firm. These writers have nothing to do with the conduct of the research, but are given a packet of materials—often with a key paragraph favorable to the drug being evaluated—from which they write an article. A medical authority, who may or may not have been involved in the research, is then invited to be identified as the author. This "guest author" is responsible for reviewing the article and giving final approval to its content, but may not always provide a critical or thorough review. However, his or her prestige gets associated with the article, and the ghostwriter's name does not appear.

Dr. Troyen Brennan, president of the Physician's Hospital Organization at Boston's Brigham and Women's Hospital, has described his experience with being invited to "guest author" an editorial. He received a call from Edelman Medical Communications, a public relations firm in New York, inviting him to write an editorial for a medical journal. The caller pointed out that such editorials can be timed to coincide with relevant new clinical developments, that the writing project would be funded entirely by a drug manufacturer, and that a professional writer would compose the article after talking with Dr. Brennan.[35]

Brennan was offered $2,500 for the project, which was estimated to take "several hours." When Brennan asked for more information, he got a mailed brochure describing how the PR firm solved negative public reactions about drugs with advertisements, medical symposiums, and managing the press. The packet included copies of editorials and articles commissioned by the firm, several of which didn't acknowledge the support of drug companies.

Brennan declined the invitation and pointed out that such offers were blurring the distinction between the best interests of patients and the financial gain of sponsors. He argued that the boundaries are becoming less distinct and that the intent of such orchestrated efforts was to blur them further. He imagined that a bland statement of drug company support would raise few eyebrows, because it is so common. But a statement that he was paid $2,500 to help a PR firm write the editorial would surely elicit more criticism.[35] That conflict of interest was exactly his point.

Some of the ghostwriters themselves have come forward, and they tell a very similar story. Ronni Sandroff is a New York medical writer and editor who once wrote two cancer pain articles "for MD signatures." Both articles were intended for peer-reviewed medical journals. Sandroff said that she "was told exactly what the drug company expected and given explicit instructions about what to play up and what to play down." She went on to note, "Once it's published, the company's point is in print.

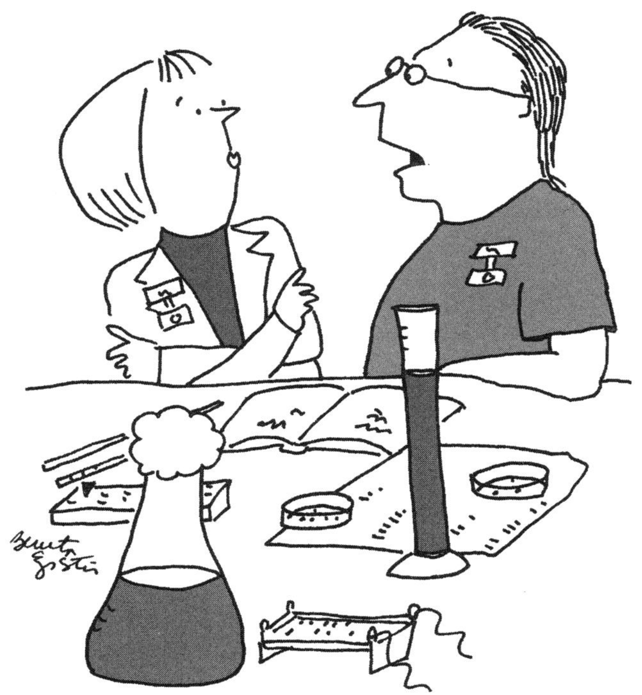

"I already wrote the paper. That's why it's so hard to get the right data."

Someone else has said it, so it looks like it's established fact—but it's basically their positioning of the drug." Another writer, Marilynn Larkin, agreed to do two reviews to appear under the names of respected "authors." She was given an outline, references, and a list of drug-company-approved phrases. She was pressured to rework drafts to be more favorable. In the end, she asked the company to reduce her fee and do the rewrites itself.[36]

In a survey of over eight hundred authors in top medical journals, researchers found that ghostwriters were probably involved in 11 percent of articles.[37] This situation reflects how pervasive university-industry ties have become. In reflecting on his experience, Brennan suggested that improving the completeness of disclosure, or other improvements in disclosure policy, might be the best option. But for the time being, ghostwritten articles and those otherwise sponsored by industry often go unrecognized by their audiences.

It was in 1994 that Brennan wrote in the *New England Journal of Medicine* about his experience.[35] At that time, the *New England Journal of Medicine* had a policy that banned authorship of editorials and review articles by professionals with a conflict of interest. Brennan predicted that this policy would become untenable because so many academic physicians and experts had ties to drug companies. He was prophetic. The *Journal* dropped its policy in 2002, citing exactly the problem that Brennan foresaw.

Ethical Review of Research

Even bioethicists are now routinely supported by the drug industry. Dr. Carl Elliott at the University of Minnesota Center for Bioethics summarized the growing trend for drug companies to support academic centers for bioethics. Such ties mute criticism of the drug companies, in Elliott's view.[38]

Furthermore, noninstitutional review boards (NIRB's) are increasingly replacing academic institutional review boards in overseeing clinical research. These boards must review and approve any research involving human subjects before the research can begin. These boards must approve plans for recruiting subjects, obtaining consent, and all research activities, then monitor progress of the projects.

The NIRBs are often for-profit ventures with major revenues coming from the drug companies. Members of the NIRBs, including ethicists, are paid for their work, often with proceeds from drug company contracts. Companies with research protocols are free to shop them around to the most lenient NIRB. Elliott concludes that from the corporate perspective, it is "better to buy a bioethicist now than to be attacked by one later." He notes ironically that the AMA is planning a huge initiative to educate doctors about the ethical hazards of accepting drug industry gifts—an initiative funded by gifts from Lilly, GlaxoSmithKline, Pfizer, AstraZeneca, Bayer, Procter & Gamble, Wyeth-Ayerst, and U.S. Pharmaceutical Group.[38]

The bottom line is that science isn't always what it seems. Be skeptical of the next breakthrough you hear announced on the evening news. The design, analysis, and interpretation of studies can be fairly easily biased, sometimes intentionally. Furthermore, any bad news can simply be withheld. Research that's industry sponsored tends to be more favorable toward the industry's products than independently funded research. Journal editors face an uphill struggle—one that is getting steeper with time—to maintain the integrity of the research they present.

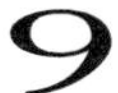

"Cancer Cured—Film at 11:00"

The Media's Role in Disseminating Medical Advances

Be careful about reading health books; you may die of a misprint. —Mark Twain[1]

No disease has been "cured" as repeatedly as cancer has.—Rick Weiss, *Washington Post*[2]

ON ALMOST a daily basis, I (Rick) have patients who bring me newspaper clippings on medical breakthroughs—breakthroughs that they want to try. Sometimes the clippings are from the *National Enquirer*, sometimes from the *Seattle Times*, and sometimes from the Internet. Sometimes they describe treatments that no one has ever tried in human beings. No matter what the source or the stage of development, all seem equally credible. When it's in print, it must be true.

When I suggest that these things aren't available, or that they aren't ready for prime time, or that it would be dangerous to try something so untested, I'm sometimes met with skepticism or assertiveness: "Well, would you call the University of Winona and see if you can get it?" "Well, maybe the government has it." "If they're testing it, I'll sign up."

You might suspect that such patients have cancer or terminal illness and are grasping at straws. But most often they're concerned about the vexations of daily life: arthritis, back pain, headaches, and the like. Such eagerness is testimony to the suffering these patients experience. Perhaps credulousness goes with desperation. But the reporting of these "breakthroughs" rarely offers the context and the caveats—or even the basic information—that would allow a reader to judge their true significance.

National news programs recently trumpeted "the very best news there has been in many years, perhaps ever, about Alzheimer's disease." The news was from a study in mice, which don't even get Alzheimer's disease. A story on creating a "smarter" mouse spawned stories about creating "baby Einsteins."[2]

Medical journalists have a big responsibility for providing accurate and unbiased information. In one survey, 75 percent of adults said that they paid great or moderate attention to health information in the news. The major sources of health news that they listed were TV (40 percent), doctors (36 percent), magazines (35 percent), and newspapers (16 percent). Undoubtedly, the Internet has grown in importance since that time. Many report changing their behavior or making treatment decisions based on media information.[1] Furthermore, many doctors get their first taste of new research developments from the mass media, and many don't have time to check out the information adequately.

In the competition for sales—of newspapers, magazines, and TV advertising—it seems that health reporting has become ever more sensational. "Making progress" pales next to "breakthrough," and journalists want to report on breakthrough science. Many health reporters have little medical

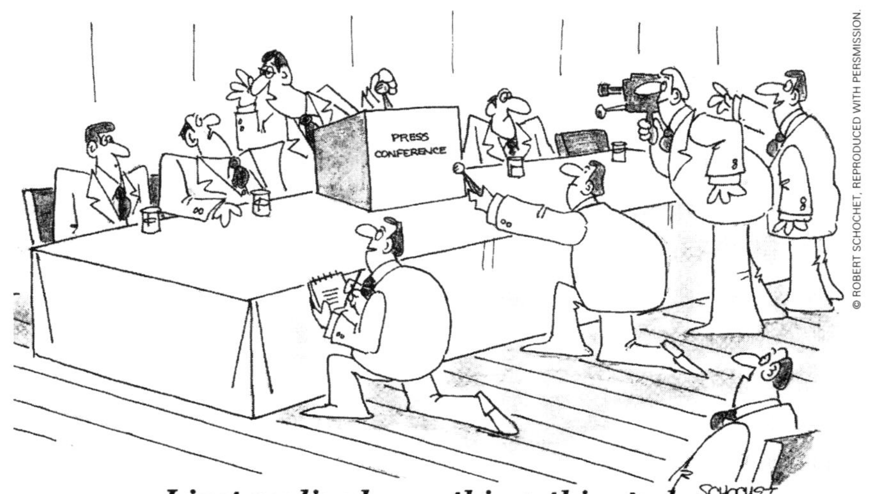

I just realized something, this study isn't that important.

background, and even experienced reporters often overstate the significance of a report. Most new research gets reported in isolation, with little context from previous or related research.

Rarely do doctors think that a single study is sufficient to determine how to manage a medical problem. Nearly every study offers only incremental information to add to an accumulating body of knowledge. Science rarely produces "the truth" as an absolute fact; instead, it achieves progressively better approximations of the truth. Furthermore, medicine has few certainties, and doctors base nearly all clinical decisions on probabilities. But the public desire, and the wish of medical reporters, is for fast, unequivocal answers. And this is often the way new research is reported. Sometimes doctors and researchers who want to promote their findings contribute to the illusion of unequivocal answers.

Robert Lee Hotz, a reporter for the *Los Angeles Times,* says, "The reality of a reporter's life is that you only exist if you're on the front page and there are several magic catchwords you can use to ensure that you get on the front page." "Cure" and "breakthrough" may be "the most likely passports to page one," but Hotz also likes "one step closer to solving" and "on the threshold of."[2] Another journalist says, "I'm in competition with literally hundreds of stories every day, political and economic stories of compelling interest. . . . We have to almost overstate, we have to come as close as we can within the boundaries of truth to a dramatic, compelling statement. A weak statement will go no place."[3]

The Publicity Machine

Doctors and scientists share the blame for hype, however. They like seeing their names in print or their faces on TV as much as the next guy, and they are prone to exaggerating the importance of their work. One researcher told a reporter that the only recognition more important to a scientist than a Nobel Prize is getting his name on the front page of *The New York Times.*[2] Egos are important, and publicity may help the prospects for research funding. Press releases are sometimes written to grab readers' attention rather than to provide a dispassionate assessment of the work. The university medical centers and research institutes where doctors work love the good PR that accompanies reports of "breakthroughs" by their own (incredibly brilliant and talented) staffs.

Doctors often like the attention of the press when they present work at major scientific meetings, and they always believe that their own work is terribly important. Indeed, Dr. Timothy Johnson of ABC News says that scientific meetings "are now becoming more like exercises in public relations organized for the benefit of the media," rather than being a place for sober discussion of science among researchers.[1] Journalists indicate that they hope researchers will be less cautious in face-to-face interviews than they are in print.[4] Johnson points out that conflicts of interest by many presenters at these meetings "increase the possibility of media manipulation."

An experienced medical journalist, Mark Schoene, notes that press offices at major meetings share complicity in this process because they labor to see studies from the conferences "placed" in the media. They promote high- and low-quality studies with equal enthusiasm. "I occasionally will get calls from five to ten PR agencies prior to a meeting," says Schoene. "At the meeting, PR representatives of the drug companies wait outside the press room, try to engage reporters in conversation, and invite them to special seminars and presentations."

Schoene also notes that studies presented at medical meetings don't get the same level of scrutiny from expert peers that published articles receive. He notes that reports on "all kinds of low-quality studies can then boast, 'based on a study presented at the Association for Interventional Radiology,' lending a veneer of respectability."

For government scientists like those at the National Institutes of Health, there's another incentive for inflating the importance of new research—increasing their budgets. This becomes especially important when their budgets are up for congressional approval. Creating the impression that they've spent tax dollars well may help to maximize their allocations.[2]

Medical journals also share some culpability. Major medical journals—especially the *New England Journal of Medicine* and the *Journal of the American Medical Association*—are closely watched by journalists on a weekly basis. Their articles are the ones that are most often reported on the nightly news or the front page of the paper. The major medical journals have become increasingly active in preparing press reports and even video material related to major studies. For the journals, this offers more control over the content and accuracy of the reporting, but the resulting publicity may inflate the importance of a new finding. Because these major journals have become important sources of revenue for the medical societies they serve, they increasingly compete to be in the media spotlight.

Furthermore, a recent study cast some doubt on the quality of the press releases prepared by major medical journals. In an evaluation of press releases from nine major medical journals, Dartmouth researchers found that only a quarter described any limitations of the studies they were reporting. A third didn't indicate how big a risk or a treatment effect was. And only 22 percent of releases on studies sponsored by industry mentioned that sponsorship. When the articles had an accompanying editorial mentioned in the press release, the editorialist's conflicts of interest were never mentioned.[5]

In the words of a medical editor and former medical writer for the *Los Angeles Times,* "Press releases, whether the work of universities, manufacturers, organizers of medical meetings, or medical journals, inherently involve self-interest."[6] The same could be said of press conferences, which often give a study the appearance of greater importance than it deserves. But in the competition for stories, no reporter wants to fail to report on something that *might* be important.[3]

As a story in *The New York Times Magazine* pointed out, the competition between the *New England Journal of Medicine* and *JAMA* "for subscribers, advertising dollars and intellectual primacy is fierce. . . . In a trend some critics consider troubling, journals are increasingly gearing their content toward general consumption, appealing directly to lay readers in a bid to increase their visibility and make themselves a 'must read' for doctors."[7] Drug makers, who supply most of the advertising revenue to these journals—and who support many of the drug studies that are published and disseminated to the media—undoubtedly benefit from the press coverage.

Medical journal editors defend the practice as improving medical journalism. But Dr. Lawrence Altman, a doctor-journalist for *The New York Times,* was quoted as saying, "All journals are increasingly playing the press. Lundberg [then editor of *JAMA*] courts the press for the same reasons that everyone does, because he wants publicity to attract advertising."[7]

The medical drug and device industries contribute importantly to the hype. Dr. Raymond Woosley, a physician and pharmacologist who is now dean at the University of Arizona medical school, is quoted by Dr. Timothy Johnson (of ABC News) as saying, "There are those who use the media for profit. They encourage stories about the faults of their competition. They leak medical stories to the press or in some cases have open press releases to boost their companies' stock values."[1]

Dr. Susan Okie, another doctor-journalist, said in the *Los Angeles Times:* "We're now being bombarded by PR people trying to push things—breakthroughs by their clients—mostly because of the profit motive. They call and fax and e-mail us and tell us, 'This is going to be very big. We have a teleconference tomorrow. . . . We'll have these experts available.'" Some of these companies provide local television stations "with ready-to-air video touting their clients' drugs," according to the *Times*.[2]

Common Reporting Pitfalls

Reporting on new drugs, in particular, is common enough that it's been possible to study the characteristics of these reports. Ray Moynihan, an Australian broadcast journalist who has spent time studying in the United States, teamed with Lisa Bero, a pharmacologist at the University of California, San Francisco, and some colleagues to analyze 180 newspaper articles and 27 television reports concerning three drugs. They studied two drugs that were new and still on patent: Pravachol for lowering cholesterol and Fosamax for osteoporosis. The third drug was an old off-patent drug, aspirin for preventing heart disease.[8]

Less than half the reports they studied mentioned side effects of the drugs, and only 30 percent mentioned cost. There were 85 stories among the 207 that cited an expert who had ties to drug manufacturers, but only 39 percent of the press reports mentioned this conflict of interest. While reports typically indicated that a drug was effective, only 60 percent indicated just how effective. In the vast majority of cases, only *relative* benefit was reported, not the *absolute* benefit. An example illustrates why this distinction is important.

On the same day in 1996, ABC, CBS, and NBC all carried stories about Fosamax, in response to a conference that had reported a major new study. All three networks reported that the osteoporosis drug reduced the risk of hip fractures by 50 percent, which one reporter described as "almost miraculous." This was the *relative* risk reduction. None reported the *absolute* risk of fracture, which was 2 percent in untreated women and 1 percent in treated women. Going from 2 percent to 1 percent is a 50 percent relative reduction, of course, but many viewers would find the 1 percent absolute difference in risk less impressive. Only one story mentioned abdominal distress as a side effect; and none mentioned that the research had been funded by the drug maker.[8]

In another example of the importance of relative versus absolute risk reduction, Marcia Angell, then editor of the *New England Journal of Medicine,* described a study showing that women who drink alcohol have a 30 percent relative increase in breast cancer risk over ten years. That sounds like a big risk, and if you multiply it times the whole U.S. population, it may be important. But for an individual middle-aged woman with a ten-year breast cancer risk of about 3 percent, a 30 percent relative increase would mean that her absolute risk would rise to 4 percent. In other words, her chance of remaining cancer-free drops from 97 percent to 96 percent. Says Angell, "Is that worth giving up your dinner wine for? Probably not."[9]

Another common pitfall in reporting is the seduction of surrogate outcomes. When a treatment lowers cholesterol, shrinks tumors, or abolishes abnormal heart rhythms, it's easy to assume that it improves longevity. However, a long and growing list of counterexamples makes it important to focus on the outcome that is of real interest. Drugs that lower cholesterol or normalize heart rhythm have sometimes paradoxically increased mortality, and tumor shrinkage is a notoriously poor indicator of real benefit.[10,11] Doctors and researchers, as well as journalists, are often seduced by these surrogate outcomes, making the reporter's job more difficult.

Of course, another problem is simply erroneous reporting. A study from the Loma Linda VA Medical Center and School of Medicine examined 587 articles from major newspapers and magazines, using two independent evaluators. They reported misleading and serious errors in 32 percent of press reports.[12] This suggests that the Mark Twain quote at the top of this chapter should include other mistakes in addition to misprints. Again, the blame for these errors may be shared by journalists and researchers.

Another pitfall in medical reporting involves the use of human interest stories. To a scientist, a single person's story is an anecdote, just one piece of data in a much larger body of information. Long-term results and typical results for an average patient may be obscured by the anecdotal case. For journalists, however, stories about individual patients make a news report interesting and may help to give the audience a vicarious sense of a disease or treatment. If the story is representative of typical cases, it can be informative, but if it's exceptional, it may mislead.

An example of misleading anecdotes comes from University of Washington researchers, headed by Dr. Wylie Burke, an internist and chair of the Department of Medical History and Ethics. Burke and her colleagues studied reports on breast cancer in popular magazines, examining 172 individual vignettes. Of these, 47 percent described women with breast cancer discovered before age forty. In reality, only 3.6 percent of all breast cancer cases occur among women this age.[13]

There's a chance that this sort of reporting might actually lead to adverse health outcomes. Burke and her colleagues noted that these stories misrepresent the age distribution of breast cancer, emphasizing atypical cases. Their concern was that this contributed to young women's fears of breast cancer and overestimates of risk. In turn, they noted that such fears may lead young women to overestimate the value of mammography before age fifty or of prevention with the drug tamoxifen. For older women, such reporting might obscure the fact that risk increases with age, reducing the motivation for appropriate mammography screening.

Yet another common error is to mistake an association for causality. For example, if a researcher found that people with lung cancer were more likely to drink alcohol than people without lung cancer, it might be tempting to assume that alcohol causes lung cancer. But this would be wrong. It's just that cigarette smokers are more likely to drink alcohol than non-smokers, and it's the cigarettes that create the risk.

Doctors, of course, sometimes make the same mistake. When they observed that women who were taking hormone replacement therapy had fewer heart attacks than those who weren't, many assumed that the hormone replacement prevented heart disease. The technology seemed to work. Only when randomized trials showed a contrary result did it become clear that healthier women were more likely to take hormone replacement—and that was the reason for their lower risk of heart disease, not the hormones.[14] So both medics and the media need to be more sophisticated in making inferences about cause and effect.

The organization and habits of health journalism sometimes contribute to poor reporting. Reporters often feel a "need for speed," to get developments into print as quickly as possible. This approach can be diametrically opposed to the need for context, a sense of incremental progress, and the scientific view that a single study is rarely definitive.

Finally, in many local newspapers and television stations, health stories are assigned to reporters with little medical knowledge. It would be unthinkable to leave the sports or financial page in the hands of someone who was unfamiliar with the field, but when it comes to medical reporting, which can directly affect people's health, inexperience is the norm. This is less a problem with national networks or newspapers like *The New York Times* and *The Wall Street Journal*, but is often a major concern with local outlets.

"Disease Mongering"

Sometimes the media distort the magnitude or the severity of a medical problem, or fail to note that it can often be self-limiting. How many stories on back pain, for example, point out that the vast majority of cases get better on their own? Some stories confidently report on the staggering human toll of conditions such as chronic Lyme disease, premenstrual dysphoric syndrome, or multiple chemical sensitivity—conditions that have no agreed-upon criteria or definitions, and that remain controversial within the medical community. We don't mean to minimize the suffering of patients who receive these diagnoses, but the ambiguity of the conditions' definitions and meanings is sometimes lost in press accounts. Catastrophic illnesses are always more newsworthy than symptoms.

Of course, doctors or commercial interests sometimes exaggerate or overmedicalize problems because it suits their purposes. Irritable bowel syndrome has long been identified as a generally mild condition with no precise criteria: It's often a "diagnosis of exclusion" when testing shows no other cause for persistent symptoms of abdominal cramping, diarrhea, or constipation. But when GlaxoSmithKline was preparing to market its new drug for irritable bowel syndrome, Lotronex, it described irritable bowel syndrome as affecting up to 20 percent of the population and posing a large burden of illness. Other estimates are that the syndrome occurs in about 5 percent of the population, and severely affects only 5 percent of those.[15]

The drug company hired a PR firm to mount a three-year "education program" to create a new perception of irritable bowel syndrome as a "serious, credible, common, and concrete" disease. The goal was to shape medical and public opinion about the condition. A leaked document indicated that "PR and media activities are crucial to a well-rounded campaign—particularly in the area of consumer awareness." A marketing magazine noted that key objectives in the period prior to drug approval were to "establish a need" for a new drug and to "create the desire" among doctors who write the prescriptions. The manufacturer marketed the drug, but then recalled it for severe side effects and deaths. The company then pressured the FDA to allow remarketing, though with new restrictions.[16]

In some cases, diseases have virtually been invented to help market drugs. "Social phobia" was not a diagnosis recognized by doctors, but it was used effectively as a way to expand the market for new antidepressant drugs. The manufacturers issued press releases, some of them picked up by the media, describing the severe impact of the "disease" and its high prevalence.[16]

On the flip side, companies sometimes exaggerate the side effects of a competitor's treatment to emphasize the putative advantages of their own. Perhaps this should be labeled "complication mongering." In any event, both reporters and readers need to be alert to the potential for disease mongering as they consider health news. Journalists should routinely question (and preferably avoid) corporate-sponsored material on the prevalence or impact of a disease.

A related concern is creating the appearance that there's no alternative to some new technology. News accounts often fail to describe older, less expensive treatments that may be equally effective for many patients. In some cases, they fail to note that patients may have an excellent prognosis without treatment at all.

Why Wait for Evidence?

Sometimes, with encouragement from manufacturers or researchers, news reports begin long before any scientifically valid data are available. Recent reporting on artificial discs for patients with spine disorders exemplifies the problems. Although artificial discs are being developed and evaluated by several manufacturers, they were only reviewed by the FDA in mid-2004 and will perhaps be approved in 2005. Until 2004, the evidence for their effectiveness had come largely from short-term case series with no comparison group, so the FDA did not regard their safety and efficacy as having been established.

But glowing press reports had already become common. An ABC report in 2000 described the case of Nancy Burall, a forty-year-old woman who had a "ruptured disc" and "paralyzing" pain in her back, legs, and arms. The story showed Ms. Burall in a wheelchair prior to surgery. She was interviewed just three weeks later: "I feel really great. It's just great." Her surgeon said, "The treatment is revolutionary."[17] For a treatment that is expected to last a lifetime, it seemed a premature assessment.

Among the many enthusiastic reports, a story on PBS was one of the few to offer any critical comments, which came from an orthopedic surgeon and researcher. Dr. Hansen Yuan of Syracuse University suggested that surgeons might be too quick to tout this experimental surgery, indicating that more study was necessary before widespread use. He noted, "Technically, this is not an easy [implant] to put in because of complication rates." He noted that "a major calamity" can result from disruption of the nerves at the back of the spinal canal or adjacent blood vessels. He also expressed concern that even if the device was approved, it might be overused in situations that hadn't been tested—such as putting more than one in a single patient, at different disc levels.[17]

Preliminary drug reports are often met with similar enthusiasm. Recently, a paper presented at the annual meeting of the American College of Rheumatology, based on just five patients, created a major media stir. One headline reported that the treatment might "cure rheumatoid arthritis," while another announced a "breakthrough as scientists discover the cure for arthritis." This extraordinary response was based on a tiny group of patients who received not only the study drug, but two other drugs simultaneously. Side effects of the combined therapy were rarely mentioned, and follow-up was just eighteen months, for what is ordinarily a lifelong disease. The $4,000 cost for three weeks of therapy went largely unnoticed. A sober observer noted that spectacular results in small, uncontrolled series of rheumatoid arthritis patients were common, but that they often couldn't be reproduced in more stringent controlled trials.[18]

Focus on Access—Don't Question Effectiveness

The problem, of course, is that false hopes are often raised in the public's mind by such reports. In the case of back pain, for example, we have a long track record of false starts and marginally effective treatments. This track record alone should be noted in reports, and should give reporters pause. Rather than acknowledging that many new treatments are unproven, however, press reports often imply that they are being held back by regulatory foot-dragging or reluctant insurance companies. Many stories focus on access to the treatment rather than on its effectiveness.

Indeed, in the era of managed care, reporting on new medical technology rarely noted that experimental treatments were unproven, dangerous, or immensely expensive. If these facts were noted, there was often an implication that ethics dictated that they be ignored. The usual slant was that these treatments were being withheld from needy patients by greedy insurance companies or managed-care companies. These human interest stories, with a David and Goliath conflict, were often irresistible.

The story of high-dose chemotherapy with autologous bone marrow transplantation for late-stage breast cancer offered a prime example of such coverage. Even though this treatment fit the description of unproven, toxic, and wildly expensive, breast cancer advocacy groups and others pressed in the early 1990s for its widespread availability. In 1991, *Sixty Minutes* did a story that was highly critical of Aetna's decision not to cover this treatment. In 1993, the media widely publicized a huge jury verdict in favor of California patient Nelene Fox. She had sued her insurance company, Healthnet, for lack of coverage. Similarly, the *Boston Globe* publicized the battle of Charlotte Turner to have her Massachusetts HMO pay for the treatment.[19]

Intense lobbying and public pressure in response to news coverage led the Massachusetts legislature to mandate insurance coverage in 1993. Similar reporting of local cases prompted several other state legislatures to require insurance companies in their states to cover the treatment. Even when laws didn't mandate coverage, most insurance carriers, facing litigation and bad publicity, caved to public demand. When definitive studies were finally reported,[20] it became clear that the fuss was over a treatment that was no more effective than standard therapy, but more toxic, at twice the cost.

In retrospect, the media could hardly claim to have protected the public interest. Undoubtedly, many reporters thought they were. Stories of the "little guy" standing up to Big Business were irresistible. And standing up for "women's rights" may have been particularly attractive. But their failure to distinguish weak from strong evidence contributed to anguish, untoward side effects, and waste of resources that would have been better spent elsewhere. They probably helped to raise insurance premiums for all of us. They were aided and abetted, of course, by zealous but misguided doctors and advocates.

Conveniently Congruent Worldviews?

Despite complaints on both sides, the media and medicine may actually share similar worldviews. They generally share an attitude that biotechnology can solve all problems and that medical researchers are heroic. They share a faith in experts and miracle drugs, as well as disdain for evil administrators and bureaucrats. Thus, the media, researchers, industry, and practicing doctors may unconsciously collude to promote an overly favorable view of new medical technology.

Whenever a medical breakthrough is announced, researchers' fame, institutions' reputations, and companies' profits are likely to be at stake.[6] Skepticism by both reporters and the public should be heightened. Joe Palca, of National Public Radio, said, "We could probably ignore 99% of the science news in a given year because its intrinsic value won't be known for many years, or may not be that great."[2] Or as a physician-editorialist suggested, "Hot findings must be handled with care."[21]

10

Doctors and Hospitals
Fueling the Drive for New and More

All professions are conspiracies against the laity. —George Bernard Shaw, *The Doctor's Dilemma (1911), Act 1*

WE LIVE in a culture that's enamored of new technology in general, and doctors are a part of that culture. Doctors are icons of technology themselves, but also advocates for technology. Doctors love new gadgets, new drugs, and new surgical techniques as much as everyone else—maybe more. Though most doctors genuinely want the best for their patients, they're just as prone as anyone else to assume that "newer is better."

As we've seen, sometimes doctors have special incentives to love new technology. In some cases, it means more patients or more income. Doctors may wish to be the first in town to offer a newly touted treatment, proving that they're in the vanguard. The practice of "defensive medicine"—the effort to avoid malpractice suits at any cost—often means providing high-tech tests and the latest treatments. And often, doctors are the ones who invent new technology, in which case they have both an intellectual and a financial investment in the new product or technique. In each of these situations, it's easy to rationalize providing more care, or more high-tech care, as improving quality. For all these reasons, doctors may be slow to put on the brakes even when new technology hasn't yet proven itself.

Jumping on the Bandwagon

Although medical doctors pride themselves on practicing scientific medicine, they're often susceptible to the same intuitive mistakes that plague us all. When a treatment makes sense, based on human physiology and risk factors for disease, doctors are often quick to adopt it, without much evidence that it really works.

The story of bone marrow transplantation for widespread breast cancer, mentioned in Chapter 9, is a case in point. The idea that bone marrow transplantation would permit higher doses of chemotherapy, and therefore would provide a better chance to cure breast cancer, made perfect sense. As a hematologist colleague remarked to us, "We just *knew* it worked."

Doctors became advocates for the new procedure right along with their patients, pressing for new transplant centers and better insurance coverage. Some prominent cancer researchers encouraged breast cancer patients and advocacy groups to take their cases regarding insurance coverage to court, then provided testimony on behalf of the plaintiffs. However, although the idea made sense, when the definitive clinical trials were finally done, they showed that the intuition was wrong. Cure rates were no better, toxicity was worse, and costs were much higher.[1] It was, in words attributed to Thomas Huxley, "a beautiful hypothesis slain by ugly facts."

When I (Rick) was in medical school, I learned that coronary heart disease was uncommon among women until the menopause, after which their risk seemed to catch up with men's. At the time, the theory was that natural estrogens in the body protected women until the menopause, when natural estrogen levels plummeted. It was a logical extension to believe that giving estrogen replacement after the menopause would help reduce the risk of coronary heart disease. Favorable changes in cholesterol levels that occurred with estrogen replacement reinforced the concept.

Many epidemiological studies seemed to support this idea, and most doctors embarked on a wholesale effort to convince women to take long-term estrogens after the menopause. Only in 2001, after decades of treating women, did it become clear from definitive clinical trials that hormone replacement didn't reduce the risk of heart disease, and might even slightly raise it.[2] Furthermore, it increased the risk of blood clots, strokes, breast cancer, and other problems, and it didn't make women youthful and energetic (an idea that had often been promoted by the manufacturers). Another beautiful theory slain by ugly facts.

Unfortunately, doctors have sometimes been guilty of using treatments or tests that "ought to work" long before there is any evidence that they really do. This evidence often must come in the form of randomized clinical trials, which are cumbersome and expensive, but which generally provide the most definitive answers.

In some cases, doctors have opposed clinical trials on ethical grounds: They "know" a treatment works, and it seems unethical to have an untreated comparison group. All too often, though, the clinical trials have yielded surprising results that ran contrary to conventional wisdom. This problem has given rise to the term *evidence-based medicine,* a concept that pushes doctors to insist on the best evidence for treatment benefits, rather than inferring or assuming that the benefits exist. The notion is gaining acceptance, but it is still not widely understood and accepted by doctors.

It's wise to bear in mind, then, that with all good intentions, doctors often advocate for new technology before its benefits (if any) are really known. In some cases, it's also convenient that the new technology has financial rewards.

Providing Unnecessary Services

We discussed some of the evidence for unnecessary testing, drug treatment, or surgery in earlier chapters. Certainly, the fee-for-service method of paying doctors gives them an incentive to do excessive tests, treatments, and surgery. In this system, insurance carriers reimburse doctors and hospitals for any bills they submit, minus some prenegotiated "discount." Patients can seek out doctors who do the most testing or provide the newest treatments. This is still the basic system used by some insurance plans, although insurance companies have negotiated ever-larger discounts. Many doctors and patients love this system because it has few restraints: Doctors and patients can provide or receive nearly anything they can think of. As we've seen, doing more and more isn't always good for patients. But it's almost always good for doctors.

In contrast to fee-for-service payments, prepaid managed care typically gives doctors a lump sum for each patient each year. If the doctors spend more than the "capitated" amount in caring for a patient, they lose money. If they spend less, they make money. They hope that inexpensive patients will balance out those who are expensive to care for, so that by the end of the year, they've made money. This reverses the incentives in fee-for-service medicine, as the doctor's financial interest is best served by doing less instead of more. While many consumers are up in arms over the incentives of managed care—for doctors to do less—the insidious incentives of fee-for-service have gone largely unnoticed.

With fee-for-service incentives, doctors are likely to do things like annual chest x-rays, cardiograms, and urinalyses. But these tests have little value for people who are otherwise healthy. As a medical resident, I (Rick) was taught to perform a similar battery of tests for every patient admitted to the hospital, even when they seemed irrelevant. These were practices that increased health-care costs, but had no benefit for patients' health. With fee-for-service incentives, if there's any doubt about the value of a test, treatment, or operation, you'll probably have it anyway. Newer insurance constraints, though they've sometimes gone overboard, have eliminated some of these practices, perhaps to consumers' benefit.

Now you're more likely to see ads for free prostate cancer screening, self-referred CT scans, or free cholesterol checks. These are great for business, because positive results always pop up when lots of people get screened. There is still enormous controversy about whether prostate cancer screening or CT scans in apparently healthy people offer any net benefit,[3,4] but that caveat is often lost in the frenzy of drumming up new business.

As an example, consider the observations of Dr. Otis Brawley, professor of hematology and oncology at Emory University School of Medicine and associate director of the Winship Cancer Institute at Emory. Among other things, he was instrumental in launching the ongoing National Cancer Institute Prostate Cancer Prevention Trial.

He was quoted in a recent interview as saying, "We at Emory have figured out that if we screen 1,000 men at the North Lake Mall this coming Saturday, we could bill Medicare and insurance companies for $4.9 million in health care costs [for biopsies, tests, prostatectomies, etc]. But the real money comes later—from the medical care the wife will get in the next three years because Emory cares about her man, and from the money we get when he comes to Emory's emergency room when he gets chest pain because we screened him three years ago."[4] Is it any wonder that health centers love to mount screening campaigns?

Brawley continued, "It bothered me, though, that my P. R. and money people could tell me how much money we would make off screening, but nobody could tell me if we could save one life. As a matter of fact, we could have estimated how many men we would render impotent . . . but we didn't. It's a huge ethical issue." Impotence is a common complication of treatments for prostate enlargement or cancer. With Brawley as head of Cancer Control, Emory doesn't do such screening.

When you get tests for no good reason—such as signs or symptoms of illness—abnormal results are far more likely to be false positives than if the test is done because of suggestive symptoms or exam findings. This is an unalterable truth, like gravity and the laws of physics. It's a consequence of the fact that no test is perfect: There are always some false positives and false negatives. Statistically, if you start with a very low likelihood of having a particular disease, a positive test is more likely to be falsely positive than if there's good reason to suspect the disease in the first place.

What's the harm, you may think. If the test is positive, maybe it will save me. And if it's a false positive, we'll find out—no harm done. But in the best case, false-positive tests mean unnecessary worry and the cost of additional testing—wasted cost in this case.

The worst case may resemble the story of Jennifer Rufer. Recall that Rufer had multiple false-positive tests for a rare form of uterine cancer. She underwent an unnecessary hysterectomy, chemotherapy, and lung surgery following false-positive tests. This was a cascade of events that meant that she'd never bear her own children.[5] Consequences that fall between these extremes are probably common: extensive testing, occasional complications, occasional useless treatment, and anxiety that interferes with normal functioning.

There are some exceptions to the rule of avoiding tests in the absence of symptoms. These exceptions are for a small number of conditions where screening healthy people can save lives. For these conditions, we know that early detection—before symptoms occur—gives better results than waiting until symptoms occur. In many cases, the early detection can actually lead to a cure. Examples are screening adults over age fifty for colon cancer and breast cancer. But screening healthy people for most other conditions doesn't have such clear benefits.

What about defensive medicine? This is the term used by doctors who order lots of tests or treatments in the hope of staving off malpractice suits, or at least of prevailing if they get sued anyway. In a litigious society, many

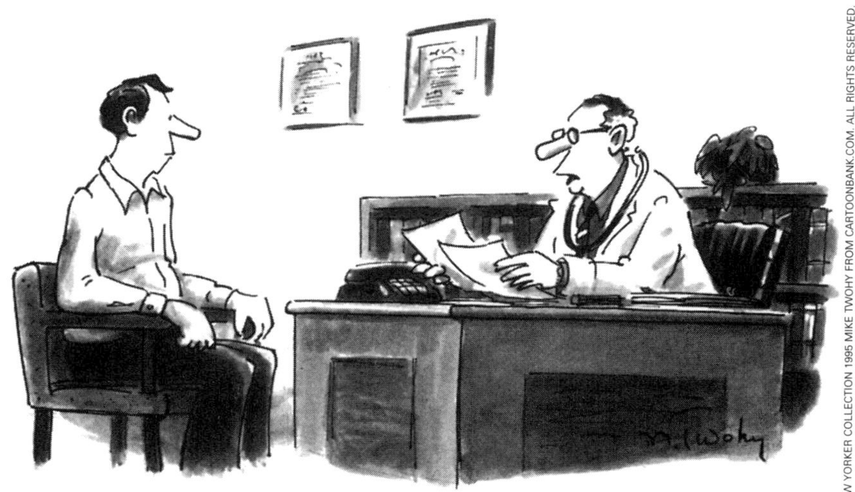

"I'll want to run a few tests on you, just to cover my ass."

doctors feel that they have little choice. Like screening programs in the local mall, this means that you get tests you wouldn't otherwise get. Your doctor is being extra careful. That can only be good, right? Actually, no. As with ill-advised screening, there are some downsides.

Even if your doctor isn't inclined to order unnecessary services, defensive practices sometimes create a "standard of care" that's hard to ignore. Obstetricians use electronic fetal monitoring almost uniformly for women in labor, although its clinical utility is dubious. Most agree that the rationale for this practice relates to the fear of malpractice suits, not the demonstrable value of the intervention.[6] And the monitoring may contribute to the unusually high rate of Cesarean sections in the United States.

A defensive standard of care may also account for the high rate of false-positive mammography in the United States. The number of false-positive mammograms is much higher in the United States than in most other countries, leading to more tests, biopsies, and anxiety. Yet breast cancer is discovered at just the same rate as in countries with fewer false positives.[6] Mammography in the United States remains a valuable screening test, but it can probably be performed in a fashion that creates less unnecessary fear and subsequent testing.

Doctors at the University of Pennsylvania conducted a formal decision analysis that demonstrated that defensive medicine can never benefit the patient, if it means doing tests without a good medical reason. Good reasons, for example would be signs and symptoms of disease, or screening in one of the situations in which benefits are proven. False positives (and false negatives) will result only in negative consequences for the overwhelming majority of people who have no disease. For those who do have disease, routine care would uncover it in nearly all cases through appropriate testing when signs or symptoms occurred. The researchers' conclusion was that defensive medicine, as it's usually understood, can only hurt patient care and not help.[7] But it increases demand for tests and patients' expectations that they should be done.

The "Little House of Horrors"

Sometimes the financial rewards of providing unnecessary care may be too much to pass up, especially in the technology-rich world of cardiology and heart surgery. Dr. Patrick Campbell at the Redding Medical Center in California had just that concern when he saw patients undergoing open-heart surgery even after cardiologists said it was unnecessary. When Campbell raised a red flag, he was told to mind his own business. But other doctors, patients, and technicians raised similar concerns, according to an account in *The New York Times*.[8]

Tenet Healthcare, a for-profit national chain, owned the hospital. According to administrators, Tenet constantly pushed the hospital for better financial performance, and the hospital consistently turned to its cardiac program for the results. Dr. Chae Hyun Moon, who reportedly billed Medicare for more cardiac catheterizations than any other doctor in northern California, became powerful within the hospital. Administrators even worried about his vacations, because a few days of absence would affect the hospital's finances. The high number of catheterizations seemed odd for Redding, a rural town of about 90,000.

But the hospital mounted advertising campaigns to bring in more heart patients. It even sponsored golf tournaments to promote its heart institute. News reports indicate that the hospital offered Dr. Moon the use of its helicopter to fly to the golf course.

After the FBI began to investigate complaints, it became clear that several patients who were advised to have surgery had gone elsewhere for second opinions, and been told that there was nothing to operate on. A Redding lawyer who came to represent several patients said, "We have over 100 clients where we have confirmed that they had unnecessary cardiac bypass surgery."

In 2003, Tenet agreed to a $54 million settlement with the government to resolve accusations that doctors had performed unnecessary heart procedures and operations on hundreds of patients. Tenet admitted no wrongdoing, but there are ongoing investigations and suits involving Dr. Moon and Dr. Fidel Realyvasquez, the hospital's top cardiac surgeon.[8,9]

Ultimately, Drs. Moon and Realyvasquez were suspended, and Moon relinquished his medical license until further investigations were resolved. A new hospital administration was also installed. One patient described the hospital as Redding's "little house of horrors."[8]

Though this case is extreme, it highlights the perverse incentives that doctors and hospitals face with regard to medical technology. It seems not to be a unique situation. In 2004, for example, the FBI raided three southern California outpatient-surgery clinics, investigating alleged unnecessary operations and endoscopic examinations. Investigators claimed that the clinics had recruiters who visited the factories and assembly lines of major companies that offered generous insurance coverage, looking for patients. In some cases, the prospective patients were offered travel costs and payments to attend the clinics, according to investigators.[10]

In response to the Redding hospital story, news reports quoted Dr. Uwe Reinhardt, a renowned Princeton health economist, as saying, "I sometimes just shake my head at the American system, where the financial intent is almost cleverly designed to create mischief."[8]

Doctors as Entrepreneurs

Sometimes doctors see an opportunity to generate some "side business" to their practices, or to gain some investment income from new medical ventures. In recent years, it has been fairly common, for example, for a doctor to invest in a new x-ray or MRI imaging center near his practice. The same thing has sometimes happened with radiation therapy facilities. Referring his patients there may be convenient, and, as an owner, the doctor gets a little return on investment every time he or she refers a patient. And what has research found about the use of these facilities? When a doctor is an owner, that doctor orders more tests and generates greater revenues.[11–13] And facilities owned by doctors who are in a position to "self-refer" often provide fewer services to the poor and the elderly.[14,15]

In certain specialties, doctors make frequent referrals to physical therapy. This is especially common in areas such as orthopedics, rehabilitation medicine, neurology, and rheumatology. So, like doctors who invest in imaging centers, such doctors occasionally invest in creating a physical therapy facility. When they do, they tend to make more referrals to physical therapy and charge more than other doctors do for similar patients.[16]

The practice of a doctor's owning an imaging center or physical therapy facility to which she refers patients is called *self-referral,* and most medical societies regard it as unethical. Certain forms of self-referral involving Medicare patients are even illegal. Nonetheless, there are some important loopholes. For example, if a doctor installs an imaging facility in his own office, its use isn't regarded as unethical or illegal.

This is exactly what's now happening in many parts of the country: Doctors are investing in CT or MRI scanning equipment. In Syracuse, New York, for example, the number of MRI scanners has increased by a third in the past three years. Patients may find it convenient, but doctors who invest in this equipment are likely to order more tests than they might otherwise order. Business people and insurers have complained that some use may be excessive, because the use of MRIs in Syracuse rose to be two-thirds higher than in Rochester, New York, and higher than the national average.

Doctor self-referral seems to result in greater "demand" for imaging. Nationally, use of imaging tests increased 23 percent in one recent year alone, even though MRI has been around for twenty-five years. Radiologic imaging is approaching a $100 billion-a-year business.[17]

Sometimes, when a new diagnostic test or treatment is developed, it's marketed to doctors with an explicit pitch that it can help them make more money. We saw the perverse incentives that can occur, for example, with cancer chemotherapy and other treatments given intravenously in the office. Similar events can occur with new diagnostic tests.

I (Rick) recently received a mailed advertisement for electrodiagnostic tests (tests that measure how well nerves can carry impulses), to be done in the office by traveling technicians with portable equipment. The mailing envelope proclaimed in large type, "We invite you to see how **technology** can change the way you diagnose your patients and **increase profits**" (emphasis in the original). The flyer inside tells how easy it is to schedule a testing day and notes, "As soon as we have verified your patients' insurance, we will be at your office."

Another recent ad that came in the mail has a mock $10,000 check enclosed. Below the check is a letter that reads, "Dear Doctor or Practice Manager: If your practice sees at least 2 dizzy or unsteady patients per week, and you don't offer Vestibular Testing and Therapy, this is the amount of revenue you have given up monthly." The rest of the message says nothing about the accuracy or benefits of the testing, but extols the financial virtues of buying the company's package of equipment, installation, and training. It concludes, "You have already missed capturing valuable revenue. I would like to help you make that up and increase your revenues this month."

Surveys in twelve cities during 2002 and 2003 confirmed that doctors are doing more tests in order to prop up their incomes. Investments in ancillary services such as laboratory testing, bone densitometry, and even PET scans have become common. A New Jersey medical director said, "Lab testing [was] off the wall," and doctor-owned ambulatory diagnostic centers were "creeping up out of nowhere."[18]

In a business, if you want to increase revenues, you increase the services that are more lucrative and drop those that are less lucrative. Doctors appear to be acting in just this way. Along with using technology-intensive strategies to increase their incomes, some doctors are dropping important but less lucrative services. In the surveys, some doctors were refusing to take emergency room calls or to accept new patients hospitalized from the emergency room. Patients who seek care in the emergency room are more likely to be uninsured than those attending a private office. Some doctors also were refusing to accept Medicare or Medicaid patients, because of lower reimbursements than from private insurance.[18,19]

Doctors as Inventors

When doctors themselves invent something new, their commitment to it is likely to be especially strong. Not only do inventors want their new products or ideas to succeed, but they're often investors in the companies that develop the new products. The risk is that their influence on medical practice may be shaped as much by personal financial interests as by good scientific data.

The rapidly changing field of cardiology is loaded with new medical devices, and it offers some good examples of the conflicts of interest that arise for doctor-inventors. Cardiac devices include artificial heart valves, pacemakers, monitoring equipment, imaging equipment, and coronary stents.

Coronary stents have been especially big business lately, with a succession of new products. These short wire mesh tubes, which look a bit like the spring inside a ballpoint pen, help to hold open narrowed or blocked arteries. They're used in conjunction with angioplasty, in which an inflatable balloon catheter is threaded through an artery and then inflated to widen a narrow segment of the artery. By inserting a stent (also done through the artery), a cardiologist makes it more likely that the artery will stay open, rather than quickly narrow again.

Because stents have been so much in the news recently, *The New York Times* reported the activities of Dr. Martin Leon, a prominent cardiologist who conducted research on the Paragon stent (a particular brand) and who was an investor in the company that manufactured the stent. Leon demonstrated the implantation of a stent to thousands of doctors on closed-circuit TV, extolling the virtues of the stent, but not mentioning his interest in the device. As the *Times* article noted, in the world of medical devices, "inventors are researchers, researchers are promoters, promoters are investors, and investors are inventors. Rare is the truly disinterested researcher, with no stake in the outcome of a study." One university cardiologist glibly remarked, "If you are working hand in glove with the companies and you might have a financial interest, what else is new?"[20]

Other doctors are less blasé. Dr. Steven Nissen, a cardiologist at the Cleveland Clinic, was quoted as saying, "How I treat a disease ought not to be decided by who's lining someone else's pockets. . . . The science has been lost in the rush for money. We've lost our way. We've terribly, terribly lost our way."[20]

Do conflicts of interest affect the quality of research? The *Times* also cited the example of Dr. Maurice Buchbinder, who was the main researcher for studies on a tiny drill used to remove plaque from clogged arteries. At the time he conducted the studies, Dr. Buchbinder also had a stake worth millions of dollars in the company that sold the device. In 1993, an FDA audit of Dr. Buchbinder's research disclosed several deficiencies, including failure to obtain proper follow-up or report some problems experienced by patients. The University of California at San Diego, where Buchbinder worked, subsequently barred him from conducting further patient research, according to the *Times*.[20]

In some cases, the *Times* reported, doctors get involved in research projects to see how a new treatment works before they buy stock in the company that makes it. In some cases, researchers sit on the boards of the companies that make the devices they're testing. As board members, they have a fiduciary obligation to shareholders that may conflict with the researcher's obligation to be objective and neutral about conducting research and reporting the results. In one case, an inventor doctor not only held shares in the company, but also stood to receive millions in honoraria if his device was approved by the FDA.[20]

Technology in the Hospital

Historians point out that the success of twentieth-century hospitals and the growth of medical specialties were both mediated through technology.[21] Hospitals are often quick to acquire new technologies, in an effort to be at the "cutting edge" and to attract patients seeking state-of-the-art care. Many hospitals have committees devoted to deciding which new imaging devices, surgical implants, or treatment techniques are worthy of investment. Often, these committees are preoccupied with return on investment, rather than with clear evidence of health benefits from the new technology. In fairness, of course, doctors and hospitals, like other businesses, have to stay in the black or they go out of business.

In recent years, cardiac technology, orthopedic procedures, and radiologic imaging have become the darlings of most hospitals, because they're cash cows. Insurance reimbursements for these services are more favorable than those for most other services. Hospital administrators report that surgical admissions are far more profitable than nonsurgical admissions, and that cardiovascular and orthopedic procedures are among the most profitable. They're also, not coincidentally, among the most technology-intensive of modern specialties.

Some critics suggest that the financial incentives may help to drive the clinical use of high technology. Cardiologist Tom Graboys of Boston has been an outspoken critic of the way cardiac technology gets used, and he has good credentials to argue the point. He is associate clinical professor of medicine at Harvard Medical School and at Boston's Brigham and Women's Hospital, has received several teaching awards, and has won a Humanism in Medicine Award from the Healthcare Foundation of New Jersey. He's also the author of numerous scientific articles and textbooks.

In a recent interview, Graboys said, "Regrettably, a large fraction of what we do in cardiology is economically based. A hospital puts up an open-heart unit or a catheterization lab. It has to get its money back, so the threshold for doing the procedures begins to lower; and the rationalization begins to increase."[22] In an editorial in the *Journal of the American Medical Association,* Graboys said,

> The growth of invasive cardiac procedures is attributable to several nonclinical factors . . . economics, overtraining of interventional cardiologists, fear and anxiety by patients and their families of imminent sudden demise, conflicts of interest between individuals and groups carrying out research in various areas, and the need of interventional cardiologists to perform a minimum number of procedures to maintain subspecialty certification.[23]

These are not reasons most of us would want to subject ourselves to invasive heart procedures.

Hospitals have also discovered the marketing value of technology. Along with conventional newspaper and broadcast ads touting their technological capabilities, some hospitals have recently begun Internet broadcasts of actual operations. Hartford Hospital in Connecticut, Brigham and Women's Hospital in Boston, and the Cleveland Clinic are among those that have hired an outside company to produce these webcasts. They typically include background piano music, camera shots outside the hospital, live audio from the operating room, close-up shots of the operation, an expert narrating—and frequent mentions of the name of the hospital.[24]

Boutique Hospitals

The handsome reimbursements for cardiac, orthopedic, and imaging procedures haven't gone unnoticed by the doctors in those specialties, who often bargain for more space and resources to be devoted to their departments. In some cases, specialists have realized that they might have greater incomes if they cut out the hospital and have started their own highly specialized hospitals, providing services in just one specialty. These are generally for-profit institutions, often owned by doctors, and sometimes belonging to national chains. They've become known as *boutique hospitals.* Doctors typically invest in these ventures, then refer their own patients to the facilities and treat them there. In a sense, this is the extreme form of doctor self-referral, with the same perverse incentives. Says John Rivers of the Arizona Hospital and Healthcare Association: "We know for a fact that these hospitals are offering phenomenal rates of return on their investment."[25]

Mainstream general hospitals and the American Hospital Association complain that these boutique hospitals are "cream skimming." They siphon off higher-paying, well-insured patients and concentrate on the most profitable procedures. This leaves the general community hospitals to shoulder unprofitable clinical services like trauma care, burn units, psychiatric services, and emergency rooms. Many fear that this may eventually drive some good community hospitals, with their more diverse range of services, out of business. Such concerns have surfaced recently all over the United States, particularly in California, Arizona, Ohio, and Indiana.[25,26]

The congressional General Accounting Office recently confirmed that boutique hospitals focusing on cardiac, orthopedic, or other surgical procedures treat fewer severely ill patients than general, full-service hospitals. Because Medicare reimbursements for a particular procedure are the same regardless of how sick the patient may be, hospitals that treat less severely ill patients are destined to be more profitable.[27] Thus, specific technologies allow the boutique hospitals to "cherry pick" the healthiest patients and the most profitable services. If such practices jeopardize the general hospitals, all of us may find it more difficult to find care for less profitable conditions, to receive appropriate care for complex conditions, or to get needed services when we have several medical problems at once.

In summary, doctors and hospitals have helped to fuel the infatuation with new technology. Many of them share the common conviction that newer and more must be better, and that technology is the solution to most medical complaints. Most doctors and hospitals are genuinely committed to providing optimal care, and many try to avoid financial conflicts of interest. But sometimes they profit handsomely from medical technology and have incentives to provide more tests, procedures, and operations. As Senator Hillary Clinton has remarked, "Our system rewards clinicians for providing more services but not for keeping patients healthier."[28]

When doctors own stock in companies that make medical products, or in hospitals that provide specialized treatments, they have financial incentives that go well beyond the lucrative reimbursements provided for many high-tech medical services. In some cases, both doctors and hospitals choose to offer new treatments or tests less because of clear benefit to patients than because of estimated return on investment.

11

Advocacy Groups

Mother Teresa's Waiting Room

Passivity and deference to scientific experts and government officials are out; publicity and in-your-face confrontation are in. —Rebecca Dresser[1]

EVERY SPRING, in the Rayburn House Office Building in Washington, D.C., public witness testimony begins before the House subcommittee that allocates medical research funding to the National Institutes of Health. The room where the hearings are held has long been dubbed "Mother Teresa's Waiting Room" because of the hundreds of sick and afflicted patients who come to testify, along with celebrities and lobbyists. So many people come that there's a lottery to decide who will get to speak. According to news accounts, those who attend represent hundreds of diseases: common forms of cancer, rare genetic diseases, and even erectile dysfunction.[2] All the speakers share a conviction that more research, and access to experimental treatments, will solve their ailments. Their stories are often heartbreaking and compelling, and sometimes influential.

Advocacy for AIDS and Breast Cancer: The Models

The modern era of patient advocacy began with AIDS activists in the 1980s. Early in the epidemic, when the causes of the disease were still obscure, AIDS activists focused on more funding for research. When research began to shift into clinical trials of new treatments, though, there was discontent with the conduct of randomized trials. Some patients in these studies didn't get the new treatment, studies took too long, some patients didn't meet the entry criteria, and new drugs were too slow to be approved. Some advocates wanted all patients to have access to experimental drugs immediately.[1]

When early treatments like AZT proved disappointing, though, another shift in focus occurred, at least among a segment of the community. Pitfalls in drug evaluation were becoming clearer, and some sophisticated advocates then began to press for higher scientific quality in the research being done. One New York AIDS advocate, Spencer Cox, said, "We pay huge amounts of money, and we suffer through major toxicities, and we have to take the drug company's word for it that the drugs work. That's supposed to be empowerment?"[3]

The advocacy efforts paid some dividends. The FDA created mechanisms to speed approval of new AIDS drugs and expanded access to some that were still experimental. Activists' arguments encouraged basic scientists to move new chemical compounds from laboratory development to clinical studies more quickly. Advocates publicized clinical trials, and ultimately encouraged enrollment in them.[1]

In her insightful book on research advocacy, lawyer and professor Rebecca Dresser summarizes the potential benefits of organized advocacy: enhanced research quality, more ethical research, and greater community involvement in the design and conduct of trials. However, she also points out some downsides of advocacy as currently practiced. Sometimes expanded access to experimental treatments results in harm to the participants, precisely because the risks and benefits aren't well known. Undue emphasis on access promotes confusion between poorly studied treatments and accepted medical care. Enhanced access to experimental treatment outside of clinical research studies may delay the studies that would determine if a new treatment is unacceptably risky or ineffective.[1]

Dresser notes: "Advocacy literature often refers to investigational agents and procedures as 'new treatments' and calls studies on terminal conditions 'life-saving research.'" The possibility that research interventions might prove ineffective or more risky than standard therapy is seldom broached. She notes that advocates stress the positive dimensions of biomedical research and often fail to draw a line between research and clinical care. Advocates typically suggest that more funding for research will inexorably lead "from cause to cure."[1]

Unfortunately, the scientific process is far from linear. There are plenty of dead ends, and many bumps in the road. Good research funding can help assure proper attention to theory, design, and planning, but it can't eliminate the bumps in the road. Clinical research isn't like the Manhattan Project to build the A-bomb, where there was a fairly clear path to be followed. As Richard Nixon's "war on cancer" showed, many cures aren't just around the corner.

Advocacy in breast cancer offers a cautionary tale that illustrates some of Dresser's concerns. Like most other grassroots advocacy efforts, breast cancer advocates followed the lead of AIDS activists. One breast cancer advocate told reporters, "We are absolutely following in the footsteps of the AIDS movement. . . . We've learned that if you want your disease to be dealt with, you go and you talk about it and you market it and you visit and you stomp and you write letters and you do it."[4]

In the 1990s, a major cause for some breast cancer advocates became access to the new treatment for advanced breast cancer: high-dose chemotherapy plus autologous bone marrow transplant. The media's influence on this new treatment was discussed in Chapter 9. In this treatment, women first store some of their own bone marrow, then undergo chemotherapy with high drug doses that would normally be fatal. This is because the chemotherapy drugs kill the normal bone marrow. But the patient is then "rescued" with her own stored bone marrow, allowing her to reestablish her immune system and to fight infections. The treatment costs $80,000 per patient and carries major risks.

Unfortunately, by 2000, there were five major randomized trials that all showed that the new treatment had no advantage over standard-dose chemotherapy in terms of survival. Editorialists and professional societies recommended that "this very toxic therapy" be abandoned except for future experimental work.[5]

However, before these results were available, breast cancer advocates had fought for access to the treatment, with considerable success. Following the example of AIDS advocates, they had won an FDA policy to increase access to experimental cancer drugs, under a "cancer drug initiative." Many saw that a logical next step was to obtain state mandates for insurance coverage for these drugs and also for the bone marrow transplant treatment. The ensuing events are nicely summarized by Harvard's Michelle Mello and Troyen Brennan in a *Health Affairs* article.[5]

By this time, breast cancer advocates had become a powerful force. There were some four hundred support, advocacy, and medical groups that were part of the National Alliance of Breast Cancer Organizations (NABCO). Skillful partnering with large corporations had helped NABCO to achieve revenues in 1999 of almost $7 million. Furthermore, doctors and researchers, with reputations, egos, and financial support at stake, provided strong support for lobbying efforts to gain access to bone marrow transplant therapy. The media were supportive, as noted in Chapter 9, and they blasted insurance companies or managed-care organizations that refused to pay for the bone marrow transplants.[5]

Insurance companies initially resisted paying for the expensive procedure, arguing that its effectiveness and safety hadn't been established. Early research studies without control groups (patients getting standard care) had seemed encouraging, although one critical reviewer noted that improvements seemed to last only a few months and came with a much higher risk of serious complications than standard treatment. However, as nearly always happens when researchers are enthusiastic, many doctors claimed that it would be unethical to do randomized trials because the value of the new treatment seemed so clear. In 1989, nearly 80 percent of oncologists thought it was appropriate to offer the treatment to patients with advanced breast cancer. Even in 1996, though, an expert panel concluded that the bone marrow transplant procedure should not yet be regarded as the standard of care.[5]

Our discussion on the media described how the media criticized insurance companies that refused to pay for the new procedure. Advocates succeeded in having many states pass laws requiring insurance coverage. In states where there were no such laws, insurance companies that refused payment often found themselves embroiled in lawsuits.

Over a hundred state and federal court decisions on the issue have been published, and many more claims resulted in settlements, were not appealed, or remain open. The case of Nelene Fox in California resulted in an $89 million verdict against her managed-care company. Court decisions were inconsistent, but sometimes challenged insurance policy language excluding "experimental" treatments because the term was impermissibly vague. When the congressional General Accounting Office surveyed twelve large health plans about coverage for the bone marrow transplant procedure, nine indicated that the threat of lawsuits was the major factor in their coverage decision—not scientific evidence.[5]

Because insurers began to cover the procedure, many women refused to participate in clinical trials, which would mean a chance that they would get standard therapy. As a result, some trials took eight years to complete, rather than three years as planned. But, starting in 1998, a series of European studies reported no benefit from the new procedures. And in 2000, a large American-sponsored trial reached the same conclusion. Besides having no greater effectiveness, the bone marrow procedure caused up to 7 percent treatment-related mortality, compared to none with standard chemotherapy.

So in the end, it appeared that some breast cancer advocates had gotten on the wrong bandwagon. In synergy with the media, politicians, and the courts, they had trumped good science to force payment for an ineffective, toxic, and expensive treatment. Some thoughtful advocates, like Fran Visco of the National Breast Cancer Coalition, had opposed wide use of the bone marrow treatment before better science was available, but others prevailed. The events pointed to one risk of advocacy: draining resources from established treatments, making access to routine care more difficult for some patients.

Advocacy for Recognition of Vague Conditions

No one disputes the major health impact of AIDS, breast cancer, and similar medical conditions. In these cases, the advocacy isn't focused on the legitimacy of the diseases, but on expansion of research and access to cutting-edge treatments. Another class of advocacy groups devotes more effort to establishing the legitimacy of their diseases, though they share the goals of ensuring access to tests, treatments, and insurance coverage.

These are conditions such as fibromyalgia, multiple chemical sensitivity, chronic fatigue syndrome, and chronic Lyme disease, all of which share certain characteristics. All have diffuse symptoms, many of which are overlapping among the conditions. All implicate many organ systems. All cause severe functional disability, despite the frequent failure of conventional medicine to identify anatomic or physiologic abnormalities.

And all are the source of ongoing controversy in the medical profession regarding their criteria and causation.[6–9] Many doctors suspect that patients with these diagnoses are mixed groups, some with true allergies or unrecognized infections, but others with depression and distress who feel they must prove that they're physically ill. If zealous advocacy refuses to recognize these complexities, it may delay good research and appropriate care for all involved.

Those advocating for disease legitimacy can be ferocious and tenacious, as Dr. Greg Simon learned. Simon is board-certified in both internal medicine and psychiatry, and is interested in the intersection of primary care with psychiatric symptoms. He works in the Center for Health Studies at Group Health Cooperative in Seattle, where he also has a faculty appointment at the University of Washington. As a research fellow, Simon began to study multiple chemical sensitivity—in part, because an outbreak had recently occurred at a local Boeing airplane factory.

Multiple chemical sensitivity has "symptoms all over the map," according to Cynthia Wilson, director of a Montana-based Chemical Injury Information Network. "Getting flulike symptoms that don't go away may be the hallmark feature," she told reporters.[10] Albert Donnay, president of another advocacy group, told newspapers that all sufferers complain of increased sensitivity to light, sound, touch, odors, and temperature changes. Other symptoms, he said, included headaches, memory loss, concentration problems, chronic fatigue, muscle and joint pain, sleep difficulty, and diarrhea. He was quoted as saying, "It looks like everything."[10]

Dr. Simon and his colleagues—one of whom later became head of the National Institute for Occupational Safety and Health—conducted a controlled evaluation of immunological, psychological, and neurological function in patients with a diagnosis of multiple chemical sensitivity. Among other things, their data cast doubt on some immunological tests that were used to support disability and liability claims. The researchers were attacked by advocacy organizations, representatives of the testing laboratories, and plaintiff's attorneys.[11]

An advocacy group, Multiple Chemical Sensitivity Referral and Resources, headed by attorney Albert Donnay, filed multiple complaints of scientific misconduct with the sponsoring institutions and the federal Office of Research Integrity. In addition, there were requests that the state medical disciplinary board revoke the researchers' medical licenses, and materials were distributed at scientific meetings accusing the researchers of fraud and conspiracy. Individual patients at Group Health were contacted and encouraged to attack Simon's credibility.[11]

The accusations were so widely broadcast that the researchers faced separate inquiries at three health-care institutions, the state disciplinary board, and the Office of Research Integrity. Extensive inquiry at all five institutions concluded that there was no basis for the complaints, but individuals and organizations continued to file complaints and accusations.[11] The researchers had unwittingly opened a Pandora's box.

Lyme disease advocates are another vocal and influential group. The conventional medical understanding of Lyme disease is that it is an infection transmitted by certain ticks that is fairly hard to acquire and easily treated with a short course of antibiotics. Untreated, it can have serious consequences, but treatment is usually highly effective.[12] Chronic Lyme disease advocates believe that there is a long-lasting form that requires months of antibiotic treatment.

But a well-designed trial of three-month antibiotic treatment for such patients had to be stopped because antibiotics were having no more effect than placebo therapy. All the patients had well-documented previously treated Lyme disease, but had persistent symptoms such as pain or fatigue.[13] Despite such studies, advocacy groups continue to argue the need for long-term intravenous antibiotic therapy and insurance coverage for it.

Dr. Allen Steere of Tufts University was the first researcher to identify the bacteria that cause Lyme disease, in the 1970s. He argues that there is no evidence for a chronic form of the disease after appropriate treatment. But he was shouted down at a 1993 congressional hearing by patients who had come to see him as an enemy.[14,15] The debate has become so painfully polarized that some researchers who are skeptical of long-term antibiotics won't speak out, for fear of being attacked by irate patients. One researcher told reporters, "I think they try to bully doctors and health care workers."[14]

This brand of advocacy seems focused on discrediting mainstream medical opinion. The advocates seek access to tests and treatments that are unproven, like long-term antibiotic use, and that may have important adverse consequences. In some cases, questions of liability and compensability are just beneath the surface.

Such advocates often find a few doctors who support their views, and selectively cite medical articles that offer even tenuous support. Sometimes the doctors and scientists who lend support are working from a biologic rationale or an interesting laboratory finding. This can lead them to believe in a clinical course of action before there's good clinical research to test their inferences. Ultimately, the advocates share a faith in technological solutions for their symptoms, and add another voice for uses of unproven tests and treatments.

The "Kept" Advocates

Pulling aside the curtain to see who's pulling the strings behind some advocacy groups can be enlightening. Although most organizations are nonprofit and maintain a public position of altruistic concern, many receive lavish funding from commercial interests that clearly benefit from these partnerships. Some "advocacy groups" are little more than front groups for commercial interests. Others have their own agendas, but may be influenced in their positions by generous donations. Though they may appear to be grassroots organizations, the term *Astroturf organizations* has been coined to indicate their artificial origins.

Citizens for Better Medicare was previously introduced in Chapter 7, in our discussion of drug company influence on political campaigns. This group is funded mostly by drug makers and the Pharmaceutical Research and Manufacturers Association America (PhRMA), the industry group representing major drug companies. In fact, PhRMA helped found the group, and a former marketing director for PhRMA, Tim Ryan, has been the director of Citizens for Better Medicare.[16] Its television campaign superficially seems to support cutting waste and reducing Medicare costs. But its main agenda is to defeat legislation that would give Medicare patients the same discounts enjoyed by other government agencies, including the VA, the military, and Medicaid. Such discounts would reduce drug company profits. And Citizens for Better Medicare is just one of many groups opposing policies that would reduce drug prices, with major support from drug companies for advertising, for toll-free phone numbers, and for surveys.[16]

Using a nonprofit group in this way puts a friendly face on corporate interests, helps to obscure the policy's true sponsorship, and may even mask the underlying intent. The tactic has been called "passion branding" or cause-related marketing.[17] In some cases, it's tied not to public issues like Medicare, but to specific diseases and specific treatments.

Some organizations promoting awareness of prostate cancer illustrate this approach. Us Too! is a prostate cancer advocacy group whose name suggests that perhaps the leadership was impressed with the success of women's groups in breast cancer advocacy. Us too! has hundreds of chapters in the United States. Despite ongoing professional controversy over the effectiveness and safety of screening and treatment for early prostate cancer, this group is firmly pro-testing and pro-treatment. Its board chair acknowledges that drug companies provide 95 percent of the funding for the organization.[17] While this is perfectly legal, remember that the makers of Lupron and Zoladex, competing drugs for prostate cancer, have been extensively investigated for more questionable marketing tactics. Using advocacy groups to indirectly boost sales appears to be one more marketing tactic.

Most contributions to advocacy groups come as "unrestricted educational grants." This means that the donors, in theory, have no control over the messages put out by the organization. But grateful organizations are unlikely to bite the hand that feeds them. Journalist Jeanne Lenzer quoted one nonprofit official as telling members, "Keep in mind, successful partnerships are built on the foundation of aligning your organization's core values and principles with those of the corporations."[18]

Schering-Plough developed a network of coalitions of doctors, community leaders, and public health officials to press state legislators for more funding to fight hepatitis C. Schering-Plough's drug for hepatitis C, Rebetron, costs $18,000 a year, according to news accounts. The coalitions, though, have toll-free numbers paid for by the drug maker, and a PR firm helped write scripts for the operators and educational materials. A Schering-paid PR executive started the first of the coalitions in Minnesota in 1997, even before the drug was approved for marketing.

Though groups such as those started by Schering-Plough may provide useful services for some consumers, their major role appears to be marketing and lobbying. Several people who became involved in the hepatitis campaign felt misled when they learned the extent of Schering's involvement.[19]

It's not just the single-disease advocacy groups, like prostate cancer or hepatitis C groups, that get major drug company support. Big groups like the American Heart Association and the American Cancer Society also benefit from this largesse. We saw earlier how Genentech contributed millions to the American Heart Association, and how those contributions raised questions about the AHA's issuance of stroke treatment guidelines favorable to Genentech's clot buster, alteplase.

But other curious arrangements are legion. Bristol-Meyers Squibb has advertised its cholesterol-lowering drug, Pravachol, with full-page ads in major newspapers that prominently feature the name and logo of the American Heart Association. SmithKline Beecham entered a licensing agreement with the American Cancer Society—worth $1 million a year—for promotion of SmithKline's nicotine patch. (The American Cancer Society may have underestimated its own value. Competitor McNeil Consumer Products entered a similar agreement with the American Lung Association for $2.5 million a year to promote McNeil's nicotine patch.[20])

The benefits of such marketing seem clear. A report from the California attorney general's office reached the following conclusions, each based on survey data:

- Consumers place a high level of trust in nonprofit organizations.
- Consumers prefer products marketed in association with a nonprofit organization.
- Consumers believe that products marketed in association with a nonprofit organization carry an endorsement by the nonprofit organization.
- Consumers believe that products marketed in association with nonprofit organizations are superior to other competing products.

But there was a potential downside to these marketing advantages: The report also noted that consumers don't expect marketing relationships between corporations and nonprofits to be exclusive, and their perceptions of the relationships change when they learn about exclusivity. When survey respondents were told, for example, about exclusive licensing agreements by the American Cancer Society, their support for such partnerships largely eroded. One study concluded, "If more people knew about the exclusive nature of ACS's 'quit smoking' partnership, they would be less supportive of the partnership program than they are now."[20]

The California attorney general's report, which was a collaborative effort by the attorneys general of sixteen states and the District of Columbia, concluded, "Commercial-nonprofit product advertisements often communicate the false and misleading messages that the products have been endorsed by the nonprofit partner . . . and that such products are superior to other competing products."[20]

Advocacy groups of whatever description play an important role in promoting new medical technology. They often skillfully harness the power of the press, the government, and the health-care industry. They've played important roles in focusing attention on the plight of certain patient groups, and sometimes they've achieved valuable policy goals that sped development of and access to therapy. Their contribution to discussions about allocating health-care resources is important, because these discussions are inherently related to society's values and priorities.

In some cases, though, advocacy groups have promoted useless technoconsumption by blurring the lines between experimental and proven treatments. In other cases, they've simply advocated for tests or treatments that haven't been validated, some of which were later proven ineffective or harmful. Concerns about legal liability have sometimes distorted any scientific discussion. Some questions—like whether a test or treatment works, or what causes an illness—are probably better answered by research than by advocacy.

And some advocacy groups, despite a veneer of grassroots legitimacy, owe their existence and allegiance to corporate sponsors. Pressure tactics have sometimes disseminated useless treatments, delayed scientific research, and given emotional appeal greater sway than scientific evidence—to no one's benefit.

12

Holes in the Safety Net

The FDA and the FTC

The culture within the FDA should welcome, not censure, differences of opinion about the impact of science on policymaking. —Richard Horton[1]

GOVERNMENT rules, regulations, abbreviations, and acronyms make our eyes glaze over faster than reading the phone book. But a couple of federal agencies have a big impact on how medical advances get introduced. Some background is important to understanding why regulatory approval may not be the "Good Housekeeping Seal of Approval" that many imagine it to be.

The Food and Drug Administration (FDA) approves new drugs and devices, as well as assuring that foods and cosmetics are safe.* It monitors more than $1 trillion worth of products, representing nearly a fourth of all consumer spending.[3] In the medical arena, the FDA's basic goal is to keep people from selling you snake oil—stuff that's ineffective or harmful. Given budget constraints, an overwhelming number of new products to evaluate, and the onus of being labeled as part of the Big Government

*The section of this chapter dealing with the FDA was published in a slightly different form in the *Journal of the American Board of Family Practice*.[2] This adaptation is published with permission.

that people want off their backs, it does a reasonably good job. Most of the drugs and devices that we have available today are effective and reasonably safe most of the time.

However, frequent recalls of drugs and devices call attention to the limitations of the approval process.[4–6] Recent news about complications of hormone replacement therapy for postmenopausal women emphasizes the gaps in the process.[7,8] Ditto for new data supporting the superiority of diuretic therapy over newer, more expensive alternatives for high blood pressure.[9]

Some of these gaps may arise because of ongoing tensions within the agency, and even conflicts of interest in the drug approval process. The FDA also faces pressures from industry, advocacy groups, and politicians. The agency's major drawbacks, in our view, are that it's underfunded for the volume of work it faces, and that it has no legislative mandate for some of the things we'd like it to do. Although most aspects of the FDA review process are highly successful despite these problems, its limitations deserve careful consideration, because they may have important implications for how we use medical advances.

Common Misconceptions

Let's start by dispelling some common misconceptions. For a new drug or device to win approval, the FDA doesn't require it to be better than already available products. It needs only to be effective, meaning better than nothing, and fairly safe. The benefit must be judged to outweigh the risks. This is all Congress allows the FDA to require. In some cases, the definition of "effective" is very narrow. A drug that lowers cholesterol, lowers high blood pressure, or improves heart rhythm can be approved without knowing if it improves life expectancy or quality of life.

Also, the studies used for drug approval aren't designed to detect important but uncommon safety problems. In some cases, approved drugs were later found to increase mortality, rather than decrease it as intended. The heart-rhythm drugs encainide and flecainide were examples. The company-sponsored trials that led to their approval showed that they were effective in suppressing the type of abnormal heartbeats that are sometimes associated with cardiac arrest. And yet, by one estimate, these drugs produced a death toll of 50,000 before their toxicity was demonstrated in a large NIH-sponsored clinical trial.[10,11] In the NIH study, the number of deaths in patients taking these drugs was twice that with placebo.

Drug approval generally requires rigorous tests of effectiveness, in the form of at least two randomized controlled trials. These types of studies are regarded as the "gold standard" for reducing many of the biases that can creep into research. But the bar for approving medical devices is lower. Medical devices include anything from contact lenses to cardiac pacemakers and MRI scanners.

The FDA approves most new devices, ironically, if the maker can argue "substantial equivalence" to a product that was marketed prior to 1976—more than twenty-five years ago. For this type of approval, a device need only do technically what it claims to do and prove reasonably safe. A device that delivers electric current to the skin might be considered effective without asking if it relieves symptoms. Devices that don't claim substantial equivalence to an older device—a tiny fraction of new submissions—are required to undergo more rigorous review. This may or may not require randomized trials.

Things the FDA Doesn't Do

There are many things the FDA doesn't do that may surprise some people. Importantly, the FDA doesn't approve old drugs and devices. Some medical products that are currently in widespread use got there before FDA approval was required, and their use is "grandfathered" in.

The FDA makes no judgment about the value for money of a new drug or device. Dr. Larry Kessler, director of the Office of Science and Technology in the FDA's Center for Devices and Radiologic Health, says that if a manufacturer wanted to market "a gold-plated biliary stent (a device for keeping the bile duct open) that costs a million dollars a pop—works great—FDA has to approve it. It's a lousy buy because the $127 version works almost as well. But the FDA has to approve it. Medicare may decide it's not cost effective and refuse to pay for it, but the FDA cannot address cost-effectiveness." In truth, even Medicare can't make reimbursement decisions based on cost-effectiveness, although private health plans and state Medicaid programs can.

The FDA can't tell you if one blood pressure drug is better than another for reducing the risk of blood pressure complications like strokes and heart attacks. It doesn't require that drugs prove this effect, nor does it require head-to-head comparisons of competing drugs. Dr. Kessler says, "The reason is that we could be seen as favoring product A over product B. And the FDA always, always, always shies away from that."

Some alarming consequences of this policy were illustrated by recent clinical trials. In one landmark study, old-fashioned diuretic therapy was found to be more effective at preventing complications of high blood pressure than newer drugs.[9] Because no adequate comparisons were previously available, and because the newer drugs were heavily marketed, diuretics had come to be used in only a minority of patients, while the newer types of drugs (at ten to twenty times the cost) had steadily gained market share.[12]

Similarly, a recent study demonstrated no advantage of an expensive drug to prevent blood clots over aspirin for preventing recurrent strokes among African Americans. This was true despite the new drug's substantially higher price and its risk of serious complications.[13]

Or consider a new drug for treating nasal allergies called Singulair. The manufacturer had previously marketed the drug for asthma, but recently it was also approved for treating seasonal allergies. *The Medical Letter,* an authoritative medical newsletter that accepts no advertising, summarized studies on the drug as showing that Singulair "might be as effective as an oral antihistamine . . . (more data are needed), but it is less effective than an intranasal corticosteroid, and more expensive than either."[14]

The FDA doesn't approve every use to which a medical product might be put. Remember Neurontin, for example, which is approved for treating seizures and for pain after shingles. But many doctors use it to treat other types of chronic pain and psychiatric problems. In fact, 90 percent of Neurontin's sales are for "off-label" uses.[15] Once a drug is approved for treating one condition, doctors can legally use it for other things.

Unfortunately, there's not always good science to support off-label uses. "When you routinely recommend some off-label use for your patients, for which there aren't data to prove this is the right thing—when does that really become experimentation without informed consent?" asks Dr. Kessler. This is an unanswered question that no one seems eager to address.

The FDA doesn't approve television or magazine ads for new drugs before they're aired or printed, although companies are required to submit ads to the agency at the time they appear. Because of their wide exposure, direct-to-consumer broadcast ads are then reviewed, but some print ads are not.[16] As a result, the FDA can request a company to pull ads that are judged misleading only after those ads are already in use. In late 2001, the Bush administration instructed the FDA not to issue regulatory letters until they've been reviewed by FDA attorneys. This has delayed letters from two to twelve weeks—long enough in some cases for misleading ads to complete their planned broadcast life cycle.

Aside from these delays, the FDA has no way to be certain that it receives all new ads from drug companies. In fact, the agency issued six regulatory letters between 1997 and 2002 citing companies for failing to submit ads when they were first disseminated. As we noted in Chapter 6, the FDA routinely sends out dozens of warning letters to drug companies each year for misleading ads, and companies sometimes replace one misleading ad with another.[16]

The FDA recalls drugs or devices if new evidence emerges that suggests that they're unsafe. However, it generally doesn't recall drugs or devices because of accumulating evidence that they don't work. The marketplace is judged sufficient to accomplish this goal, and it sometimes does—but slowly. As a consequence, tests and procedures often continue to be used for years after they've been found to be ineffective or inferior to alternative products.

The FDA doesn't regulate new surgical procedures in any way. It does regulate devices, such as surgical implants. Examples would be metal hip replacements or cardiac pacemakers. It also regulates new surgical instruments, such as the fiber-optic scopes that are increasingly being used for minimally invasive surgery. But if a surgeon develops a new approach or technique for surgery that doesn't involve a new device, it falls outside the jurisdiction of the FDA.

Medical Devices

The FDA's approach to approving medical devices differs substantially from its approach to approving drugs. In some ways, it's both more complex and less stringent.[17] The FDA's authority over devices dates only to 1976, when I (Rick) was a medical resident, and therefore seems to us relatively recent. This legislation was a response, in part, to public outcry over some well-publicized device failures. The most prominent was the Dalkon Shield, an intrauterine contraceptive device that was associated with serious infections.[18] In contrast, the FDA's authority over drug safety dates to 1938, although its authority over truth in labeling dates to 1906.[19]

With few exceptions, given the timing of the FDA's authority, devices introduced prior to 1976 were never required to undergo rigorous evaluation of their safety and efficacy. With the huge number of things that suddenly fell under its purview, the FDA had to prioritize its resources and efforts.

One way of prioritizing device review was to focus first on safety. Evaluation of effectiveness, in many cases, was reduced to engineering performance: Does the device hold up under its intended uses, does it deliver an electric current as advertised? The potential benefits in terms of relieving pain, improving function, or ameliorating disease generally didn't have to be demonstrated.

Another way of prioritizing was to assign categories of risk associated with the devices. Rubber gloves seemed less risky than cardiac pacemakers, for example. So the agency assigned devices to one of three levels of scrutiny. Class I devices have low risk, and the purpose of oversight is to maintain high manufacturing quality standards, assure proper labeling, and prevent adulteration. Latex gloves are an example. Let's not dwell on Class I.

At the other extreme, Class III devices are the highest risk. These include implantable devices, things that are life supporting, or diagnostic and treatment devices that pose substantial risk. An electrical catheter for burning a tiny section of heart muscle to interrupt abnormal heart rhythms would be an example. An artificial heart valve is another.

In general, these devices require a "Premarket Approval," including data on their performance in people, not just in the laboratory or in animals. This approval requires extensive safety information and extensive data on effectiveness. This evaluation comes closest to what's required of drugs. In fact, Dr. Kessler says, these applications "look a lot like drug applications: big stacks of paper. They almost always require clinical data—almost always. And they often require randomized trials. Not always, but often." These devices are often expensive and are sometimes controversial because of their cost.

Class II devices are perhaps the most interesting. They make up an intermediate group and generally require only performance standards. Examples would be biopsy forceps, used to snip polyps out of the large intestine during colonoscopy; some surgical lasers; and some artificial hips. The performance standards focus on the engineering characteristics of the device: Does it deliver an electrical stimulus if it claims to, and is the stimulus in a safe range? Is it made of noncorrosive materials? Most of these devices get approved by the "510(k)" mechanism. The 510(k) approval requires demonstrating substantial equivalence to a device marketed prior to 1976. "And," says Kessler, "the products that have been pushed through 510(k) are astonishing."

This may strike you as bizarre. As Kessler points out, "For the first five to ten years after 1976 this approach made sense. But in 2001, twenty-five years after the Medical Device Amendment, does it make sense? There was a lot of stuff on the market that wasn't necessarily great in 1975—why would you put it back on the market now?" The new device need not prove superiority to the older product—just functional equivalence. If a company wants to tout a new device as the latest and greatest, why would it claim substantial equivalence to something that's twenty-five years old?

The reason is that the 510(k) process is much easier and cheaper than seeking a Premarket Approval. The 510(k) process usually doesn't require clinical research. In the mid-1990s, a 510(k) application, on average, required three months for approval and about $13 million. A Premarket Approval required, on average, about a year and $36 million. Both are modest compared to the time and cost for new drug approvals. The process by which the agency decides if something is "equivalent enough" to be approved by the 501(k) mechanism is subjective.

Because pre-1976 devices were not subject to any rigorous tests of clinical effectiveness, a newly approved device may be equivalent to something that has little or no therapeutic value. Doctors, patients, and payers therefore often have little ability to judge the value of new devices. As an example, the FDA still receives 510(k) applications for intermittent positive-pressure breathing machines—devices for assisted breathing for patients with emphysema and similar lung disorders.[17] Their use was common practice when I (Rick) did my residency training. But a thorough review by the federal Agency for Health Care Policy and Research found that these devices offer no important benefits.[20]

How much do manufacturers take advantage of the easier 510(k) approach? Since 1976, nearly 98 percent of the devices entering the market have been approved through the 510(k) procedure.[15] In 2002, for example, there were 3,708 approvals through the 510(k) process and only 41 through the Premarket Approval process.[21]

Pressures for Approval

Perhaps the biggest challenge and source of friction for the FDA is the speed of approvals for drugs and devices. Protecting the public from snake oil would dictate a deliberate, cautious, thorough process. On the other hand, getting valuable new technology to the public—to save lives or improve quality of life—would argue for a speedy process. Some consumer protection groups argue that the agency is far too hasty and lenient, bending to drug and device company pressure. On the other hand, manufacturers argue that the agency still drags its feet and kills people who are waiting for new cures. Says Kessler: "That's been the biggest fight between the industry, the Congress and the FDA over the past decade: getting products out fast."

To help speed up the review process, Congress passed a law in 1992 that allowed the FDA to collect "user fees" from drug companies. This was in part a response to AIDS advocates, who demanded quick approval of experimental drugs that might offer even a ray of hope. These fees, over $300,000 for each new drug application, now account for about half the FDA's budget for drug evaluation and 12 percent of the agency's overall $1.3 billion budget.[22]

The extra funds have indeed accelerated the approval process. By 1999, average approval time had dropped by about twenty months, to an average of a year. In 1988, only 4 percent of new drugs introduced worldwide were approved first by the FDA. By 1998, FDA was first in approving two-thirds of new drugs introduced worldwide. The percentage of applications ultimately approved had also increased substantially.[22] Nonetheless, industry complained when approval times slipped to about fourteen months in 2001.[23] In 2002, device makers announced an agreement with the FDA for similar user fees to expedite approval of new devices, and congressional approval followed.[24]

Critics, like two former editors of the *New England Journal of Medicine,* argue that the user fees create an obvious conflict of interest. So much of the FDA budget now comes from the industry it regulates that the agency must be careful not to alienate its corporate "sponsors."[25] FDA officials claim that they remain careful, but they concede that user fees have imposed pressures that make review more difficult, according to *The Wall Street Journal.*[26]

An internal FDA report in 2002 indicated that a third of FDA employees felt uncomfortable expressing "contrary scientific opinions" to the conclusions reached in drug trials. Another third felt that negative actions against applications were "stigmatized." The report also said that some drug reviewers stated "that decisions should be based more on science and less on corporate wishes."[26] *The Los Angeles Times* reported that agency drug reviewers felt that if drugs were not approved, drug companies would complain to Congress, which might retaliate by failing to renew the user fees.[22] This, in turn, would hamstring FDA operations and probably cost jobs. However, Congress reapproved the fees in 2002.

Another criticism is that the approval process has allowed many dangerous drugs to reach the market. A recent analysis showed that of all new drugs approved from 1975 to 1999, almost 3 percent were subsequently withdrawn for safety reasons, and 8 percent acquired "black box warnings" of potentially serious side effects. Projections based on the pace of these events suggested that one in five approved drugs would eventually either receive a black box warning or be withdrawn. The authors of the analysis, from Harvard Medical School and Public Citizen Health Research Group, suggested that the FDA should raise the bar for approval of new drugs when safe and effective treatments are already available or when the drug is for a non-life-threatening condition.[4]

According to *The Los Angeles Times,* in the approval process for seven drugs that were withdrawn between 1993 and 2000, the FDA had disregarded "danger signs or blunt warnings from its own specialists. Then, after receiving reports of significant harm to patients, the agency was slow to seek withdrawals." These drugs were suspected in 1,002 deaths reported to the FDA. None of these were lifesaving drugs. They included a heartburn drug (Propulsid), a diet pill (Redux), and a painkiller (Duract). The *Times* reported that the seven drugs had U.S. sales of $5 billion before they were withdrawn.[22]

After analysis, FDA officials have concluded that the accelerated drug approval process is unrelated to the drug withdrawals. They point out that the number of drugs on the market has risen dramatically, the number of applications has increased, and the population is using more medications.[5] In their view, more withdrawals are not surprising. Dr. Janet Woodcock, director of the FDA's drug review center and one of the analysts, argues, "All drugs have risks; most of them have serious risks." She believes that the withdrawn drugs were valuable and that their removal from the market was a loss, even if the removal was necessary, according to *The Los Angeles Times.*[22]

Nonetheless, many people believe that the pressures for approval are so strong that they're contributing to employee burnout at the FDA. In August 2002, *The Wall Street Journal* reported that 15 percent of the agency's medical officer jobs were unfilled.[26] The attrition rate among medical officers at the FDA is higher than that for medical officers at NIH or CDC. The journal reported that the reasons, among others, included pressure to increase the pace of drug approvals and an atmosphere that discourages negative actions on drug applications. Attrition due to employee burnout is now judged to threaten the speed of the approval process. In 2000, even Dr. Woodcock reportedly acknowledged a "sweatshop environment that's causing high staffing turnover."[22] FDA medical and statistical staff have echoed the need for speed, describing insufficient time to master details.[22,23]

An opposing view of the FDA's function, though, has been articulated in some biting editorials. An example is one from *The Wall Street Journal,* by Robert Goldberg of the Manhattan Institute. He wrote that the agency "'protects' people from the drugs that can save their lives" and needs to shift its role to "speedily put into the market place . . . new miracle drugs and technologies." He argues that increasing approval times for new treatments are a result of "careless scientific reasoning" and "bureaucratic incompetence," and that the FDA should monitor the impact of new treatments after they are marketed, rather than wait for "needless clinical trials" that delay approvals.[27]

Thus, the FDA faces a constant "damned if you do, damned if you don't" environment. No one has undertaken a comprehensive study of the speed of drug or device approval to determine the appropriate metrics for this process, much less the optimal speed. It remains unclear how best to balance the benefits of making new products rapidly available with the risks of unanticipated complications and recalls.

Postmarketing Surveillance of New Products

Although user fees have facilitated preapproval evaluation of new drugs, the money needed to evaluate the safety of drugs after they're marketed has generally not been available. But experts point out that roughly half of approved drugs have serious side effects that are not known prior to approval, and that only postmarketing surveillance can detect them. This can happen because drugs are often tested in hundreds or thousands of patients, but not in millions, so side effects that are infrequent may not become apparent. The other reason is that drugs are often tested in patients who are younger or healthier than the patients for whom they are typically prescribed after approval.

But in the opinion of some experts, the FDA lacks the mandate, the money, and the staff to provide effective and efficient surveillance of the over five thousand drugs already in the marketplace.[28] Even in situations where approval of a drug has been contingent on conducting postmarketing studies, the studies are often seriously delayed. The FDA has acknowledged that in some cases, it didn't fix a completion date, and that record keeping has sometimes been lax.[29]

Although reporting of adverse effects by manufacturers is mandatory, late reporting and nonreporting of cases by drug companies are major problems. Some companies have been prosecuted for failure to report, and the FDA has issued several warning letters as a result of late reporting. Spontaneous reporting by practitioners is estimated to capture only 1 to 13 percent of serious adverse events.[30]

And aggressive promotion of new drugs—before some of the serious side effects are known—increases patients' exposure to the unknown risks. Nearly twenty million patients (almost 10 percent of the U.S. adult population) were exposed to five drugs that were recalled in 1997 and 1998 alone.[31] Fortunately, the new law allowing user fees for device manufacturers doesn't have the same restriction on postmarketing surveillance that has hampered drug surveillance.

Conflicts of Interest in the Approval Process

Another problem that has come to light in the FDA approval process is the conflict of interest among some members of the agency's eighteen drug advisory committees. These committees have about three hundred members and are influential in recommending whether drugs should be approved, whether they should remain on the market, how drug studies should be designed, and what warning labels should say. The decisions of these committees have enormous financial implications for drug makers.

A report by *USA Today* indicated that roughly half the experts on these panels had a direct financial interest in the drug or topic they were asked to evaluate. The conflicts of interest included stock ownership, consulting fees, and research grants from the companies whose products they were evaluating. In some cases, committee members had helped to develop the drugs they were evaluating. Although federal law tries to restrict the use of experts with conflicts of interest, *USA Today* reported that the FDA had waived the rule more than eight hundred times between 1998 and 2000. The FDA doesn't reveal the magnitude of any financial interest or the drug companies involved.[32]

Nonetheless, *USA Today* reported that in considering 159 advisory committee meetings from 1998 through the first half of 2000, at least one member had a financial conflict of interest 92 percent of the time. At more than half the meetings, half or more of the members had conflicts. At 102 meetings that dealt specifically with drug approval, 33 percent of committee members had conflicts.[32] *The Los Angeles Times* reported that such conflicts were present at committee reviews of some recently withdrawn drugs.[22]

The FDA official responsible for waiving the conflict-of-interest rules pointed out that the same experts who consult with industry are often the best for consulting with the FDA, because of their knowledge of certain drugs and diseases. But according to *USA Today*, "even consumer and patient representatives on the committees often receive drug company money."[33] Consumer protection groups like Public Citizen argue that "the industry has more influence on the process than people realize." And in 2001, congressional staff from the House Government Reform Committee began examining the FDA advisory committees to determine whether conflicts of interest were affecting the approval process.[34]

The FTC and Free Markets

What about another federal agency, the Federal Trade Commission (FTC)? This agency deals broadly with antitrust and consumer protection laws. In the health-care arena, its activities have focused on promoting competition among manufacturers and trying to minimize the extent of misleading advertising. As we saw earlier, the FTC plays an active role in trying to assure fair use of patents and allowing generic drugs to emerge when patents expire.

FTC Chair Timothy Muris, a Bush appointee, told a Senate committee in 2002 that brand-name drug companies had used a variety of "illegal tactics" to impede generic drug competition, "costing consumers millions or even billions of dollars without valid cause." He indicated that the agency was dramatically increasing investigations in the health-care industry, including drug companies.[35]

The FTC is alert to noncompetitive practices on the part of doctors and hospitals, as well as manufacturers. In 2002, for example, doctor groups in both Dallas and Denver settled FTC charges that they had worked together to keep prices artificially high. In Dallas, the 1,250-member Genesis

Physicians Group was involved. In Denver, it was eight practice groups of obstetrician/gynecologists, composed of over eighty doctors. In both cities, the groups admitted no wrongdoing, but agreed to avoid future price fixing, according to *USA Today*.[36] The FTC is also investigating some hospital mergers to determine if their increased market power accounts for some rapid price increases.

The FTC also monitors advertising for health products, though the FDA does much of the surveillance of prescription drug ads. Advertising for medical procedures, diet supplements, and alternative medicines all fall under FTC scrutiny. As an example, in 2001 the FTC cracked down on six dietary supplement companies that were advertising their products as cures for cancer, AIDS, arthritis, and Alzheimer's disease. One company sold a Zapper Electrical Unit to "treat and cure" Alzheimer's disease and AIDS.[37] In some cases, the FDA and the FTC have joined forces in an effort to broaden enforcement against fraudulent Internet advertising.

In summary, these federal agencies, despite some bad-mouthing from politicians and the industries they regulate, are generally doing a credible job of trying to protect the public. But politicians and corporations frequently portray the FDA, in particular, as plodding and bureaucratic, sarcastically suggesting that it is preventing access to new cures rather than protecting the public from snake oil. Critics of the agency seem to assume that new technology can only be good, and that serious safety considerations are rarely an issue.

But pressures for speed, conflicts of interest in decision making, constrained legislative mandates, inadequate budgets, and often limited surveillance after products enter the market mean that scientific considerations are only part of the regulatory equation. These limitations can lead to misleading advertising of new drugs, promotion of less effective over more effective treatments, delays in identifying treatment risks, and perhaps unnecessary exposure of patients to treatments whose risks outweigh their benefits.

Regulatory approval provides many critical functions. However, it alone doesn't identify the best treatment strategies. Doctors, patients, and the public should realize that new drugs may not be as effective as old ones, that new drugs are likely to have undiscovered side effects at the time they're marketed, that direct-to-consumer ads are sometimes misleading, that new gadgets are generally not as well tested as new drugs, and that value for money isn't considered in the approval process. If you're relying on these federal agencies to protect you from harm or from wasting your money, you should realize that there are substantial holes in the safety net.

PART III

USELESS, HARMFUL, OR MARGINAL

Popular Treatments That Caused Unnecessary Disability, Dollar Costs, or Death

13

Ineffective, Inferior, or Needlessly Costly New Drugs

The enthusiasm with which these were at first received appears to have been unwarranted by fuller experience and may be taken as another instance of ill-judged medical faith in a remedy which is often one of the misfortunes of the profession. —Editorial on arsenic compounds in the *Journal of the American Medical Association, 1903*[1]

HAVING CONSIDERED some of the players in disseminating medical advances, it may be helpful to study how they've acted and interacted over specific drugs, devices, operations, and other products. The goal of this section is to describe some illustrative events, first considering new drugs, then surgical procedures, medical devices, and the weight loss industry. For this purpose, probably nothing is better than some good stories. Those recounted here are illustrative, but hardly exhaustive.

More Cost for Less Benefit? Calcium-Channel Blockers for High Blood Pressure*

On a March day in 1995, Dr. Bruce Psaty ascended the podium to present a scientific paper, as he had done many times before.[2] At a hotel in San Antonio, he was speaking before the Epidemiology and Prevention Council of the American Heart Association, a small meeting of academic

*This section adapted and reproduced with permission from the BMJ Publishing Group from *Quality and Saftey in Health Care* 2002; II: 294–296.

researchers. Psaty and his colleagues had been studying complications associated with drugs for treating high blood pressure. The paper seemed innocuous. "I had no idea it would do anything," he says. But a hostile question-and-answer session presaged a relentless attack from drug manufacturers. And the apparent controversy piqued the interest of journalists attending the meeting.

Psaty had found that a class of relatively new and expensive drugs—calcium-channel blockers—was associated with a higher risk of heart attacks than older, less expensive drugs.[3] This was especially true for short-acting calcium-channel drugs. As soon as he returned home to Seattle, Psaty found himself at the center of a maelstrom. Press reports had already appeared, doctors and patients were alarmed, and drug makers were surly.

Psaty's office was inundated with phones calls and faxes, requiring him to divert staff from research to public relations. The press reports were generally accurate, but they lacked the caveats and context needed for a clear perspective on the findings. They offered little help for patients who were taking the drugs and wondered what to do. In his interviews, Psaty consistently recommended that patients see their own doctors rather than stop taking their current medications. He recommended that physicians follow the current guidelines from the Joint National Committee on the Detection, Evaluation, and Treatment of High Blood Pressure, which recommended the older, cheaper diuretics and beta-blocker drugs unless they were poorly tolerated or couldn't be used because of other medical problems.[4]

Furthermore, Psaty was already under attack by the makers of calcium-channel blockers. In his office, he found a fax to the medical school dean from Pfizer Corporation, a manufacturer of calcium-channel blockers, complaining about Psaty's presentation. Psaty remembers a call from a vice president of Pfizer, who "was very angry and wanted to see the data." He also recalls that the dean of the School of Public Health was contacted by a state legislator to complain about the activities of this University of Washington professor of medicine. "I felt vulnerable," says Psaty, "because this was such an unfamiliar and uneven playing field. I was schooled in a scholarly style of debate, not in marketing hyperbole and character attacks."[5]

Psaty became one of a growing number of researchers who have been besieged by drug companies for getting the "wrong" results. In other cases, researchers have had publication of their work blocked for several years, universities have been sued, journal editors have been threatened, and faculty have had their careers stymied. These battles have moved well beyond legitimate scientific debate into character attacks, "spin doctoring," and legal action. Sometimes inadvertently, researchers with unfavorable results about profitable drugs find that they are sticking their necks out, risking ostracism and threats to their careers. "Fortunately, I suppose," Psaty said, "one sometimes decides to take a scientific path unaware of what may lie ahead."

Psaty fits the stereotypical image of a professor in demeanor and appearance, with his salt-and-pepper beard, balding forehead, large spectacles, and ready smile. In addition to his medical degree and epidemiology training, he has a PhD in English, so he is a lover of words as well as of statistical methods. His intellectual and research interests are broad, and they are certainly not fixated on the adverse effects of calcium-channel blockers. Fortunately for patients with high blood pressure, though, Psaty has been willing to pursue work on drug safety, sometimes in a chilly atmosphere. Other experts credit Psaty with doing more than anything in the past decade to stimulate rigorous clinical-trial research on high blood pressure.

In the ensuing days, the dean of the School of Public Health was called by company officials, who suggested that Psaty's work should not be published because it might prove to be wrong. News stories began to focus on the media's seemingly alarmist handling of the report, and this diverted attention from the basic question of drug safety. Psaty wondered if the PR staffs of certain of the manufacturers had helped in this deflection. A blistering "Dear Doctor" letter attacking Psaty's work was distributed nationwide by a prominent expert in high blood pressure. Only later was it clear that this was sponsored by Bayer, the manufacturer of another brand of calcium-channel blockers.[6]

According to an article in the British journal *The Lancet,* in 1995 Bayer was already under investigation by the Department of Health and Human Services for a "kickback" program, in which pharmacies received $35 for every new prescription of Bayer's brand of calcium-channel blocker. In 1994, the company (then known as Miles) had paid a fine of $605,000 and agreed to drop the scheme.[7]

Psaty received requests from several drug companies that he found intimidating—for documents, tables, manuscripts and new analyses. Pfizer's attorneys made use of Washington State's Freedom of Information Act to:

> . . . request all records, reports, data, analyses, correspondence, and any other documentation related to the design, conduct, results and

> conclusions of this study. This includes but is not limited to, records relating to the following: study design and methodology; study protocol(s); individual data for all study subjects including study and control populations; case report forms; tabulations of study results and data; data sets; statistical calculations, methodologies and analysis; correspondence, meeting minutes, notes and other documentation of Dr. Psaty and any other University researchers, faculty or staff and of any departmental, staff or other research committees; meeting minutes, reports and other documentation of evaluation by Institutional Review Board and/or other oversight committees or bodies within or outside the University.

Psaty noted that at the time of this work, roughly 20 percent of patients with high blood pressure were taking calcium-channel blockers, so the findings were potentially of major public health significance. The drugs were heavily marketed to physicians and enjoyed a growing market share. They were fifteen times more expensive than older alternatives, which were known not only to reduce blood pressure, but also to reduce the devastating complications of high blood pressure, such as strokes, heart attacks, and heart failure.

Despite the attacks, Psaty's work has withstood the test of time. His report in San Antonio had been a case-control study, a research design that is more susceptible to certain types of inadvertent bias than randomized trials.[3] Thus, it was regarded as potentially important, but not definitive. Other studies, using different research designs, have generally confirmed Psaty's findings, which seem to hold for several drugs in this class.[8–12] Recent studies combining the results of many randomized trials indicate that calcium-channel blockers are less effective at preventing heart attacks and heart failure than other drugs for high blood pressure.[9–12] The calcium-channel blockers are better than a placebo for high blood pressure, justifying the manufacturers' claims that they are safe and effective. They just aren't as effective at preventing complications as less expensive alternatives such as low-dose diuretics.

This appears to be true despite effective lowering of blood pressure by the calcium-channel drugs. Thus, Psaty's work helped to establish a more fundamental point: that blood pressure drugs may be very different in their benefits, despite equal success at controlling blood pressure.[13] This in turn suggests that researchers should evaluate new drugs not just for their effects on blood pressure, but for their effects on its many complications as well.

Much of the controversy focused on short-acting preparations of calcium-channel blockers, which Psaty's initial report had associated with the greatest risk. Manufacturers correctly pointed out that the FDA had never approved short-acting drugs for the treatment of high blood pressure (they were approved for use in angina). Nonetheless, short-acting drugs were widely used for this purpose, a fact that was evident in Psaty's data and acknowledged by the FDA. In February 1996, after an advisory committee meeting, the FDA issued a letter to makers of calcium-channel blockers, requiring new labeling that warned against such use.

An independent review in 2001 concluded that short-acting calcium-channel blockers "should be avoided in the routine treatment of hypertension."[14] Drug makers argued that the evidence didn't implicate the longer-acting calcium-channel blockers. In fact, Pfizer continued to market its long-acting calcium-channel drug, amlodipine (Norvasc), which became the fifth-largest-selling drug in the world by 2000, with global sales of $3.3 billion.[15]

However, recent studies suggest that, compared to other drugs for high blood pressure, even the long-acting calcium-channel blockers may be less effective at preventing heart attacks and congestive heart failure.[8–11] Finally, in 2002, the largest study of blood pressure medicines ever conducted (with over 33,000 patients) found that diuretics were just as effective as amlodipine in lowering blood pressure, and more effective in preventing heart failure.[12]

Referring to amlodipine and other new drugs that were studied, one of the researchers, Dr. Curt Furberg of Wake Forest University, said, "If everyone were switched to diuretics, we would have 60,000 to 70,000 fewer cases of heart failure and stroke each year."[16] Making the strategy even sweeter, a separate estimate is that such changes would save $1.2 billion a year over current prescribing patterns.[17]

Additional problems have recently come to light. Studies published in 2001 found that, compared with other drugs, amlodipine was associated with worse effects on kidney function in patients with diabetes or with kidney disease due to high blood pressure.[18,19] Guidelines prepared by a national expert committee continue to recommend the older, cheaper drugs as first-line therapy for "uncomplicated" high blood pressure, reserving calcium-channel blockers for special situations.[20]

Psaty concludes, "I'm indifferent toward calcium-channel blockers. However, I'm a big fan of low dose diuretics which are inexpensive, safe, and effective." His advice to patients is, "If you have drug-treated high blood pressure and you're not on a low-dose diuretic, consider asking your doctor 'why not?'"

Trends in drug use suggest that Psaty's work had at least some impact. A study in British Columbia demonstrated a decline in new prescriptions for calcium-channel blockers, comparing the years before and after Psaty's study. Though several other factors were also at play, the researchers attributed part of this change in clinical practice to Psaty's research and the ensuing publicity.[21]

The controversy over Psaty's research spawned a unique investigation of conflict of interest among medical authors. A group of Canadian doctors identified articles on the controversy that appeared in the medical literature during the eighteen months after Psaty's presentation in San Antonio. They contacted the authors of each article to inquire about funding from the makers of calcium-channel blockers—including research grants, employment, consulting fees, honoraria, and travel expenses. They found that 96 percent of authors who supported the use of calcium-channel blockers had financial ties to manufacturers, as opposed to just 44 percent of neutral or critical authors.[22]

Through the investment of a substantial amount of time, good communication with the media, and support from senior collaborators, Psaty has weathered the storm with his reputation and sanity intact. On the positive side, the attacks by the drug companies raised the visibility of Psaty's research, and may paradoxically have helped his career. "In a sense, Pfizer did more to promote the findings of our unwanted study than I could ever have done on my own. And maybe Bayer, too. I don't want to give Pfizer all the credit," he notes. "The whole effort to discredit our work helped to create the calcium-channel blocker controversy. Their confrontational methods only served to publicize it widely to physicians and patients alike."

The risk for society is that other researchers may shy away from controversial but important questions after watching doctors like Psaty be intimidated by vested interests. For his part, Psaty sees himself as neither crusader nor watchdog. "I don't see myself as a risk taker. I'm just a country scientist," he says. "I delight in doing new stuff and trying to anticipate important questions."

Thyroid Supplements

Psaty's experience may seem extraordinary, but other stories suggest that it's business as usual. Consider Betty Dong, a pharmacologist at the University of California at San Francisco. Her research on thyroid hormone preparations might have reduced drug costs for millions of patients with an underactive thyroid gland. But it might also have caused the industry leader's sales to plummet and disrupted a billion-dollar corporate buyout. Facing an abyss of potential financial losses, the manufacturer who had asked Dong to do the work blocked publication of the results for seven years.

In 1987, Dong was approached by the predecessor to Boots Pharmaceuticals, the maker of Synthroid, to conduct a study comparing its product with the generic drug competition. Synthroid is a synthetic version of thyroid hormone that is prescribed for patients who have an underactive thyroid. Synthroid had dominated the market for years, thanks to concerns that other thyroid hormone preparations were not as well absorbed or as consistent in their potency. They were considered by many doctors not to be "bioequivalent" to Synthroid, which was regarded as a superior preparation.[23]

However, the high cost of Synthroid led some states to consider substitutes for their formulary lists, allowing doctors and pharmacies to substitute a cheaper version. Threatened with a loss of business (Boots had 84 percent of the market), an executive approached Dong to do a study comparing Synthroid with two generic versions and another brand-name version of thyroid hormone. Executives and scientists at Boots, as well as Dong herself, expected to find that Synthroid was superior.[23]

Beautiful theories, though, are still sometimes slain by ugly facts. Dong's study was completed in 1990, and it unexpectedly showed that the four preparations of thyroid hormone were in fact equivalent.

Boots had hand-picked Dong to do the work, perhaps because her earlier work on the hormone content of different thyroid preparations had been favorable toward Synthroid. The contract between Boots and Dong specified in advance the study design and data analysis plan. The company made regular site visits, about three each year, to assure that the work was being done properly. The study was well designed, and it later received favorable reviews by both internal UCSF investigators and external reviewers at the *Journal of the American Medical Association*—a top research journal.[23,24]

But when Boots executives saw the results, they suddenly objected to nearly all aspects of the study. For the first time, they expressed numerous concerns about the conduct of the study, challenging the way patients were selected, how well patients took their medicines, the length of time blood samples were stored, the statistical analyses, and (according to the research team) 136 concerns about case-report forms alone. The list of objections filled a thick binder, according to *Wall Street Journal* accounts.[24]

The company sent its complaints to the university chancellor, the vice chancellors, and several department chairs. Two investigations by the university found only minor and easily correctible problems. The head of one review noted in 1992 that "It would be extreme hyperbole to question the scientific merit of the study on the basis of these deficiencies." UCSF also had the work reviewed by an outside expert on comparative drug analysis, who concluded that the criticisms were unwarranted. *The Wall Street Journal* quoted the expert as saying, "The Boots people were deceptive and self-serving."[24]

This was merely a prelude to legal threats that blocked Dong and her colleagues from publishing the results. The company cited a restrictive clause regarding publication in the contract, which Dong had naively signed, even though its provisions were contrary to university policy. University attorneys were initially supportive of Dong's right to publish, citing academic freedom and university policy. In 1994, Dong's team submitted a report to the *Journal of the American Medical Association* (JAMA), and the article was accepted for publication. But two weeks before its scheduled publication, in January 1995, Dong withdrew the manuscript. A new university attorney had reversed positions, urging the researchers not to publish and to comply with the publishing rights clause. If they published, they were warned, they would have to defend themselves in court, without university help.[24]

While this legal maneuvering played out, Boots was negotiating to sell its drug division to Germany's BASF AG. The deal was completed in April 1995; BASF paid $1.4 billion for the company, which became part of BASF's Knoll Pharmaceutical subsidiary. According to a drug industry analyst interviewed by *The Wall Street Journal,* publication of Dong's results would have been disastrous for Boots, lowering its sale value and "accelerating the decline of the brand."[24]

In May, *JAMA* received a letter from Boots/Knoll, disparaging both the study and Dr. Dong. In an astonishing move, employees of Boots/Knoll then proceeded to publish the results of Dong's study with no acknowledgement of the actual researchers, including a reanalysis that came to the opposite conclusion and a table of "eighteen major study limitations." The effect was to strengthen Synthroid's position. And ordinarily such publication would preclude subsequent publication in a peer-reviewed journal.[23]

Eventually, under pressure from the FDA for alleged misleading claims and in the face of negative publicity, Knoll agreed not to block publication of Dong's manuscript. In April 1997, despite the earlier publication of data, *JAMA* published the article.[25] With it appeared an apology from Knoll for blocking publication, a letter with Knoll's continued objections to the article, a rebuttal from Dong's team, and a lengthy editorial describing the events.[23]

Knoll subsequently faced a class action lawsuit by consumers, alleging that they were overcharged for medication because the data on bioequivalence were unavailable. Knoll denied any efforts to suppress publication, but offered $135 million to settle the suit.[26] Dong and her colleagues had estimated that if generic drugs were substituted for Synthroid, $356 million might be saved annually.[25]

Taxol and Cancer Chemotherapy

If you wanted to sell a product in a competitive economy, you might choose a low price, to undercut the competition. Perversely, as we saw in Chapter 7, if you made cancer chemotherapy drugs, you might instead choose a high price and expect to sell more. Dr. Scott Ramsey learned this the hard way when he conducted an economic trial of competing drugs for lung cancer. His results were attacked not by the drug makers, but by his professional colleagues.

Ramsey is a rare breed: an MD who also has a PhD in economics. He works at the Fred Hutchinson Cancer Research Center in Seattle, studying the cost-effectiveness of cancer tests and treatments. He is tall, athletic, and clean-cut, with wavy blond hair. He routinely braves downtown Seattle traffic to ride his bike to work.

In 1998, he began work with the Southwest Oncology Group (SWOG) on a comparison of two treatment approaches for lung cancer. The study compared two competing treatment regimens: a standard regimen of Navelbine plus cisplatin and a new combination of Taxol and carboplatin. Ramsey succeeded in getting the makers of both Navelbine and Taxol to fund an economic analysis, figuring that dual funding would preempt concerns about conflict of interest. The makers of Taxol seemed confident that their drug would be less toxic and more effective, and "would be a slam-dunk from a cost-effectiveness standpoint," says Ramsey. The makers of Navelbine, he thinks, felt that their drug was equally effective and was priced far lower.

The treatment results were published in the *Journal of Clinical Oncology* in 2001 and showed identical survival results.[27] Says Ramsey, "If you look at these survival curves, they're so on top of each other, you almost wonder if either drug works! I mean, they're just identical. And the data also showed no difference in quality of life—no difference whatsoever." The different drugs showed differences in their side effects, but overall measures of quality of life were indistinguishable. The Taxol group had fewer reports of nausea and vomiting, but Ramsey checked for use of antinausea drugs in each treatment group. He found "there was actually more antiemetic use in the Taxol group than in the Navelbine group." This leaves some uncertainty as to the real advantages of Taxol.

With such minimal differences between treatments, we might expect cancer specialists to stick with the less expensive treatment program. Instead, Ramsey says, the researchers proposed at an oncology society meeting that they "eliminate Navelbine from the next trial, effectively making it no longer the standard of care." The stated rationale was the apparent advantage of Taxol in reducing nausea, but the stance was sharply criticized at the meeting.

With the researchers sensitized by this response, Ramsey prepared his economic results for the next meeting of SWOG. He recalls, "So I come along and do the economic study, and guess what? Vastly more expensive in the Taxol group. One of the main people for the trial tried to get me to change slides the night before my presentation, and I refused. So I present this data at the plenary session, and I got attacked by the audience, and I really didn't understand why." The person who asked Ramsey to change his slides "started attacking me and grilling me about intricacies of the clinical trial that he knew I didn't know as well as he did—such as intricate details of drug dosing—and actually was only shut up when the chairman of SWOG, Charles Coltman, stood up and said 'this doesn't matter!'"

Ramsey was puzzled. "Why were people attacking me? I couldn't figure this out. What I learned later was that oncologists keep their own pharmacies. They purchase drugs at a discount and then by law are reimbursed at Average Wholesale Price minus 5%, which is much higher than the discounted prices . . . so the profit they make by prescribing Taxol is huge compared to Navelbine. In addition, the Taxol regimen is somewhat simpler for the oncologist to deliver. And you know lung cancer is a big part of most oncology practices. So when you publish this, I'll get killed. But I think what has happened is, it's a lot about money."

Ramsey is quick to point out that this is speculation on his part, but other events give credence to his hunch. During 2000, Medicare prompted a congressional inquiry into drug pricing that affected Medicare and Medicaid costs. The focus was on cancer drugs that are administered in a doctor's office because they must be given intravenously rather than orally. The investigators noted that drug companies sometimes *raise* prices over those of their competition, increasing the spread between an oncologist's discount price and the reimbursement from Medicare. Internal corporate documents found by the congressional investigators indicated that in several cases, companies raised prices to make their drugs more attractive to doctors.[28]

In an example cited by *The Wall Street Journal*, a doctor might buy fifteen units of the cancer drug Bleomycin for $140. The "sticker price" would result in a Medicare reimbursement of $294, resulting in a profit for the doctor of $154.[28] Similarly, press reports indicated that doctors' reimbursement for Lupron, a prostate cancer drug, typically exceeded their costs by $100 to $150 for a monthly dose.[29] Even more striking, the Minnesota attorney general claimed that doctors in Minnesota paid $7.75 per dose of the cancer treatment Vincasar, while the average wholesale price was listed as $742. This resulted in typical payments from Medicare of $564, plus $141 from the patient.[30] In most cases, the higher the cost of the drug, the higher the profit for the doctor.

Doctors argue that the expense is justified because Medicare and Medicaid don't adequately reimburse them for the costs of administering treatment to their patients. But at the same time, cancer specialists sometimes refer to the generous reimbursements as the "chemotherapy concession."[31] The inspector general of the Department of Health and Human Services says, "Publishing an artificially high AWP is used as a marketing device to increase a drug company's market share."[32]

The congressional investigators focused on some fifty drugs made by over a dozen companies—mostly for cancer and for AIDS. The investigators suggested that Medicare and Medicaid might be overpaying $1 billion per year for such drugs. Subsequently, in 2001, several drug companies, including Bayer, Abbott, and TAP Pharmaceuticals (a joint venture between Abbott and Japan's Takeda Chemical Industries Ltd.), reduced drug prices or reached multimillion-dollar settlements with federal and state investigators. TAP settled a related fraud case for $875 million, the largest criminal fine ever levied by the government for health-care fraud.[33,34]

Equally alarming, congressional investigators suggested that some doctors may overprescribe certain drugs because of the big reimbursements.[28] Ramsey echoes this concern. In the lung cancer trial, patients entered the study with advanced cancer and poor prognoses. Nonetheless, Ramsey notes, "These patients were getting second, third, fourth line chemotherapy, and yet it did nothing. People who failed Navelbine were turned around and getting Taxol as a second line therapy. And it was just going on and on, and I thought 'why are they doing this to these people?' I think it has a lot to do with economics. It's sort of a third rail, though, to bring this up, because you can argue patients are desperately ill and willing to try anything."

But these concerns appear to be more than speculation. In a study of Medicare payments for cancer chemotherapy, researchers found that chemotherapy was being continued into the last three months of life for many patients. This was true even for cancers that doctors generally consider unresponsive to chemotherapy, such as pancreatic, liver, and kidney cancer. Although this may be the result of desperation on the part of patients and families, efforts to palliate symptoms, or uncertainty as to prognosis, it raises concern about overuse of chemotherapy at the end of life.[31,35]

What about the bottom line on costs for the two lung cancer treatment regimens that Ramsey studied? Considering the number of people with late-stage lung cancer and the higher cost of Taxol, he estimated that making Taxol the standard of care would cost almost an additional $1 billion per year. A senior researcher on the clinical trial threatened to block publication of the economic analysis if Ramsey kept the billion-dollar figure in the manuscript. But in the end, the article was accepted for publication in the *Journal of the National Cancer Institute*, where the editor insisted on including the billion-dollar implication.[36]

When Treatment Causes Harm: The Story of Encainide and Flecainide

The stories of calcium-channel drugs, Synthroid, and Taxol all raise questions of added cost with no benefit over alternative drugs. But the story of encainide and flecainide is one of outright harm from a new technology. An estimated fifty thousand people died from taking these drugs, which were intended to prevent cardiac arrest. As Thomas J. Moore, author of *Deadly Medicine,* notes, this exceeded U.S. casualties in the Vietnam War.[37]

Moore's book details how this happened and why there was so little public outcry—a common theme with the introduction of wasteful or harmful new technology. Rather than recount the full history, we'll focus on the hazards of surrogate markers of drug benefit and the reasons for the meager professional and public response.

A surrogate marker is some physiological effect—in this case, eliminating abnormal heartbeats—that we hope is a marker for some more important result, such as improved survival. In other words, counting abnormal heartbeats becomes a "surrogate" for measuring how long people live. But the two don't necessarily go together. In some other examples, researchers might look at the effects of a drug on tumor size, cholesterol level, or immune cells. Just because a drug affects these measures doesn't necessarily mean that it improves survival, and there are several counterexamples. But drug companies prefer to study surrogate markers because they can be measured more quickly than waiting to assess the effects of a drug on survival.

In 1985, the 3M Company marketed a new drug called Tambocor—a trade name for flecainide. The drug was very effective at suppressing a type of abnormal heartbeat known as premature ventricular contractions. In advanced form, these abnormal heartbeats sometimes become life-threatening. They occur in healthy people, but they are much more common among persons who have had a heart attack. Some ten million prescriptions had been written the year before for other drugs to treat these abnormal heartbeats.

At the time, it was an article of faith that suppressing such beats must be good, must prevent cardiac arrest, and must save lives. But subsequent events made this a classic example of the fallacy of assuming that surrogate markers (like the suppression of ominous heartbeats) necessarily translate into tangible benefits like improved quality of life or longer survival.

Even as Tambocor was being marketed, the NIH was starting an ambitious clinical trial to test the efficacy of Tambocor, a closely related drug called encainide (Enkaid, Bristol-Myers), and a somewhat different drug called Ethmozine. The study was to examine not only the ability of these drugs to suppress abnormal heartbeats, but whether they actually saved lives. The drug companies hadn't undertaken such studies because they weren't required for FDA approval. The conviction that suppressing extra beats must be good was so strong that demonstrating this was sufficient for approval. Indeed, many doctors thought that conducting a randomized trial was unethical, because we knew that these drugs must save lives—it only made sense.

But the NIH trial showed just the opposite.[38] Patients taking encainide and flecainide had a death rate more than twice that of the patients taking placebo! Patients who were randomly assigned to take the sugar pills could thank their lucky stars, because they were more likely to live to hear the main results announced in 1989. Later results also suggested, less definitively, that Ethmozine caused excess deaths.[39]

Because the results were so important, and because so many patients were taking the drugs, Dr. Claude Lenfant, director of the National Heart, Lung, and Blood Institute, felt obliged to announce the results quickly and directly to the press. FDA Commissioner Frank Young joined in the effort. By doing so, they probably saved thousands of lives. However, the press conference was almost cancelled at the last minute as a result of pressure from the White House. According to Moore's account, this was a consequence of calls from drug company attorneys.[37]

The response to the press announcement was remarkable. Rather than being hailed for forthright and timely disclosure of lifesaving news, Lenfant and Young were vilified by the medical profession. Doctors reported that some patients' lives might be threatened by stopping the drugs—a largely hypothetical concern. The proven dangers of the drugs were minimized by many, and cries for professional autonomy were overwhelming. Medical societies condemned both men for not notifying doctors before notifying the public. Manufacturers of competing drugs (which had never been tested for their effects on patient survival) immediately began aggressive advertising campaigns to take the market share that was being vacated by encainide and flecainide. Subsequent studies have suggested that they shared similar risks, and prescribing of all drugs in this class eventually fell substantially.

Doctors, drug makers, and the FDA shared responsibility for what was, in retrospect, a debacle. All the embarrassed parties had an interest in spin control, so their messages to the media emphasized not the thousands of deaths caused by these drugs but, instead, the largely hypothetical risks of stopping them suddenly. The media, accused of alarmism and endangering patients, covered the story only briefly. The professional bias for action seemed to make stopping these drugs feel dangerous. No public outcry over the widespread use and aggressive marketing of deadly drugs ever emerged.

The FDA chose not to recall the drugs, but to add more restrictive warnings and leave their use to doctors' discretion. Except for Enkaid, they remain on the market, though their use now is far less than it was in the 1980s. They are still considered for patients with more life-threatening disorders than run-of-the-mill premature beats—although there's no rigorous proof that they help even these patients.

The incident vividly illustrated the risks of accepting surrogate markers in judging drug efficacy. In the end, no one disputed that suppression of premature ventricular beats was a poor marker of drug benefit. It led to exactly the wrong conclusion about the outcome that was of real interest: patient survival. It was similar to assuming that all drugs that lower high blood pressure are equally effective at preventing its complications—a theory disproved in the calcium-channel story. However, this experience hasn't been translated into policy at the FDA.

Drug makers dislike the idea of having to prove that their drugs save lives or prevent strokes. It takes too long and requires too many patients, so they view it as too expensive. It's easier to show the drugs suppress abnormal heartbeats or lower blood pressure.

It seems that the FDA wasn't impressed by the encainide and flecainide story. Thanks to pressure from drug makers, doctors, and politicians, the FDA subsequently proposed *greater* use of surrogate markers after the encainide disaster. In essence, showing theoretical benefits (instead of proven benefits) was sufficient. The proposed regulation, as reported by Moore, said that "approval of a drug on the basis of a well-documented surrogate endpoint can allow a drug to be marketed earlier, sometimes much earlier, than it could be if a demonstrated clinical benefit were required."[37]

Again, doing something—even if it later proves harmful—seems more politically acceptable than doing nothing. And marketing new drugs is implicitly equated with benefit to patients, despite the harsh lessons of encainide and flecainide.

The stories of calcium-channel blockers, Synthroid, Taxol, and encainide and flecainide may seem like exceptional cases: Surely they are not representative of day-to-day events, you may imagine. Indeed, most drugs are reasonably safe and effective.

But we could go on and on with similar examples of widely used but ineffective, marginally effective, or needlessly expensive drug treatments. We listed some of these in the chapter on the FDA. Others appear to include intravenous albumin for critically ill patients, Remune for HIV infection, low-dose dopamine for preventing kidney failure in critically ill patients, drugs for maintaining normal heart rhythm in patients with a condition called atrial fibrillation, and some drugs for Alzheimer's disease. And don't forget hormone replacement therapy for preventing heart disease in postmenopausal women. All of these were widely used standard treatments, or in late stages of testing, before accumulating data suggested that they were minimally effective, ineffective, or harmful.[40–45]

Careful surveillance of the news media reveals a steady stream of such stories, although most of them never make the nightly news or achieve widespread public awareness. Nonetheless, intimidating researchers, delaying bad news, and influencing the editorial process appear to be business as usual. This is sometimes true for drug companies and doctors alike. The FDA's procedures and the gaps in its authority mean that regulation alone won't protect you. In this environment, the best scientific evidence sometimes must struggle to emerge, even when it would save consumers money and improve their health.

14

Medical Devices That Disappoint

If you have a screwdriver, everything looks like a screw. There will be a lot of people doing the wrong thing for back pain for a long time, until we finally figure it out. I just hope that we don't hurt too many people in the process. —Dr. Seth Waldeman[1]

DEVICE MANUFACTURERS offer a steady stream of innovations that's growing into a torrent. Recently introduced medical devices include coronary stents, which prop open narrowed arteries; implantable defibrillators, which shock faltering hearts back into a normal rhythm; and the "gamma knife," which uses highly focused and precisely targeted radiation to treat certain brain tumors instead of cutting with a steel blade. On the near horizon are implantable insulin pumps that continuously adjust to changes in a diabetic's blood sugar, robots that can perform precise biopsies inside an MRI scanner, and pacemakers for the heart that can alert doctors to blood pressure changes or fluid buildup in the lungs.[2] Some of these sound like gadgets from *Star Trek*, and these are the things that many people think of as "medical technology."

Medical devices include a huge range of products, including things like artificial joints, heart pacemakers, and MRI scanners. They also include more prosaic products like tubes, catheters, and contact lenses.

Although devices pervade medical practice in every specialty, the biggest markets are for cardiovascular and orthopedic devices.

The medical device industry, at $74 billion in the United States, is about half the size of the drug industry. But as former Senator Everett Dirksen said, "A billion here, a billion there, pretty soon you're talking about real money." And sales are rising almost as fast as they are in the drug industry. Among the largest device companies, average annual revenue growth for the past decade was 23 percent. Like that of the drug industry, the profit margin in the device industry runs around 18 percent.[3] This is a big, lucrative business.

As with new drugs, some new devices are wonderful, some are only so-so, and a few prove to be outright harmful. Like drugs, they're all aggressively promoted to doctors and hospitals. As with new drugs, many of the risks aren't clear until after the devices are in widespread use. And like those of new drugs, costs for new devices often seem to make them more precious than South African diamonds. Here are some stories that may promote a healthy skepticism about many of the new device claims you hear.

The Bjork-Shiley Heart Valve: Earn as You Learn

In 1988, fifty-six-year-old Carol Barbee of Monong, Wisconsin, had what seemed to her husband like a heart attack. He rushed her to the nearest hospital, where the emergency room doctor made the same diagnosis. Within forty-eight hours, Carol was dead. Only during those forty-eight hours did Fred Barbee learn that when his wife had received an artificial heart valve six years earlier, she'd received a model that was prone to breakage. Carol's valve had had just such a breakage, and the result was fatal.[4]

The manufacturer of the valve, Shiley Incorporated, and its parent company, Pfizer, had known about the fracture problem for years and had withdrawn the valve from the market in 1986, but they hadn't notified patients or primary care doctors. Only her surgeon, whom Carol had not seen for six years and who had moved his practice, had been notified. Lawsuits by other patients had not been publicized because of "protective orders" in their settlements.[4]

Patients get artificial heart valves for a variety of reasons: rheumatic heart disease, congenital heart valve abnormalities, degenerative changes that occur with aging, and infections that damage the heart valve. Carol Barbee had received a Bjork-Shiley convexo-concave heart valve, which was intended as an improvement on earlier models. The Bjork-Shiley valve had a clever design, with a tilting disc mounted inside a ring, held in place by metal struts. The ring around the disc had a Teflon collar so that it could be sutured in place.[5,6] The original version was quite reliable, but the company sought to improve on it with the convexo-concave version. It was approved because the risk of blood clots forming on the valve was thought to be lower than for other artificial valves.

This version of the Bjork-Shiley valve quickly became the most popular model of artificial heart valve, and surgeons implanted 86,000 worldwide. But by 1990, over six hundred of the valves had failed, with two-thirds of the failures resulting in the death of the patient; the remainder survived because of emergency surgery to replace the defective valves. It's generally agreed that the actual number of fractures was even higher, because many deaths were probably erroneously attributed to heart attacks. Autopsies are rarely performed to show otherwise.[5]

The first fractures of the Bjork-Shiley convexo-concave valve occurred during testing in 1978. However, these were thought to be anomalous, and the valve was quickly approved by the FDA. The fractures consistently occurred where one of the struts that held the disc in place was welded to the ring. Valve failures continued to occur after the FDA approved the valves in 1979, so the company initiated a series of modifications in the design, without success.[5]

In 1980, Dr. Viking Bjork, the Swedish cardiologist whose name was given to the valve, was planning to publish a paper concerning the valve failures, but the company, Shiley, sent him a telex: "We would prefer that you did not publish the data relative to strut fractures. We expect a few more and until the problem has been corrected we do not feel comfortable." When the situation was reviewed during congressional hearings, Oregon Congressman Ron Wyden said, "I read something like this, and it doesn't sound to me like it's in the public interest."[4]

Then in 1982, Bjork complained to the company. He indicated that other doctors were frequently asking him about valve fractures, that the manufacturing process was "unacceptable," and that Shiley had not given him "trustworthy data" about its plans. And by 1984, the FDA no longer believed that the convexo-concave valve had any advantages over the earlier Shiley model. Statistical analysis showed no reduction in blood clots, and strut fractures were more common than had previously been realized. The delay in reaching this conclusion occurred partly because the FDA had been short of statistical staff until 1982 and partly because of frequent valve modifications that the company had made.[4]

By 1986, the FDA pushed to have the valve withdrawn, and Shiley removed it from the market. The congressional investigation, an FDA task force, and personal damage lawsuits turned up other irregularities. Rather than reporting adverse events—like strut fractures—within ten days, as required by the FDA, the company had delayed its reporting by three weeks to two years.[5,6] After inspections, certain valves were supposed to have been rewelded. In some cases, though, the rewelding wasn't done, and a worker simply polished out the crack instead. Up to 1,700 valves were involved, and records were apparently falsified to indicate that rewelding had been done.

Studying fracture rates was difficult because the actual percentage of recognized failures was small. Fewer than 1 percent of the valves had failed by 1990, but the proportion was statistically greater than that seen with other valves. The acting commissioner of the FDA eventually testified, "The fracture rate is real. It is above most other valves."[4]

In 1990, an FDA task group report concluded that during the valve's history, "Shiley engaged in efforts to thwart the FDA's intervention by untimely reports of fractures, unreported changes in quality control and manufacturing procedures, failure to correct known poor manufacturing procedures, and minimization of the overall problem through misleading and confusing communications to the FDA and the medical community."[4]

A congressional report, also in 1990, concluded, "Shiley, Inc.'s decision to continue to market the valve despite its unsuccessful attempts to identify or correct the cause of the strut fractures illustrates a common practice of conducting clinical trials while continuing full scale marketing. This 'earn as you learn' philosophy has prematurely cut short the lives of hundreds of implantees."[4]

Though Shiley repeatedly and vigorously denied the various allegations, its parent company, Pfizer, was found liable for making false statements. In 1992, Pfizer agreed to a settlement that included $10.75 million for deaths caused by the faulty valves and $9.25 million to monitor patients who had received the valve at Veterans Administration hospitals.[5] Some critics argued that this was too small a penalty; a company statement announced that the settlement is "expected to have no material adverse financial effect on Pfizer."[7]

The events surrounding the Bjork-Shiley valve led to several reforms at the FDA, where oversight of medical devices had just begun when the valve was first considered. Among other things, the episode forced the FDA to develop a guidance document specifying the types of valve testing that the agency would deem adequate; this document came to be used internationally. The FDA also implemented new rules for reporting adverse effects of medical devices after the Safe Medical Devices Act of 1990.[5]

In a recent follow-up, the device industry is trying to protect itself from liability for faulty products. Leaders in the Senate recently slipped a proposal for industry protection from lawsuits into a draft of patient rights legislation. It would have prohibited lawsuits against makers of any body implants, even if the devices were defective. It was championed by the Health Industry Manufacturers Association (now called AdvaMed) with the support of its members, including Pfizer. The clause was killed when it became widely known.[8]

Many patients still have the Bjork-Shiley convexo-concave valves in place, and fractures are still being reported. These patients and their doctors now face a difficult decision about whether and when to consider open-heart surgery to replace the valves, in an effort to avoid disastrous valve failures. Open-heart surgery itself poses substantial risks, of course. James Willems, a cardiologist at the University of Washington, says, "Some of these patients can easily choose between these options and are content. Others, though, carry a tremendous psychological burden from the 'ticking time bomb' versus 'the cure can kill you' struggle."

Ironically, the convexo-concave valves were introduced as an improvement on the predecessor valve, which has had a very low failure rate. This seems to be yet another example where "tried and true" proved better than "latest and greatest."

Patients with Back Pain: Getting Screwed?

If you haven't had low back pain, you probably will. About two-thirds of adults get back pain at some time in their lives. If you seek medical care for the problem, you may discover that nearly every aspect of care for back pain—the terms that are used, the diagnostic tests performed, and the treatments provided—is controversial. With our colleague Dan Cherkin, we once wrote a medical journal article on variations in back pain diagnosis that we titled, "Who you see is what you get."[9] In the words of Dr. Seth Waldman, a New York doctor who heads a referral center for chronic pain,

"Each approach to diagnosis and treatment is essentially a franchise, and there are too many franchises battling for control."[1]

One of the most controversial treatments for back pain is spinal fusion, an operation in which adjacent vertebral bones are "welded" together with bone grafts in an effort to reduce pain. These fusion operations are sometimes performed with plates and screws to immobilize the bones while the bone grafts heal.

An example of how politics, advocacy, commercial interests, and doctors' interests converge to affect the use of technology arose from our own research on results of spinal fusion surgery. I (Rick) was the head of a back pain research team at the University of Washington, supported by the federal Agency for Health Care Policy and Research (AHCPR). Our studies suggested that spinal fusion surgery had few scientifically validated indications and was associated with higher costs and complication rates than other types of back surgery.[10,11]

I also participated in a multidisciplinary AHCPR-sponsored panel to develop evidence-based guidelines for managing acute back problems, meaning those of recent onset. The panel recommended nonsurgical approaches in most circumstances.[12] Our research and the guideline effort inspired a letter-writing campaign to Congress by the North American Spine Society (NASS). This group consists largely of spine surgeons, who alleged that our research team and the guidelines were biased against their preferred forms of therapy.[13]

Much of the controversy seemed to hinge on the use of pedicle screws, a type of metal screw with attached plates or rods that is often used in spinal fusion surgery. A member of the NASS board founded a lobbying organization to eliminate funding for the AHCPR and curtail the powers of the FDA, which had restricted its approval of pedicle screws to a small number of very specific situations. The organization, labeled an "ersatz grassroots organization" by National Public Radio, was cleverly dubbed the "Center for Patient Advocacy."[13,14] A manufacturer of pedicle screws, Sofamor Danek, unsuccessfully sought a court injunction to prevent publication of the guidelines.[13]

The AHCPR came under attack not just because of the back pain research, but also because it had a new director who was mistrusted by Republican leaders in the House of Representatives, and because of general budget-cutting fervor. Many medical and hospital professional groups came to the support of the AHCPR in the Senate, in an effort to prevent its outright elimination.

In the end, the AHCPR survived, but with a 25 percent budget cut. And it stopped producing clinical guidelines, even though that had been part of its original mandate from Congress.[13] Political pressure related to the back pain guidelines, and earlier pressure related to cataract guidelines, seemed to weigh heavily in this decision.

NASS later faced lawsuits alleging that some of its continuing education courses were thinly disguised promotions for pedicle screws. These suits arose from product liability claims from thousands of patients claiming injury from the devices. The plaintiffs argued, among other things, that manufacturers sponsored "educational seminars" that were really sales events, which the plaintiffs likened to "Tupperware parties."[15]

Many of the suits against NASS were dismissed for lack of evidence, although suits against the manufacturers proceeded. In 1996, one manufacturer, AcroMed, agreed to a $100 million settlement for thousands of lawsuits, without acknowledging any liability.[16]

But sales of pedicle screws, which typically add thousands of dollars to the cost of a single back operation, have increased steadily. In fact, the annual number of spinal fusion operations increased 77 percent between 1996 and 2001, despite ongoing uncertainty as to who should have a fusion operation, and when.[17] And the proportion of these operations that involve pedicle screws or similar hardware has steadily increased as well.[18] In contrast, hip and knee replacement surgery increased by only about 14 percent during that time.

Some surgeons, like Dr. Edward Benzel at the Cleveland Clinic Spine Institute, believe that too much spinal fusion surgery is being performed. Benzel estimated to *The New York Times* that less than half the spinal fusions being performed were appropriate. "The reality of it is, we all cave in to market and economic forces," he was quoted as saying, adding that the current system of paying doctors is "totally perverted." Dr. Zoher Ghogawala, a Yale neurosurgeon, agreed that too much fusion surgery is done, saying, "I see too many patients who are recommended fusion that absolutely do not need it."[19]

Stan Mendenhall, the editor and publisher of an orthopedic newsletter, said, "A lot of technological innovation serves shareholders more than patients . . . the money is driving a lot of this." Mendenhall said that the national bill for spinal fusion hardware alone is $2.5 billion a year.[19]

Former employees of Medtronic, the largest maker of spinal fusion hardware, claim that Medtronic offered surgeons enticements to use its products, including first-class plane tickets to Hawaii, nights in the finest hotels, and large consultation fees.[19] One former employee provided *The New York Times* with a list of about eighty surgeons who received consulting fees of up to $400,000 a year from Medtronic. Another employee claimed that some of these contracts were a "sham" because they involved little or no work. Medtronic disclosed in 2003 that the federal government was investigating whether it gave illegal kickbacks to surgeons.[19]

Leaving aside the controversy over who should have spinal fusion, what's the evidence that adding pedicle screws to the operation helps? Pedicle screws were introduced to the market with no randomized trials to test their effectiveness; in fact, they were first approved for use only in the long bones of the arms or legs. Nonetheless, they were widely used "off label" in the spine, a practice that's legal for doctors, but that companies aren't allowed to advertise. Over the past twenty years, there have been several skirmishes among the manufacturers, surgeons, and the FDA over the marketing and use of these devices, in addition to thousands of lawsuits from patients.[15,16,20]

However, several randomized trials have been completed since the controversy involving the AHCPR. Randomized trials are generally regarded as the most rigorous way to evaluate treatment effectiveness. These studies compared spinal fusion using bone grafts alone with fusions performed with pedicle screws. They overwhelmingly indicate that bone grafting alone gives results—in terms of pain relief and daily functioning—that are just as good as those from fusions that add the pedicle screws. Some studies even suggest better results without the screws. Furthermore, when screws are used, patients have longer operations, more blood loss, more nerve injuries, and more complications, and are more likely to need another operation later.[17]

A recent article in *The New Yorker* quoted a surgeon as saying that he had previously recommended that patients with back pain avoid fusion surgery unless it was absolutely necessary—because of severe fractures or dislocations, for example. But he found that most of the patients he turned away ended up having operations with other surgeons. He then figured that if patients were going to have surgery anyway, he might as well be the one to do it. He figured he'd at least do it right. So the reason for doing this type of operation may not necessarily be a biological need, but the fact that "if I don't, someone else will."[1]

The Saga of the Pulmonary Artery Catheter

Like the drawbacks of drugs, as seen in the story of diethylstilbestrol for preventing miscarriage or hormone replacement therapy in menopause, the drawbacks of new devices sometimes aren't apparent for decades. The pulmonary artery catheter is a case in point. This is a long, thin plastic tube that's inserted into a vein, then threaded through the heart and into the main artery of the lung. It was introduced in 1970—before FDA oversight of medical devices—and current estimates are that 1.2 million are sold per year. The costs of the device and the associated supplies and personnel for its use are estimated at $2 billion a year.[21] But recent studies suggest that some patients receiving one of the catheters are worse off than they would be without it.

The so-called Swan-Ganz catheter was introduced when cardiologists devised a balloon-tipped catheter that could be inserted at the bedside and allowed to travel with the blood flow through the right side of the heart and into the pulmonary artery. In that position, the catheter could be used to monitor several pressures that indicated cardiac output, heart failure, and shock, and also blood oxygen in a key part of the circulation. It could be left in place for several days, allowing doctors to monitor heart function and directing the choice of intravenous fluids or powerful medications to optimize heart function.

The catheter came to be routinely used in intensive care settings for patients with heart attacks, heart failure, lung failure, severe trauma, and high-risk surgical procedures. It became almost a hallmark of being in an intensive care unit.

As a recent editorial in the *New England Journal of Medicine* noted, "A layperson might assume that if a form of medical technology is so widely used, there must be clear cut indications for its clinical use. Unfortunately, that would be an incorrect assumption. . . . No clinical trials were conducted to determine whether patient outcomes were altered by the data derived from insertion of these catheters or the associated therapeutic interventions. Benefit was simply assumed."[22]

In 1987, seventeen years after the catheter was introduced, a study was completed among patients who had had heart attacks and experienced heart failure or shock. Patients who had received a pulmonary artery catheter were compared with patients who hadn't received one. Mortality was unexpectedly higher among those who got the catheter.[23] A similar study in 1990 got similar results, but doctors remained uncertain as to what to do.[24] The problem was that because patients weren't randomly assigned to get a catheter or not, there remained a possibility that those who got catheters were sicker than those who didn't, and that that might explain their higher death rate.

In 1996, a carefully designed study matched up patients with comparable diagnoses and severity of illness, and studied almost six thousand ICU patients from five hospitals. Once again, patients who got the catheter had worse mortality after one month and three months of follow-up.[25] In 2001, another study examined older patients undergoing major surgery and undertook detailed statistical adjustment for factors that might affect the results. Patients who got the catheters were twice as likely to have cardiac complications after surgery.[26]

Several possible explanations were suggested. Perhaps some doctors had a poor understanding of how to use the data from the catheter. Perhaps using the catheter was a marker for an aggressive style of care that contributed to worse results. And perhaps the greater mortality was a result of complications caused by the catheters, which include infections, blood clots, and dangerous heart rhythms.[26]

These studies led to calls for randomized trials to provide more definitive information. But as in other situations in which medical technology is already in wide use, practicing doctors resisted, arguing that it was unethical to withhold the catheters from critically ill patients.[21] This should sound familiar by now: It's the same argument that was made for the heart rhythm drug encainide, for bone marrow transplants in women with breast cancer, and for many other treatments that already enjoyed a market share. In fact, an early attempt to conduct a randomized trial of pulmonary artery catheters failed for just this reason. Doctors were unwilling to have their patients enter the study because they were so convinced of the value of using the catheters.[21]

Finally, in 2003, two randomized trials of pulmonary artery catheters were completed. One was a study of older patients undergoing high-risk surgery. Almost two thousand patients were randomized to have surgery with or without use of the catheter. There was no difference in survival rate, but the catheter group got more blood clots in the lungs. The catheter group also got more heart medications, blood pressure medications, blood transfusions, and intravenous fluids—yet had no better results.[27]

The use of more medicines, transfusions, and fluids suggests that part of the problem with pulmonary artery catheters may be that they lead to tampering. Because they monitor various pressures, blood gases, and heart function, they may detect a variety of random fluctuations. If doctors respond to these, they may inadvertently make things worse instead of better. This phenomenon is recognized in manufacturing processes, where quality control efforts must be designed to detect important variations in temperature, for example, but not trivial changes.

The second randomized study involved adult patients of any age with shock or with a form of severe lung failure. Although use of the catheter didn't increase complications, it didn't reduce them, either. And patient survival was the same with or without the catheter.[28]

The trial in elderly patients was published in the *New England Journal of Medicine,* with an accompanying editorial by Dr. Polly Parsons, professor of medicine and chief of critical care services at the University of Vermont School of Medicine. She concluded that routine use of the catheters in high-risk surgery patients is unwarranted. Use of the catheters in other situations is still being examined, and the studies have continued to face the concerns of practicing doctors who are convinced that the catheters help. Dr. Parsons concluded, "These debates represent. . . . the difficulty posed by the legacy of an over-enthusiastic embracing of technology without adequate assessment. I hope that we are learning from our experience."[22]

Endografts for Aortic Aneurysms

The aorta is the huge artery that receives blood from the heart and then travels downward through the chest and the abdomen, giving off branches that supply the vital organs, arms, and legs. With aging, parts of the aortic wall can weaken, and the aorta may begin to bulge, creating a dilated section with a weak wall—a condition called an aneurysm. This happens most often in the abdomen, where it's called a "triple A": abdominal aortic aneurysm.

If an aortic aneurysm ruptures, internal bleeding can be rapid and severe, and many patients die before they even reach the hospital. Happily, the risk of rupture is fairly small when the aneurysm is small. So when doctors discover a small aneurysm, they typically follow it with ultrasound every six or twelve months to see if it enlarges over time.

When an aneurysm reaches a certain size, the risk of rupture increases greatly, and surgery is often done to repair the aneurysm before it ruptures. In most cases, the diseased section of the aorta is removed, and a tubular Dacron graft is sewn in as a replacement. Under the best of circumstances, this is risky surgery, with mortality of 3 to 6 percent.[29] So no one wants to jump the gun and perform surgery unnecessarily.

In 1985, an article by a Russian researcher first described so-called endovascular repair of aortic aneurysms. In this technique, a stent-graft system is slid into an incision in the major artery of the thigh, then threaded upward into the abdominal aorta, where a self-expanding stent is used to trap a Dacron wall in place inside the aorta. This avoids cutting into and removing the diseased section of the aorta and provides a new reinforced wall for the diseased segment. Some devices use hooks and barbs to hold the device in place. Unfortunately, leaks from fabric tears sometimes lead to rupture of the devices.[29]

When the endovascular stent-graft systems emerged, surgeons were extremely enthusiastic, imagining the high death rate from conventional aneurysm surgery might be reduced. Patients for whom the conventional surgery was too risky might be candidates for the new procedure. The new devices were quickly embraced, but problems were also quick to emerge.

One of the devices was made by the Guidant Corporation and was introduced in 1999. Within four months, a patient died because a device got stuck in the wrong position. Within nineteen months of the device's hitting the market, 2,628 of the 7,600 devices sold had had malfunctions of the delivery system used to insert the device into the aorta. The company failed to report the problem to the FDA, and also failed to report that fifty-seven patients had had to have emergency surgery and twelve people had died from bleeding or from heart attacks.[30]

In these early months of using the device, Guidant sales representatives were required to be in the operating rooms when the devices were used. When the delivery system malfunctioned, some sales reps tried to persuade doctors to avoid emergency surgery by breaking off the handle of the device and removing the system piece by piece. This procedure had not been approved by the FDA, and it sometimes caused damage to the arteries and even death.[31]

In mid-2000, the FDA made an inspection at the company and asked to be told of all malfunctions. The company reported only 172 cases. But three months later, seven anonymous employees of Guidant wrote to the FDA alleging fraud and cover-up. In 2001, the company voluntarily recalled the device and revealed to the FDA the true magnitude of the malfunctions. When the situation was brought to court, company officials acknowledged that they had intentionally misled the FDA, doctors, and the public. News accounts reported that an FBI special agent claimed that the bottom line for the company had been making money. The devices sold for about $10,000 each.[30]

In June of 2003, Guidant pleaded guilty to ten felonies and agreed to $92.4 million in criminal and civil penalties. This was the largest penalty ever imposed on a medical device maker for failing to report problems to the FDA. The company still faces individual lawsuits.[30]

Although the Guidant endovascular device has received the greatest publicity, other manufacturers' devices have had problems of their own. In 2001, the FDA issued a Public Health Notification regarding the devices, citing the problem with Guidant's graft, but also problems with a device made by Medtronic. For the Medtronic system, the FDA had received reports of aneurysm ruptures, suboptimal placements of the grafts, leaks, slipping out of place, fabric tears, suture breaks, and fractures in the metal frame.[32] Newer versions of these devices have been returned to the market, and the companies believe that they're safe. Nonetheless, Guidant decided to stop selling its device entirely in 2003.

A 2003 review article in the *New England Journal of Medicine* concluded that it was still unclear whether surgical risks with the endovascular devices were less than those with conventional aneurysm surgery. The authors noted that in addition to the FDA warning about two devices, the Medical Devices Agency in the United Kingdom had issued similar alerts about three additional devices. They also noted that there's still no evidence that the risk of aneurysm rupture is reduced after endovascular repair. The reported risk of rupture is 1 percent per year, which is similar to that observed in patients with no surgery.[29] And finally, the endografts are too new to know how they'll hold up over a patient's lifetime.

Randomized trials of conventional surgery versus endovascular repair are now underway, and improvements in the new devices are likely. With more experience and longer follow-up, the technique may become the standard approach. But the problems and deaths encountered with the early models are reminiscent of the "earn while you learn" strategy associated with the Bjork-Shiley heart valve. We can hope that this device continues to improve, but it demonstrates yet again the risks of jumping at the "latest and greatest" technology.

Like our stories about drugs and operations, these cautionary tales about medical devices may be the tip of an iceberg. There is at least controversy and conflicting evidence about the effectiveness or safety of other devices for treating back pain, such as intradiscal electrothermal therapy;[33,34] other heart valves such as the St. Jude Silzone heart valve;[35] and treatments for heart disease like transmyocardial laser revascularization.[36] Some diagnostic devices, like electronic fetal monitors used during childbirth, also appear to be of dubious value.[37] Even FDA officials write that "new devices are less likely than drugs to have their safety established clinically before they are marketed."[38]

Manufacturing defects are reported with some regularity, resulting in patient complications and recalls of devices. In 2002, the FDA received over 120,000 reports of deaths, injuries, and specific malfunctions related to medical devices. Furthermore, around one thousand devices are recalled every year, although only ten to twenty are judged to be for "high-risk" problems.[38] The learning curve associated with both the design of devices and their use argues in most cases for a "wait and see" approach unless your hand is forced.

15

Ineffective or Needlessly Extensive Surgery

A minor operation is one that is performed on the other fellow. —Russell Pettis Askue[1]

FOR MANY people, surgery exemplifies what we mean by high-tech medicine. You might suppose that before doctors start cutting into your body, they're damn sure that what they're doing will work. Most of the time, that's true. But not always. While commercial interests and regulatory practices heavily influence drug prescribing, tradition and authority perhaps more heavily influence surgery. Recently, researchers have looked more closely at some operations that have been done for years. Old practices die hard, and tradition has sometimes overwhelmed convincing evidence. Other research has focused on new operations that seemed to have great promise. The results have occasionally been surprising, and doctors have gone back to the drawing board.

We've already seen how devices used in surgery—like heart valves or spine screws—are sometimes introduced before we understand their limitations. At least devices are subject to FDA review. But a surgeon can perform any new procedure he wishes, assuming he can find a willing patient.

The risk of dying after major surgery seems to be generally higher than published research studies indicate. Two doctors at Dartmouth, Emily Finlayson and John Birkmeyer, recently examined Medicare records nationwide to determine mortality rates after various operations. They counted deaths that occurred either within thirty days of the operation or while patients were still in the hospital.[2]

A typical finding was that, overall, replacement of one type of heart valve resulted in 7 percent mortality among Medicare patients, compared to the 2 to 5 percent reported in the surgical literature. For esophagectomy (removal of part of the esophagus, usually for cancer), mortality was almost 14 percent, compared to literature estimates of 2 to 7 percent. For nearly every operation they examined, Finlayson and Birkmeyer found a higher risk of death among Medicare patients than what is reported in the medical literature. For older patients (beyond age seventy-five), the discrepancies were often large. This means the risks of surgery may be greater than you or your surgeon realize.[2]

Finlayson and Birkmeyer speculated that the research literature is dominated by studies from major referral centers, which may have better results than many community hospitals. They also suspect that many research studies excluded the highest-risk patients—those who were older and sicker. Finally, it may simply be that surgeons with worse results are less likely to publish their scorecards than surgeons with better results.[2]

Another problem is that new technologies are introduced into surgical procedures if they seem like a good idea, often without rigorous evaluation. Dr. David Flum, a general surgeon at the University of Washington, cites the example of using lasers to make incisions and to stop bleeding in abdominal surgery. Says Flum,

> In the early 90's that was where it was at. Everybody had a laser. We were going to take out your gallbladder with a laser, cure all bleeding with a laser, do liver biopsies with the laser. Ultimately, we came to realize it wasn't any better than older techniques, it was cumbersome, and it got in the way in the operating room. And it did have some collateral damage. If you fired that laser in the wrong spot, you just put a hole in the intestine. We kind of realized soon after we bought them, there was very little use for them beyond showing them to people and saying you had a laser.

There were powerful forces that promoted the use of technology like the laser in the 1980s and more recently surgical robots to assist in the operating room. According to Flum, "Every surgeon wants to be seen as cutting edge. Add to that an industry that pours millions into product promotion and a naturally competitive spirit among surgeons, and you have a recipe for disaster when it comes to using evidence-based practices in the operating room."

There's also the problem of doing surgery for iffy reasons. The last chapter described an interview with a spine surgeon who found that many patients he turned away (because they didn't need surgery) ended up having surgery done by someone else. Eventually, he concluded that if the patients were going to have surgery anyway, he might as well be the one to do it.[3]

In this situation, the reason for doing surgery would be that someone else will do it anyway, not that there's a clear medical reason to do it. This may be a risk for many types of "elective" surgery—surgery that isn't necessary to save a life or prevent obvious disability.

It's also more important when the surgery is at the patient's discretion. An operation to remove a cancerous lump may be elective, but everyone agrees it's necessary. Flum asks,

> What about surgery for knee pain, back pain, or obesity? Patients may be desperate with their conditions, perhaps depressed, and often unrealistic about the risks associated with surgery. Surgeons are in an awkward position when it comes to these patients seeking "quality of life" operations. Are they supposed to send away patients who don't have insight into risk? Decision-making can pose conflicts of interest.

Surgery also offers a lesson in how low-tech aspects of care have a big influence on the high-tech results. Even the best surgeon with the best technology relies on good old-fashioned bedside nursing to achieve good results. A study in 2002 showed just how much by examining the effect of nursing workload on surgical mortality. Dr. Linda Aiken and her colleagues assessed data from over 100,000 nurses and 230,000 patients (from general surgery, orthopedic surgery, and vascular surgery) in 168 hospitals. Each additional patient that a nurse had to care for was associated with a 7 percent increase in the likelihood of death. For example, increasing a nurse's patient load from four to six would be accompanied by a 14 percent increase in mortality.[4] High-tech or no, medical care works only as a team sport.

Aside from these general problems, there are often problems associated with specific operations. Researchers have discovered that some popular operations simply aren't effective, or are more destructive than they need to be. These stories offer some examples.

Radical Mastectomy for Breast Cancer

Radical mastectomy is extensive and disfiguring surgery with a host of complications. It's done for women with breast cancer, and it involves removing the entire breast, two large chest wall muscles, and a number of lymph nodes, mostly from the armpit. This leaves the chest looking almost excavated on one side and is usually accompanied by lymphedema of the arm on the affected side. Lymphedema is swelling that's often uncomfortable, interferes with functioning, and is sometimes severe and unsightly.

In the 1950s, a somewhat less radical operation, the modified radical mastectomy, began to gain favor. This operation removed only one of the chest wall muscles, the pectoralis minor, leaving the larger muscle, or pectoralis major, in place. Although surgical authorities sometimes vilified early advocates of the modified procedure,[5] it became a fairly standard operation. Though somewhat less disfiguring than the original radical mastectomy, the modified radical mastectomy still had a dramatic impact on the body.

The radical mastectomy or modified radical mastectomy remained the standard treatment for nearly all women with breast cancer until the past decade, despite growing evidence that a smaller operation, combined with radiation therapy, works just as well. The smaller operation involves simply removing the tumor, a small amount of surrounding breast tissue, and a small number of lymph nodes. This operation, often called a lumpectomy, has been avoided by some surgeons, who feared that it was inadequate. But two key studies, published together in 2002, reported twenty-year follow-up of women who had had either the radical mastectomy or a breast-conserving operation, and found survival to be just the same.[6,7] Lymphedema is half as common with the less extensive types of surgery.[8]

So why did the more disfiguring operations hold sway for eighty years? In large measure, it was because of the extraordinary influence of William Halsted, a pioneering surgeon at Johns Hopkins Medical School in Baltimore, who developed the technique and described it in the *Annals of Surgery* in 1898. Halsted was a giant in the early field of surgery. He made a host of enduring contributions, including the need for sterile technique, gentle handling of tissues, and procedures for treating cancers, hernias, aneurysms, and thyroid enlargement. More than other great surgeons of his time, Halsted trained many future surgeons, who spread his gospel to other medical schools and taught it to further generations of surgeons.[5,9] More than his peers, Halsted was destined for surgical sainthood.

Halsted thought the radical mastectomy could prolong women's lives, and for his disciples, the procedure symbolized the possibilities of "scientific" surgery. The goal was to operate extensively in order to remove every last cancer cell. Halsted's early results seemed to support the notion. Despite the evolution of some variations, the radical mastectomy became the treatment of choice for breast cancer, regardless of size or type of cancer or patient age, until the 1970s.[5] When I (Rick) was in medical school in the 1970s, I participated in some of these operations, and I learned what was still common dogma: This operation gave patients the best chance of survival, and cosmetic concerns shouldn't override the curative goal.

Dr. Barron Lerner, an internist and medical historian at Columbia University's medical school in New York, has detailed the course of this approach and subsequent shifts in thinking in his popular book *Breast Cancer Wars*. He describes the important impact of the women's movement in the 1970s, as women demanded more information from their doctors and a bigger role in decision making. In many ways, women pushed doctors to treat the disease both more humanely and more scientifically.[5]

Lerner also suggests the unfortunate impact that the combat metaphor of a "war on cancer" may have had on the thinking of doctors and patients alike. He says, "That notion of getting it all, of the surgeon coming out of the operating room and saying, 'We got it all,' has such cultural resonance in the entire cancer experience and the entire way we treat and understand cancer."[10]

Finally, in the 1970s, Dr. Bernard Fisher, a surgeon at the University of Pittsburgh, doggedly persuaded his colleagues to subject radical mastectomy to a rigorous scientific comparison with less aggressive surgery. His theory was that breast cancer had often spread widely through the body by the time it was diagnosed, making the extent of local treatment relatively unimportant.

Several randomized controlled trials, some of which Fisher directed, have now shown that for most women, lumpectomy yields survival results equivalent to those of radical mastectomy.[6,7] Not every patient may be a good candidate for the less aggressive surgery, but most are. Women who undergo lumpectomy avoid loss of the breast, although most require local radiation and sometimes chemotherapy. Women who choose mastectomy avoid the need for radiation and have a somewhat lower risk of local recurrence. But they must deal with the loss of a breast and have no better survival rate. Except for patient preference, Fisher believes, "there's no reason to get a mastectomy today."[11]

So here's an example of overtreatment that had enormous physical, emotional, and psychological impact on women. In 1968, some 70 percent of women with breast cancer still received Halsted's original operation. In a more recent survey, assessing women treated in 1994, about 57 percent of women who were candidates for breast-sparing surgery were still receiving some form of mastectomy.[12] With the studies from 2002, this situation may change rapidly. But the persistence of a century-old operation has been remarkable testimony to the power of tradition and authority, which delayed the emergence of rigorous scientific evidence.

Boosting the Blood Supply to the Heart

In the 1950s, before coronary bypass surgery had become commonplace, another type of surgery was sometimes done, in hopes of relieving pain and preventing heart attacks. The operation was called internal mammary artery ligation, and it involved making small incisions in the chest and blocking two arteries by tying sutures around them. These arteries, which travel along each side of the breastbone, supply blood to the bones, cartilage, and soft tissues of the chest wall. Modern surgeons often connect this artery to the coronary arteries to improve blood supply, a strategy that's usually very successful.

But in the 1950s, surgeons found that the arteries could be tied off completely without endangering the crucial blood supply to any organs. The rationale behind blocking them was that if less blood circulated through these arteries, more would be diverted to circulate through the coronary arteries to supply the heart muscle. Furthermore, it was thought, blocking these arteries would cause the body to form collateral vessels—new or enlarged arteries that follow a different route and might supply more blood to the heart. In other words, one could do without the internal mammary arteries, and blocking their circulation might decrease chest pain and heart attacks.

This operation was performed for patients with angina—chest pain that results from insufficient blood supply to the heart, usually because of narrowing in the coronary arteries. People with angina are the ones who are most likely to sustain a heart attack, where part of the heart muscle actually dies, to be replaced by scar tissue. Internal mammary artery ligation was a big success, it seemed, because up to 90 percent of patients reported less angina after surgery.[13] Early results were described as "spectacular."[14]

But some cardiologists were skeptical, among them Dr. Leonard Cobb. Cobb, then a young cardiologist, is now professor emeritus at the University of Washington in Seattle. Among other things, he's largely responsible for the fact that more citizens in Seattle than in any other major city are trained in cardiopulmonary resuscitation. He also helped develop Seattle's pioneering emergency medical system, and he still has an office with the "Medic I" program. In the late 1950s and early 1960s, he began to question the value of internal mammary artery ligation, and he designed a study that seemed radical: Patients would be randomly assigned to have the regular operation or a fake operation that involved just making incisions in the chest, but not tying off any arteries.[15]

This may seem unethical, and performing sham surgery in research studies is still a topic of spirited debate. But a growing number of ethicists argue that sham surgery may be justified for research purposes when the main purpose of the real operation is a subjective result (like pain relief) rather than saving life. Also, of course, the risks must be minimal, and patients must agree ahead of time to the possibility of receiving a fake operation. If a fake surgery group helps to make it clear that a real operation is ineffective, thousands of patients may be spared unnecessary treatment and complications.

To the surprise of many, the real operation proved no better than the fake in Cobb's study. A majority of the patients in both groups reported far less angina than before the operation. Some, even in the fake surgery group, reported no angina at all afterwards.[15] The study was reported in the prestigious *New England Journal of Medicine,* and another similar study reported strikingly similar results.[16] The use of internal mammary artery ligation declined quickly after these articles were published.

Many people find the results puzzling and surprising. Why would patients who got a fake treatment improve so much? The answers remain complex, but it's increasingly clear that in treating pain, there can be a substantial placebo effect. Although no one really knows how the placebo effect works, an important component seems to be the patient's *expectation* of getting better. With a dramatic treatment like surgery, many people believe that expectations and the placebo effect may be more powerful than those from just taking pills.[17] Even with dummy pills, the placebo effect can be huge, with 35 to 75 percent of patients reporting improvements.

Other factors may enter into the results as well. For many painful conditions, the natural course is to improve gradually over time. Natural healing processes occur, and this alone may account for some improvement in trials like this one. In essence, as Ben Franklin quipped, "God heals and the doctor takes the fee."[1]

Statisticians also point to a phenomenon that they call regression to the mean. The idea is that researchers may enroll patients while their symptoms are at their worst. This is, after all, when patients are most likely to be seeking medical care, and perhaps when they are most willing to participate in research. Symptoms wax and wane, though, so it's understandable that if we start treatment when symptoms are waxing, they're more likely to be waning when we follow up. Random fluctuation creates the impression of improvement. The flaring symptoms regress toward their average level, or mean—hence the term.

These factors—the placebo effect, natural healing, and regression to the mean—help to explain why patients often improve even with ineffective treatment. And they also help to explain why randomized, controlled trials are so important. Simply treating patients and seeing that they improve may be very misleading. Although they get better, this may have little to do with the treatment. Only by having a placebo group or an alternative treatment group (the so-called control group) can we figure out how effective a new treatment really is, above and beyond these nonspecific improvements or some competing treatment.

Arthroscopic Surgery for Arthritis of the Knee

Dr. Nelda Wray is a little shorter than average, with short, dark curls and an intense demeanor. She has a penchant for navy blazers and scarves, and her speech gives away her Texas roots. In 1995, she became the first woman to be named professor in Baylor University's Department of Medicine, and she also became professor of medical ethics. At one time, she served as health policy adviser to Senator Robert Dole, and she was appointed by then Governor George W. Bush to several state medical boards and councils. Most of her career has been in Houston, and she still has a small ranch outside the city. For a time during the Bush presidency, she was director of research for the entire VA medical system, and she moved to the nation's capital. She's an internist and a researcher in health-care delivery, and she asks lots of good questions. In 1995, she began asking whether a popular operation for knee arthritis really works. She and an orthopedic colleague, Dr. Bruce Moseley, decided to find out.

Some patients with knee arthritis are offered surgery through an arthroscope, a fiber-optic tube that allows some cutting and manipulation. The surgery involves "rinsing out" the joint with several quarts of fluid and shaving any rough cartilage (the smooth cushioning where bones come together in the joint). Sometimes the surgeon also shaves torn fragments of the meniscus, the tough, fibrous tissue that helps to stabilize the knee. The theory is that rinsing gets rid of fragments of cartilage, crystals, enzymes, and cells that cause inflammation, and that smoothing the rough surfaces should reduce mechanical stresses. This type of surgery doesn't involve repairing torn ligaments, a different type of knee surgery. But the arthritis operation has been done on about six hundred thousand people a year, at a cost of roughly $5,000 a pop. That's a total tab of about $3 billion a year, if you do the multiplication.[18]

Like Nelda Wray, Dr. Bruce Moseley is no loose cannon. A Dallas native, he's now a clinical associate professor of orthopedics at Baylor and team doctor for the Houston Rockets basketball team. In 1996, he was team doctor for the U.S. Olympic basketball "Dream Team" in Atlanta. But in the early 1990s, Moseley was skeptical about the benefits of the arthroscopic knee procedure, and he approached Wray about designing a study to evaluate it.

What they came up with may be surprising. They designed a study in which patients were randomly assigned, after giving their permission, to get one of three treatments: the rinse-out of the knee, the rinse plus shaving the cartilage, or a fake operation. For the fake operation, patients came to the operating room and underwent all the same rigmarole as patients getting the real operation. They even had three half-inch incisions made in the skin of the knee, to mimic the real thing. Like Len Cobb studying internal mammary artery ligation, the researchers were concerned that without a fake operation, they might get a biased impression of treatment effectiveness—which might make the research unethical if it mistakenly supported an ineffective operation.

To make a long story short, the real knee operations—both rinsing alone and rinsing plus shaving—proved to be no better than the sham operation. As reported in the *New England Journal of Medicine,* all three groups got better.[18] A patient who had the sham operation told reporters that his knee now has no pain; he can mow the lawn and walk wherever he wants. He said, "The surgery was two years ago and the knee never has bothered me since."[19]

In fact, the study suggested that results might even be slightly worse among patients who got the shaving operation than among those who got the fake procedure. An ethicist who helped design the study, Dr. Baruch Brody, reflected on standard practice and said, "Here we are doing all this surgery on people and it's all a sham."[20]

An editorial that accompanied the research report noted that the rationale for the operation was appealing. But, the editorialists noted, problems like bad knee alignment, muscle weakness, instability of the joint, and obesity might be more important in determining how much trouble knee arthritis would cause. They concluded that the surgery "may simply remove some of the evidence while the destructive forces of osteoarthritis continue to work."[21]

When results of the study were publicized, a *New York Times* reporter asked the vice president and chief executive of the American Academy of Orthopedic Surgeons for his reaction. He indicated that he had questioned the operation, and he said that he himself had osteoarthritis of the knee. He said, "I'm not going to have arthroscopy done. I recognize that it's not going to help." Paradoxically, though, he said that he would hate to see insurance companies refuse to pay for the operation. Other orthopedists questioned the results and felt that the study was not indicative of their own results.[20]

Dr. David Felson, one of the editorialists, told reporters that he thought it was a wonderful study, but he wasn't sure whether doctors and patients would abandon the operation. *The New York Times* quoted him as saying, "There's a pretty good-sized industry out there that is performing this surgery. It constitutes a good part of the livelihood of some orthopedic surgeons. That is a reality."[20] In other words, the best scientific evidence isn't necessarily going to be embraced by doctors who have something to lose.

Bypassing Clogged Arteries to the Brain

By now, most people are familiar with coronary artery bypass surgery. This operation is done to bypass clogged arteries that supply blood to the heart muscle. It's clear that this operation, in the right patients, can prevent heart attacks and extend peoples' lives. A heart attack occurs when the blood supply gets so small that a piece of heart muscle dies and is replaced by scar tissue.

A stroke is caused when arteries to the brain are clogged, and some people have suggested calling it a "brain attack," analogous to a heart attack. In a stroke, a piece of the brain dies, and nerve cells are replaced by scar tissue. It seems logical, then, to think about bypassing the clogged arteries, just as we do for coronary arteries. In 1967, some neurosurgeons began doing just that. An artery that was clogged before it entered the skull ("extracranial") could be bypassed, and another artery could be hooked up with an artery inside the skull ("intracranial") that wasn't narrowed. Most often, this was done by using an artery in the scalp to "plug into" the artery inside the skull, improving its blood flow. The operation was called an extracranial-intracranial bypass operation, or EC/IC bypass.

This operation was performed on thousands of patients for almost two decades. It made perfect anatomical sense. It was generally offered to patients who had had "transient ischemic attacks" (TIAs), sometimes called "mini-strokes." These are warning signs of inadequate blood supply to a part of the brain and are often harbingers of a full stroke. The symptoms can include sudden blindness in one eye, difficulty speaking, weakness of part of the body, or dizziness, depending on the part of the brain affected. As is often the case, the operation became popular because it made sense and it seemed to work, but studies were small and didn't include a comparison group with optimal nonsurgical treatment.

So in 1977, an international trial involving seventy-one medical centers began, with funding from the National Institutes of Health. The study enrolled 1,377 patients who had had TIAs or small strokes, and was headed by Dr. HLM Barnett at the University of Western Ontario. One of the key proponents and designers of the trial was Dr. David Sackett, then at McMaster University in Ontario.

Sackett is an original. Now a professor emeritus, he has a shock of white hair and a full white beard. At medical meetings, where most doctors wear their mandatory uniforms of navy blazers or dark suits, Sackett can be spotted in Western shirts, without a coat or tie. In a profession that takes itself too seriously, his books on research methods are written with refreshing humor. Among his many honors, Sackett was recently appointed an Officer of the Order of Canada, which he describes as "the Canadian equivalent of a knighthood, but without the swordplay." But he's better known as the father of evidence-based medicine, an approach that we'll discuss in detail later. Among other things, he and his colleagues were the first to show that aspirin could prevent strokes and heart attacks.

Aspirin works to prevent strokes because it paralyzes platelets, the tiny particles in the bloodstream that initiate clotting when you get a cut. In other words, aspirin acts as a blood thinner. Because it was known to help prevent strokes, aspirin was a key part of the treatment given to the control group in studying EC/IC bypass surgery. The study compared patients who got surgery to patients who got just aspirin and careful attention to blood pressure control.

The results of the trial, published in 1985, were clear-cut and stunning. The surgical patients had more strokes and more deaths than those who just got aspirin. Even after eliminating the strokes and deaths caused immediately by the surgery (in about 1 percent of patients), the surgery group fared worse.[22] For several months after treatment, patients in the surgery group had worse ability to speak, dress, get in and out of bed, and prepare food than patients in the nonsurgical group.[23] Follow-up was continued for four and a half years to see if the surgery group did better in the long run, but it didn't. Results were better in the nonsurgical treatment group throughout the study. Dr. Murray Goldstein, director of the NIH institute that funded the study, told reporters, "The data are crisp. There are no ifs, ands, or buts. The EC/IC bypass is not efficacious."[24]

Surgeons largely abandoned the operation after this study was publicized, but there were sour grapes among some neurosurgeons. Even today, some of them talk about EC/IC bypass as a "good operation that was taken away from us."

But a resurgence of the operation may be starting. In 1998, researchers reported that with PET scanning (a new technique that involves radioisotopes), they could identify specific areas of the brain that were at highest risk in patients with narrowed arteries.[25,26] They believed that this would help surgeons to identify the best candidates for EC/IC surgery, and they suggested that a new trial be performed, using PET scanning to identify the patients who are most likely to benefit. Although such a trial hasn't yet been done, some centers have eagerly begun performing EC/IC bypass again, convinced that it simply must be helpful. You can count us among the skeptical, but until a new trial demonstrates an unequivocal benefit, we would regard this as speculation—as it proved to be the first time around.

Fetal-Cell Therapy for Parkinson's Disease

In 1988, Dr. Curt Freed at the University of Colorado Medical Center first offered a novel treatment to a man with Parkinson's disease. The treatment involved injecting fetal cells into the part of the brain affected in Parkinson's. This was on the cutting edge of fetal-cell research, offering the promise that healthy fetal cells could take over from diseased and dying cells. The treatment seemed to offer great hope for patients with a progressively disabling condition. Some doctors began to offer the treatment routinely to patients before definitive studies were done. The procedure cost about $40,000.[27]

Many patients, desperate for hope, figured that they'd take their chances and that they had nothing to lose. As it turned out, they were wrong. More than a decade after he began doing the procedure, Dr. Freed's own research showed disappointing results for most patients and some devastating side effects.

Parkinson's disease is a degenerative condition that affects a certain part of the brain, resulting in tremor, stiffness, difficulty moving, and a halting, shuffling gait. It occurs most often in older adults, past the age of sixty-five, and it usually causes progressive disability. The part of the brain affected is called the substantia nigra, where cells that produce dopamine begin to die. Dopamine is one of several substances that transmit impulses between nerve cells, and in this case, the nerve pathways affected are those that make our movements fluid.

Freed and his colleagues obtained dopamine-making nerve cells from fragments of fetuses that were aborted just seven or eight weeks following conception. These cells were then grown in the laboratory, and the researchers proved that the cells were making dopamine. The treatment involved drilling four small holes in a patient's forehead and inserting long needles through the holes into the brain. The exact location of the needles was guided by MRI scanning, so that the needles would be placed in the right location within the brain. The fetal cells were then injected through the needles.[27,28]

The researchers designed an ambitious study to test the effectiveness of the injections. Just as in the studies of internal mammary artery ligation and arthroscopic knee surgery, they compared the real treatment to a fake operation. This involved drilling the holes in the forehead, but not inserting needles. A year after beginning the study, patients who had had the fake surgery were offered the real thing, if they wanted it. All the patients were then followed out to two years. Forty patients took part in the study.[28]

Overall, there were no differences in treatment results between the real surgery and the fake surgery. When younger patients were compared with older patients, it looked as if the younger patients (under age sixty) benefited from the real operation after one year, but there was no benefit for the older patients. Tests showed that the transplanted cells were surviving. So initially, it seemed that at least younger patients would benefit from the new, high-tech procedure.

But there were two problems. First, the great majority of patients with Parkinson's disease are over age sixty—the group that showed no benefit from the operation. Second, after two years of follow-up, several of the younger patients had developed severe side effects. These were bad enough that the researchers began to advise patients who had started in the fake surgery group not to have the real operation.[28]

The side effects that showed up after two years were sometimes devastating, involving uncontrollable movements. One of the researchers, Dr. Paul Greene, described the situation: "They chew constantly, their fingers go up and down, their wrists flex and distend." Some patients would writhe and twist, jerk their heads, and fling their arms around. Greene said to reporters, "It was tragic, catastrophic. It's a real nightmare. And we can't selectively turn it off."[27] The problem seemed to be that in some patients, the new cells grew too well and led to an excess of dopamine.

Several conclusions emerged from the study. First, Dr. Greene said that his position was, "No more fetal transplants. We are absolutely and adamantly convinced that this should be considered for research only. And whether it should be research in people is an open question." Second, Dr. Gerald Fischbach, head of the National Institutes of Health program that funded the research, pointed out that early, poorly controlled studies of any technology can be misleading. He said, "Ad hoc reports of spectacular results can always occur. But if you do these studies systematically, this is the result you get."[27] Third, it became clear that one year of follow-up may not be enough to see the end results of a treatment. In this case, the adverse effects were apparent only after two years of follow-up.

As with EC/IC bypass surgery, advocates remain enthusiastic about the treatment and believe that modifications and refinements of the technique may eventually prove successful. Research in the field should continue, but any new techniques should be subjected to equally rigorous evaluation before they're widely accepted. And patients should understand that if they enter research of this sort, there are significant risks.

Episiotomy During Childbirth

As with breast cancer, it's women who endure the pain and the complications of childbirth. And like the traditional use of radical mastectomy, women have frequently been subjected to a traditional minor operation during childbirth: the episiotomy. And as with radical mastectomy, only recently has anyone seriously challenged well-established dogma.

An episiotomy is an incision that's made to widen the vaginal opening during childbirth, to give the baby's head more room to pass through. The incision is typically an inch or two long and goes through the skin and muscle behind the vaginal opening. The rationale was that if the opening were made wider, women would be less likely to have tears in the tissue that could extend to the anus, causing long-term incontinence of the bowels. It was also assumed that episiotomy helped to prevent weakening of the pelvic floor muscles, which sometimes led to incontinence of the bladder. Finally, doctors figured that by speeding up delivery, it might prevent injuries to the baby. After delivery, the obstetrician would have a clean surgical incision to sew up, rather than a possible ragged tear in the muscle and skin.

Superficially, this all seems like sound reasoning. But as with many of the treatments we've described, the reality doesn't match the expectation. And it took decades to find out.

Episiotomies were first introduced in the 1920s. In the 1940s, when most women began to have babies in the hospital rather than at home, they became routine. By the 1960s, a majority of women who delivered in the hospital would have an episiotomy.[29] Only in the 1970s did patients and doctors begin to challenge its value and start doing systematic research on the procedure. Rates subsequently began to fall, but by 1997, almost 40 percent of women having vaginal deliveries still received episiotomies.[30]

When the research finally began to yield results, what did it show? A review of high-quality randomized studies was done in 1999; it included six studies conducted during the 1980s and 1990s. Most of these studies compared "liberal" use of episiotomy to "selective" use of the procedure. Doctors performing deliveries in the "liberal" group were typically told to do episiotomies in order to prevent any kind of tear. Those in the "selective" group were told to do episiotomies only if they believed that the baby was in danger or that a severe tear below the vagina seemed imminent.[31]

The results were clear: Women who had the more selective use of episiotomies actually had fewer complications. They were less likely to have injuries close to the anus, were less likely to require suturing, and had fewer healing complications after a week. In other words, women who had episiotomies were actually *more* likely to have serious tears, not less likely. There were no differences between the study groups in bladder incontinence or vaginal pain during sexual intercourse after recovery.[31]

As one doctor put it, "Routine use of episiotomy only increases the incidence of serious lacerations involving the rectum and the anal sphincter." Another obstetrician said of episiotomy, "It's a procedure that has been over utilized, whose benefits are not as pronounced as some would claim."[29]

In fact, episiotomy rates have fallen by a third in the last two decades. In 1998, the rate in the United States was just under 40 percent, compared with almost 64 percent in 1980.[30] But according to news reports, some hospitals perform episiotomies in less than 10 percent of mothers,[29] suggesting that even lower rates may be appropriate. Perhaps this is another case of "less is more."

What Can We Learn from Surgical Miscues?

As with drugs, there are other examples of surgical procedures that became widely used or widely sought after before we knew whether they worked. Other operations that have probably been overused in the past include tonsillectomies and sacroiliac joint fusion for back pain. Today, surgeons are becoming more conservative about removing injured kidneys or livers after abdominal trauma, repairing hernias in the groin, and certain types of sinus surgery.[32] Some new procedures, like pancreas transplants for diabetes, may decrease survival compared to nonsurgical treatments.[33] In other cases, it's becoming clear that older surgical techniques may be as good as or better than newer "minimally invasive" techniques.[34]

Several conclusions seem to emerge from these stories. First, many people have probably been subjected to unnecessary or unnecessarily aggressive surgery. Even when patients seem to get better, it's not necessarily because of the surgery, and sometimes the results of nonsurgical treatments are even better. Second, high-tech treatments (surgery in this case) aren't always better than lower-tech nonsurgical treatments. Third, many operations are done because of charismatic authority, tradition, or marketing by companies promoting new technology, not because of good evidence that they really help. Fourth, we should be wary of new operations before they've been rigorously tested. Even when it seems that there's nothing to lose by trying a new operation, and even when the operation seems to make perfect sense, there are some devastating possibilities.

Don't get us wrong. We're not calling for less research on surgical procedures, but for more. If radical mastectomy and episiotomy had been subjected to modern randomized trials when they were introduced, many women might have been spared their complications. At the time, of course, modern research methods such as randomized trials were unknown, and hindsight is always 20-20. But there's no reason why most new operations can't be subjected to the rigorous scrutiny undergone by internal mammary artery ligation, knee arthroscopy for arthritis, EC/IC bypass surgery, and fetal cell implants for Parkinson's disease. Although these operations didn't pan out, the research was extremely successful in giving us clear answers about their ineffectiveness. And research like this is still rare. So perhaps a final conclusion is that it may be better to clamor for good research studies—recognizing the risks—than to clamor for automatic insurance coverage of every new operation that sounds promising. "Just doing it" may be even riskier.

16

Weight Loss Technology

Shedding Pounds from Your Waistline or Your Wallet?

Lose 30 Pounds in Just 30 Days.
Lose Weight While You Sleep.
Scientific Breakthrough . . . Medical Miracle.
Lose All the Weight You Can for Just $39.99.

—Claims that the FTC suggests are misleading[1]

IN 2003, a twenty-three-year-old Baltimore Orioles pitcher, Steve Bechler, arrived at baseball camp in Florida weighing 249 pounds, noticeably heavy to his manager and teammates, even at his height (6 feet 2 inches). On a Sunday morning, a sunny day with temperatures in the low 80s and humidity around 70 percent, Bechler came for a regularly scheduled workout. After about 60 percent of the light running workout was completed, he became faint and collapsed near the outfield fence. He was rushed to the training room, where he received treatment for about twenty minutes until emergency personnel arrived. His body temperature temporarily reached 108 degrees, and heat was blamed for his loss of consciousness. At the hospital, Bechler's condition declined, and he was placed on a respirator. From that point on, medical staff fought a losing battle to stabilize him, and he died, according to a team physician, from "multi-organ failure due to heatstroke."[2,3]

The medical examiner who conducted the autopsy on Bechler found ephedra in his system and concluded that the toxicity of ephedra had played a significant role in his death. According to Bechler's family, he had used Xenadrine RFA-1, a diet supplement that contains ephedra. Bechler's widow, who was seven months pregnant when her husband died, filed a lawsuit against Nutraquest, the maker of the supplement sold by Cytodyne.[4] According to *The New York Times,* Xenadrine's label describes it as a "rapid fat loss catalyst," and says, "Lose weight fast."[3] It has been implicated in 155 deaths.[5]

In April 2004, ephedra was removed from stores and web sites that sell diet supplements, by order of the Food and Drug Administration. The ban targeted ephedra supplements that were advertised for weight loss, muscle building, and athletic performance. This doesn't mean that ephedra will disappear entirely. Herbal medicine preparations containing ma huang, the type of ephedra grown in China, will still be available from acupuncturists and herbalists. These are often recommended for conditions such as colds, asthma, cough, and headache.[6] Further, manufacturers of some ephedra products are seeking to reverse the FDA ban.[5]

Steve Bechler was one of millions of Americans who are struggling to lose weight. Like many, he pursued a course that was heavily promoted, but somewhat risky. Ephedra earned $1.3 billion at its peak, and an estimated 13 million people had tried the supplement.[7] Like many, Bechler apparently hoped for a quick solution to a lifestyle problem.

Previous chapters have dealt with conventional medical treatments for conventional diseases. Treatments for excessive weight offer an opportunity to examine how conventional drug therapy, surgery, and even diet supplements are promoted and used for a common lifestyle problem. Although dietary supplements may not strike you as medical advances or high technology, their promotion and risks have similarities to those of new pharmaceuticals.

Over 50 percent of Americans are overweight or obese. For those who are, and even for many of those who aren't, finding a way to get slim or stay slim commands plenty of attention. Weight loss and diet aids are touted everywhere—on TV and radio, on the Internet, in magazines, and even on flyers that appear on car windshields and telephone poles. Ads describe miraculous ways to lose weight quickly.

But as the American Obesity Association notes, if there really were a miracle cure, our weight problems wouldn't be so severe. Rates of obesity have risen at an epidemic rate during the past twenty years. Despite the advent of the South Beach Diet and the ever-growing marketing of low-carb snacks, trends indicate that rates of overweight and obesity are likely to increase.

Everyone knows that being overweight is bad for your health. Overweight individuals are more susceptible than average to high blood pressure, high cholesterol, diabetes, heart attacks, heart failure, stroke, gallstones, gout, arthritis, sleep apnea, some types of cancer, complications of pregnancy, menstrual irregularities, infertility, bladder control problems, and kidney stones. They also are at higher risk for depression, eating disorders, distorted body image, and low self-esteem. Obesity can be embarrassing and demoralizing. Even this list is probably incomplete, as more studies appear every day.

Diet and Exercise Programs

About 40 percent of women and 25 percent of men are trying to lose weight at any given time. Nationwide, another 55 percent of Americans are actively trying to maintain their current weight. Some 45 million Americans diet each year.

Consumers spend about $30 billion per year trying to lose weight or prevent weight gain.[8] This includes spending on diet sodas, diet foods, artificially sweetened products, appetite suppressants, diet books, videos and cassettes, medically supervised and commercial programs, and fitness clubs.[8,9]

There are thousands of diets that promise to shed pounds. The low-fat and high-fat camps and the advocates of low-carbohydrate diets compete for credibility. There's rarely a week when there aren't one or more diet books on the bestseller list. But the evidence that these diets can produce long-term weight loss for most people is slim at best. In the weight-loss market, separating truth from promise is nearly impossible.

Almost as popular as "how to" diet books are commercial and noncommercial weight-loss programs. Most of these programs involve restricted-calorie diets coupled with individual or group counseling. Few participants keep the weight off for long. In fact, the Federal Trade Commission has brought action against some companies, challenging their weight-loss and weight-maintenance claims.[8]

It may be that the most successful weight losers are do-it-yourselfers. In a survey of more than 32,000 dieters conducted by *Consumer Reports*, nearly a quarter had lost at least 10 percent of their starting body weight and kept it off for at least a year.

About 12 percent were "superlosers": those who had maintained their weight loss for five years. The superlosers usually did it on their own, without programs or drugs. Most identified exercise as the main factor in their success.

Only 14 percent of the superlosers ever signed up with Weight Watchers, Jenny Craig, or other commercial programs, and only 6 percent used dietary aids like Metabolife or Dexatrim. A *Consumer Reports* editor said that the report "overturns the long-held conviction that to lose weight, you have to enroll in an expensive program, buy special food, or follow the regimen of a particular diet guru."[10]

Magic Bullets: Diet Supplements

Nowhere is the hype more evident than at your local drugstore. Herbs and supplements that claim to control weight include green tea extract, chitosan, psyllium, chromium and chromium picolinate, 5-hydroxytryptophan, soy isoflavones, ma huang (a.k.a. ephedra), guarana, kava, St John's wort, spirulina supplements, white willow bark, l-carnitine, pancreatin, fiber, dehydroepiandrosterone, coenzyme Q10, dandelion leaves, hydroxycitric acid, betaine, calcium, docosahexaenoic acid, eicosapentaenoic acid, glutamine, vitamin B5 (pantothenic acid), vitamin C (ascorbic acid), vitamin D, zinc, glucomann, pectin, cat's claw, blessed thistle, and probably many others. For almost every one of these "diet supplements," there have been claims that it facilitates weight loss.

Americans spend huge sums on these products, with estimates ranging from $6 to $10 billion each year. Sadly, there's little evidence regarding the efficacy of these herbs and supplements. The FDA doesn't authorize or test dietary supplements. This leaves room for a wide range of claims, both fraudulent and legitimate.

The 1994 Dietary Supplement Health and Education Act freed the manufactures of diet supplements from having to prove that their products were safe and effective. Under this act, the companies aren't required to report adverse reactions or deaths resulting from their products to the government or to consumers. Some advisory groups are working with Congress to try to change this legislation.[11] Both the FDA and Congress are considering initiatives to require makers of diet supplements to test their claims and show supporting evidence. In the upcoming months, debate between government and manufacturers should be lively.

Ephedra, which played a part in the death of Steve Bechler, was well known to have problems. In 2003, *The New York Times* reported that the Food and Drug Administration received more than a hundred reports of deaths among ephedra users, as well as 16,000 reports of other problems, including strokes, seizures, heatstroke, heart disorders, and psychotic episodes.[12] Even so, only the worst cases draw attention. The FDA itself estimates that it gets reports on fewer than 1 percent of severe adverse effects linked to dietary supplements.

The allure of these treatments affects not just overweight people but also those who are trying to stay slim. A friend recommended some tablets to Jennifer Rosenthal, age twenty-eight, a truck dispatcher and the mother of a four-year-old in Long Beach, California. The pills sounded wonderful: They were supposed to increase the metabolism to help the body burn off fat. "It was like you're doing aerobic exercise while you're just sitting there," said Jennifer. The capsules were sold over the Internet for $39.95 for ninety and contained only one ingredient—usnic acid, a chemical found in some lichen plants. Jennifer took half the maximum dose recommended on the label for two weeks, skipped two weeks as the label directed, and then started again for a total of seventeen days.[13]

In less than a month, Jennifer was in a coma with liver failure, connected to a respirator. Her rapid deterioration prompted the hospital to put her at the top of the waiting list for a liver transplant, which she got within days. Doctors observed that her own liver was so badly damaged that it had shriveled to about a third of what it should have weighed. They concluded that almost certainly the liver damage was related to usnic acid, because there was no other explanation for her illness.

Her surgeon told reporters, "This is a young woman who almost lost her life. Although she's got her life back now, she has to be under life-long medical care. Her life has been altered forever. The fact that you can get these things over the Internet is mind-boggling."[13]

Over the years, various treatments have been found ineffective, and products such as ephedra are coming off the market. In the early 1990s, ineffective diet patches were also removed from the market. The Federal Trade Commission warns against other ineffective weight loss products: magnet diet pills that purportedly "flush fat out of the body," bulk fillers like guar gum that can cause intestinal obstruction, electrical muscle stimulators, "appetite suppressing eyeglasses," and "magic weight-loss earrings."[8] You can probably still find these products being touted for sale. It's not illegal to sell ineffective treatments that aren't regulated by government.

More Magic Bullets: Weight-Loss Drugs

No one has yet developed a highly effective prescription drug for long-term weight loss. By far the most common prescription diet pills are appetite suppressants, a family of drugs that includes Meridia (sibutramine) and Adipex-P (phentermine). These drugs increase the amount of serotonin and catecholamine in the brain, and these brain chemicals modulate mood and appetite. At sufficient levels, they reduce hunger and create a feeling of fullness. Most people taking these drugs lose no more than ten to fourteen pounds. Many regain the weight when they stop taking the drug.[14]

Another drug, Xenical (orlistat), blocks the absorption of dietary fat in the intestines. Up to a third of all ingested fat may be blocked. But there are sometimes unpleasant side effects like urgent bowel movements, gas, and irregular menstrual periods.

Dexfenfluramine (Redux), phen-fen (a combination of fenfluramine and phentermine), and fenfluramine (Pondimin) were withdrawn from the market in 1997 because of side effects involving the heart and lungs. Doctors wrote 18 million prescriptions for these drugs in 1996, and six million people in the United States reportedly used Pondimin or Redux.[15,16]

Wyeth, the manufacturer of phen-fen, has subsequently faced tens of thousands of claims. In 1999, Wyeth settled a class action lawsuit for over $3 billion.[15] In April of 2004, a Texas jury awarded over $1 billion to the family of a woman who died of lung disease allegedly caused by phen-fen. According to *The New York Times*, the company has set aside nearly $17 billion to cover its liability.[17]

Wyeth had used the strategy of placing ghostwritten articles in the medical literature to help promote the drug, according to news accounts. According to a lawsuit, the company tried to play down or remove descriptions of side effects from the articles. At least one guest author said that he was unaware that Wyeth had financed or edited his article.[16]

Many people continue to hope that such drugs will offer a one-stop solution to weight control—the technological fix. Most evidence indicates that any weight-loss drug must be used along with diet and physical activity to have any substantial effect. However, several major pharmaceutical companies are developing new prescription drugs for obesity, so the story is far from over.

Surgery for Weight Loss

Some people turn to surgery for a cure. The NIH suggests that only men who are about one hundred pounds overweight or women who are at least eighty pounds overweight should consider surgery. Those who have diabetes or life-threatening cardiopulmonary problems might consider surgery at slightly lower weights.[18]

Gastric bypass surgery, also called bariatric surgery, has become the most common type of weight-loss surgery. The operation certainly works, and many patients lose about a hundred pounds. Successful surgery can improve obesity-related health complications, psychological well-being, and quality of life. Furthermore, after a year of recovery, even patient survival is improved.[18]

But just as with every other treatment, there are drawbacks. Unlike drugs, though, surgery can't easily be reversed at a later date. The International Bariatric Surgery Registry puts the thirty-day mortality rate at a reassuring 1 in 300. The real mortality rate, however, may be far higher than that—possibly as high as 1 in 50 cases, close to the death rate from coronary surgery.[19] *The New England Journal of Medicine* notes: "Bariatric surgery is not cosmetic surgery. It is major gastrointestinal surgery performed in extremely large patients whose obesity puts them at risk for complications and death—both from the medical problems with obesity and from the surgery itself."[20]

The high estimate of mortality comes from research by David Flum, a University of Washington surgeon who analyzed data for over three thousand patients who underwent gastric bypasses. Flum attributes the high complication rate, in part, to inexperienced surgeons who are eager to add the lucrative but demanding surgery to their repertoire. "You have lots of obese patients, insurers willing to pay, and doctors just learning the operation. It is the perfect storm for bad outcomes," he says. The operation can work wonders, Flum admits, "but patients need to go in with their eyes open."[19,21]

With growing demand for the surgery, it has become big business, and many medical centers are scrambling to start programs. In Massachusetts, the state Department of Health had to investigate widely publicized reports of surgery-related deaths.[20,22] The president of the American Society for Bariatric Surgery notes: "All of a sudden there has been this explosion of people doing the procedures, and some, quite honestly, are not doing the operation the right way or do not follow up the right way."[22] Experts say that some doctors have even encouraged obese patients to gain more weight so that they would become heavy enough to qualify for the surgery.[21]

Even successful surgery isn't a magic bullet. Dr. James Ostroff at the University of California–San Francisco, says, "many patients are misled into thinking that bypass surgery will solve weight problems forever without any effort on their part."[21] Without proper follow-up, including dietary and often psychological counseling, patients often gain back all the weight they lost or, conversely, become malnourished. The head of one nutrition center says, "We consider these people our patients for life."[22]

Yet another surgical "cure" for overweight is liposuction. Liposuction is the removal of fat deposits under the skin using a hollow stainless steel tube with the assistance of a powerful vacuum. Although generally safe, liposuction is expensive, and removing subcutaneous fat doesn't address the causes of excessive weight. It's primarily a cosmetic procedure, and it's most effective for those who aren't severely overweight. Of major concern for those considering liposuction is finding practitioners with the qualifications to do the procedure, as serious complications can arise.[23]

The Epidemic of Obesity

Obesity experts, the surgeon general, and public health officials argue that individual efforts and technology alone won't solve the broader obesity epidemic. Individual treatments for overweight and obesity need to be considered in the context of the culture and the physical and social environment in the United States.

For example, the bestseller *Fast Food Nation* describes how Americans have come to frequent high-volume, high-fat restaurants.[24] Use of the automobile is often invoked in explaining the obesity epidemic, as is the overuse of television. In addition to reducing the need to walk, cars have changed the built environment. There are fewer sidewalks, little opportunity for safe bicycling, and little attention to attractive environments for exercise. Changes in entire social and physical systems may be needed in order to induce a largely inactive and overweight population to control their weight effectively.

For a condition that is so prevalent, with health impacts that are so great and a public that is so willing, far more resources might be put into environmental change, as well as evaluating various weight-loss treatments and disseminating the results. It's startling that the first randomized trials of popular diets have been published only recently.[25,26]

A realistic expectation for individuals needs to be coupled with a realistic expectation for populations. Even a small weight loss on a population basis could yield many health benefits at a societal level. Like the war on smoking, the war on obesity will take decades, with many ups and downs in different population segments. Helping the public sort out the dangerous from the benign, the effective from the ineffective, and "waste of money" from "worth the investment" should be a high priority for public health and medicine.

PART IV

CROSSING THE THRESHOLD

Improving the Transition from "Experimental" to "Standard Care"

17

For Doctors

Evidence-Based Medicine

Supposing is good, but finding out is better. —Mark Twain[1]

It seems unlikely that the results of the Women's Health Initiative trial of estrogen and progestin replacement will transform the interventionist mind-set of American medicine. "Don't just stand there, do something!" will continue to be the battle cry of most doctors and patients. On the other hand, it's going to be a little bit harder from now on to say of interventions aimed at improving health that they're so obviously beneficial that only a compulsive fussbudget could demand proof. —David Brown, *Washington Post* journalist[2]

WE'VE DISCUSSED many common medical practices that proved to have no basis: long-term hormone replacement therapy after menopause, episiotomy for childbirth, pulmonary artery catheters for high-risk surgery patients, encainide for abnormal heart rhythms after a heart attack, expensive new drugs for high blood pressure instead of old-fashioned diuretics, bone marrow transplants for late-stage breast cancer, radical mastectomies for breast cancer, and many others. If these treatments were useless or wasteful (and sometimes harmful), why did doctors use them? How did their use get started in the first place? How can we avoid similar mistakes in the future?

We'll argue in these final chapters that we can improve the process of technology adoption if all parties are willing to make some changes. There's no single solution to this problem, and there's no single stakeholder whose choices will be decisive. Instead, any improvements are likely to come through a combination of changes in doctors', patients', the media's, and manufacturers' behavior; better research; new regulatory approaches; and better educational approaches. New insurance or financing arrangements will also be important, although we'll largely avoid a discussion of health-care financing. Dealing with medical advances will be a challenge under any financing scheme. But a unifying theme might be the need for more *evidence-based* approaches to the adoption of new treatments.

The evidence-based approach argues that it isn't enough to know that a particular treatment ought to work, that it makes sense, that it's common practice, that we learned it in medical school, that we've always done it that way, that an expert vouches for it, or that it works in mice. Even further, this approach says that it's nice, but not enough, to know that treatment lowers blood pressure, improves cholesterol, normalizes heart rhythms, or has similar physiological benefits. These are all common reasons why doctors do things, and one or more of these reasons explain the wide use of each of the inappropriate treatments listed earlier. The newer evidence-based approach asks instead, what's the best evidence that a new treatment actually extends lives or improves quality of life, and what are the risks?

Advocates of evidence-based medicine argue that the best evidence available to answer questions about effectiveness comes from multiple

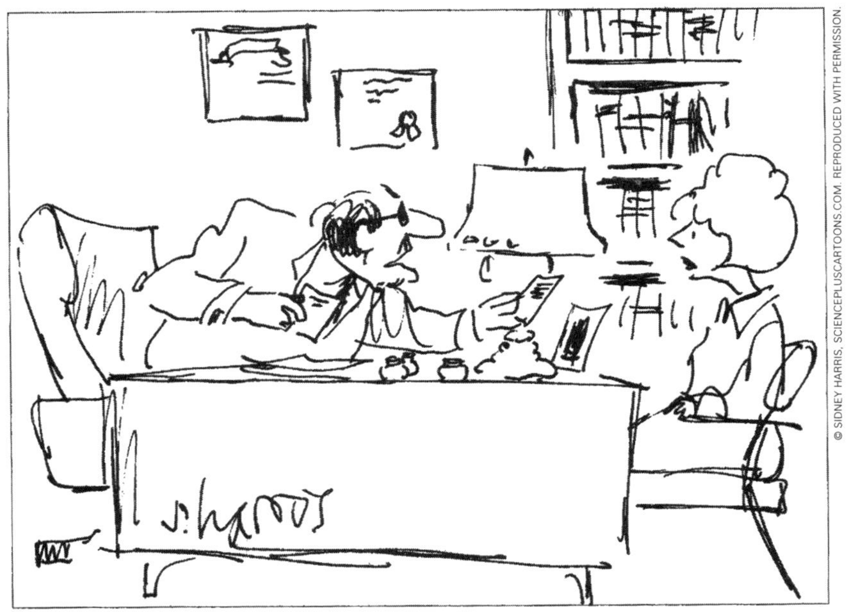

"Take these pills three times a day, unless you read in the paper that they've been proven ineffective."

randomized controlled trials. When these aren't available, we still have to make clinical decisions, but they're based on less rigorous information and may be more prone to error. The basic idea behind randomized trials is to compare a new treatment with the standard treatment or—when there's no proven alternative—with a placebo, or sham treatment. Randomly allocating patients to the alternatives is the best way to assure that we're comparing apples with apples, and not apples with oranges. That's because it ensures that a researcher's or patient's biases, whether conscious or unconscious, don't result in cherry-picking the best patients for one treatment or the other. The use of a placebo treatment that mimics the real thing is valuable because it helps minimize the effects of researchers' biases and patients' expectations.

Randomized trials aren't infallible, by any means. Designing and analyzing them is often complex, and there are many ways to go wrong. This is why one randomized trial is rarely enough. Multiple trials, if they give consistent results, are more likely to provide a valid answer. These trials can be cumbersome and expensive. But over and over, they've proven to be our most powerful tool against faulty reasoning.

The rise of evidence-based medicine concepts doesn't negate the need for more fundamental biomedical research. Basic biological research is still our best hope for understanding why and how heart disease, arthritis, cancer, diabetes, and other common conditions occur. And this understanding is our best hope for developing effective treatments or prevention strategies. These strategies will become more effective than the rear-guard action of simply replacing or repairing organs after the damage is done. But while basic science will provide these insights, randomized trials will still be the best way to determine the benefits of the resulting treatments. Randomized trials will be essential to show how effective these treatments are when they're actually used in people, with all their individuality.

The Backlash Against Evidence-Based Medicine

Evidence-based medicine is a hot topic right now among doctors, insurance companies, planners, and the public. There are frequent workshops on how to practice and teach it, as well as workshops on its role in insurance coverage and policy making. Medical schools and residency programs are figuring out whether and how to incorporate it into their curricula. New centers and new medical journals have been launched with this as a central theme.[3]

But there's also been a backlash against the idea. Many doctors argue that we've always practiced evidence-based medicine, that medicine has always been based on science. But "science" has often meant inferences drawn from what we know of human physiology and disease behavior, information from studies of animals, or expert opinions. It's sometimes based on the observation that "I tried treatment X and my patients got better." Even lawyers recognize the fallacy in this line of thinking, embodied in the phrase "post hoc, ergo propter hoc." Just because patients get better, doesn't mean that they are getting better *because* of the treatment applied. As we saw earlier, they may have improved because of natural healing, regression of symptoms to their mean, or placebo effects. It's easy for both doctors and patients to be fooled about the real benefits of treatment just because someone gets better after the treatment is given.

The new model argues that these older methods are often a good basis for designing and testing a treatment, but they aren't enough. They're necessary, but not sufficient. The biological inferences, animal models, opinions, and clinical impressions must generally be subjected to the purifying heat of randomized trials to reveal the true benefits and risks of a new treatment.

Any hope that doctors are already consistent about practicing evidence-based medicine is dashed by the repeated observation of huge variations in practice from doctor to doctor, hospital to hospital, and place to place. Unless all treatments and clinical strategies are equally effective, the different approaches can't all be right. If we were all practicing evidence-based medicine, the litany of ineffective treatments that began this chapter wouldn't have been used for years or decades. And even with the best of intentions, it's almost impossible for any doctor to keep up with all the latest scientific advances in any specialty.

Other doctors complain that evidence-based medicine amounts to "cookbook" medicine. Some complain that it's "a dangerous innovation, perpetrated by the arrogant to serve cost cutters and suppress clinical freedom."[3] They argue that it denies the value of clinical judgment, specialized expertise, and patients' unique personal preferences.

But advocates of evidence-based medicine argue just the opposite. They argue that clinical judgment is critical in deciding how to apply evidence that comes from other people to each individual patient. Without that ability to generalize, we'd be lost. Advocates also argue that doctors must always consider patients' preferences in making clinical decisions. Rather than slavish adherence to top-down dictates, evidence-based practice integrates the best evidence, clinical judgment, and patient preferences in every clinical situation. The hard part for most doctors is finding, evaluating, and interpreting the best evidence.

As for costs, evidence-based practice may in some cases decrease costs, but in other cases it can increase costs. Eliminating useless operations or choosing less expensive and more effective drugs will decrease costs. On the other hand, we know that many types of effective screening and treatment are underused. If we start doing all the screening for colon cancer that's recommended, or treating every diabetic with the full cocktail of drugs and monitoring that are recommended, costs are likely to increase. The approach isn't inherently cost saving, though in some situations it may be.

Requiring evidence of the sort advocated here places a burden of proof on the advocates of a new treatment. In areas of medicine where there isn't a long history of rigorous research design or where research funding is scarce, these criteria are often unwelcome and are seen as an obstacle to innovation. Some opponents of evidence-based principles argue that new treatments should be adopted and paid for unless they're proven ineffective, reversing the burden of proof. As our examples in earlier chapters suggest, though, both safety and cost considerations make this position untenable. Too many people have been hurt by blind faith that new treatments have to be better.

Leave it to the Aussies to recognize pomposity and pretense, which are sometimes associated with the resistance to evidence-based medicine. With tongue in cheek, two Australian doctors summarized some of the alternatives to evidence-based medicine,[4] all of which still operate widely:

> *Eminence-based medicine:* Grey hair and years of experience are the basis for recommendations. The faith of such physicians in their clinical experience has been defined as "making the same mistakes with increasing confidence over an impressive number of years."
>
> *Vehemence-based medicine:* The louder and more strident the advice, the easier it may be to browbeat colleagues.
>
> *Eloquence-based medicine:* Here, a fine suit and verbal eloquence supercede evidence.

Providence-based medicine: When the doctor has no idea what to do, decisions can be left in the hands of the Almighty.

Diffidence-based medicine: Doing nothing from a sense of despair. Of course, just standing there may often be better than just doing something, but it's unsatisfying.

Nervousness-based medicine: Fear of lawsuits drives excessive testing and overtreatment. "The only bad test is the one you didn't think of ordering."

Confidence-based medicine: Especially common among surgeons, of whom it's sometimes said, "they're often wrong, but never in doubt."

What Is the Evidence?

Even for doctors, hospitals, and insurance carriers who buy the idea, evidence-based medicine is surprisingly hard to practice. Simply knowing the evidence is hard, because of the enormous size of the medical literature and the rapid pace of its change. Busy doctors don't have the time to do even electronic searches of all the relevant literature, identify the most useful articles, read them, evaluate the quality of the results, and integrate the pieces into a coherent whole every time they see a patient. They'd be lucky if they were able to do this once a month.

Fortunately, doctors can get help with this. A growing number of medical journals focus on high-quality, clinically relevant articles and provide quick summaries. There also are a growing number of clinical guidelines, which at their best provide a doctor with summaries of the literature that have been extensively researched and evaluated, to help guide the doctor's decisions, but not dictate them.

One hazard is that guidelines are sometimes promulgated by organizations with a self-interest in the recommendations or with commercial influences lurking in the near background. For this reason, doctors can't accept guidelines uncritically. The other major hazard is that guidelines can be cumbersome and time-consuming to construct, so they risk being outdated before they're released or shortly thereafter. Nonetheless, they're generally far more current than what doctors learned in medical school, and they're often both more rigorous and more current than medical textbooks.

Having found the relevant medical research or guidelines, evaluating their quality is the next challenge most doctors face. This requires a strong knowledge of research design and statistical methods, which are rarely taught well in medical schools. If they're included at all, they usually are treated as side dishes to the main courses of biochemistry, pathology, microbiology, and the like. Although the latter remain integral to training effective doctors, the principles of evidence-based medicine need to be taught with equal rigor, enthusiasm, and high expectations.

As Dr. Drummond Rennie, deputy editor of the *Journal of the American Medical Association,* remarked, "If you are not trained to think statistically, if you are not trained to think epidemiologically, it's extremely difficult to grasp 'risk' and a whole lot of other things like that. You have to have years of training before you really get into the habit of thinking of risks rationally."

In other words, doctors need somewhat different training if they are to distinguish high-quality from low-quality evidence for clinical interventions. Incorporating principles of evidence-based medicine into the medical school curriculum may help the next generation of physicians to become more critical consumers of medical research. It needs a higher priority than it often receives.

Rennie also notes that the practice of evidence-based medicine will require constant updating and questioning throughout a doctor's career. He has prepared journal articles, a book, a CD, and a web version of guides for doctors, because he believes "it's the only way ahead."

The Cochrane Collaboration database is another underutilized resource for doctors, patients, and insurance companies. Its organizers named the effort for Archie Cochrane, a British physician and researcher who died in 1988, who argued that society could afford to pay for all effective treatments, if we would just stop paying for the ineffective ones. The Cochrane Collaboration is an international effort to systematically review the medical literature on all treatments, evaluate the quality of individual studies, summarize the results, and pool data from the best randomized trials. The program leaders also intend to update the reviews on a regular basis. All the results are available online, and the number of topics reviewed (already in the thousands) is rapidly growing.[5,6] One advocate has argued that the Cochrane Collaboration will prove to be as pivotal in modern medicine as the human genome project.[7]

Outside the United States, the Cochrane Collaboration has acquired enormous influence among doctors, scientists, and those who pay for medical care. This is true in Canada, Europe, Australia, and most developed countries. In the United States, though, it's still only modestly familiar and modestly used, perhaps because commercial, political, and media influences often outweigh scientific ones. If we decide that science should play a bigger role, there are resources to help.

Computers in Medicine

Another source of help in practicing evidence-based medicine, one that's increasingly available to doctors and hospitals, is computer technology. *Medical informatics* is the term that is applied not only to the use of electronic medical records, but also to so-called decision support programs that can be integrated with electronic medical records. Many doctors recognize the difficulty they have keeping up with the literature, and would welcome authoritative, evidence-based information just at the moment they're making decisions. The computer makes this increasingly possible.

Suppose the doctor has just admitted an elderly patient from a nursing home into the hospital and has diagnosed pneumonia. She doesn't yet know exactly which bacteria (or other microbes) are causing the pneumonia, and in many cases it never becomes clear. But she has to choose an antibiotic and a dose based on what infections are commonly acquired in nursing homes, what the local patterns of antibiotic resistance may be, how well the patient's kidneys are functioning, what drugs the patient is allergic to, how each antibiotic may interact with the other six medicines the patient is taking, the patient's age and weight, what spectrum of bacteria each drug will kill, the common side effects of each antibiotic, and the particular clinical pattern of this patient's illness.

In most cases today, she has neither the time nor the knowledge to look up each of these factors and somehow integrate them into a precise solution. Instead, she'll choose an antibiotic based mostly on habit, local convention, or what she recently heard from a drug rep she likes. She'll prescribe a standard dose that she uses for most adults. Because there's a good margin for error in many medical judgments, the patient will usually do just fine—but not always.

Wouldn't it be nice if this doctor could simply enter her interview and examination findings into the computer and have the computer automatically look up the most common kinds of pneumonia among patients recently admitted to this hospital from nursing homes; consider the antibiotic resistance patterns of bacteria tested by the lab in this hospital over the last six months; check the lab results for the patient's kidney function;

check the nursing notes for the patient's height and weight; check the pharmacy records to identify the patient's other drugs; run an automated check for serious interactions with any of those drugs; check the pharmacy, previous hospital records, nursing notes, and doctors' notes for any record of drug allergies; and make a recommendation for an antibiotic and a dosage based on all these factors plus the best research evidence, embodied in a current clinical guideline. The computer might even list two or three alternatives, with the pluses and minuses of each. The doctor is then free to choose one of the recommendations or to ignore them, perhaps because of other factors that were not considered by the computer.

Even with this scenario, there are no guarantees the patient will improve, but the chances are probably better. The doctor's and patient's autonomy haven't been usurped. The doctor isn't practicing cookbook medicine; she's had to gather the patient's symptoms and exam findings, make the right diagnosis, decide on hospitalization, and make dozens of other decisions. But she's grateful for the more complete assessment of antibiotic choices she's gotten. It's saved her time, and she's been able to use that time to talk with the family and reassure the patient. The recommendations aren't based on commercial interests, personal biases, or local habits.

This scenario isn't quite reality today, but it may be in the near future. A few hospital systems have decision support programs with several of these elements already. Early indications are that these systems reduce errors in the hospital and can save money at the same time; their potential in other aspects of medicine is enormous.

So the computer is one technology that we think has been underused in medicine. Given the huge amount of information that we now gather on every patient, the complexity of decision making, and the volume and volatility of medical knowledge, it may be our only hope for effectively using the technological progress available to us. We think that the investment in information technology by American medicine should increase substantially, and the Bush administration is moving to support such initiatives.

As with the construction of guidelines, one caution is that these decision aids must be developed in an evidence-based fashion by someone who doesn't have a financial interest in the clinical recommendations. Also, the decision aids will have to be continuously updated. These tasks, like the hardware, will be expensive, but they may prove to pay for themselves. Ultimately, the real benefits and risks of information technology will need to be evaluated as carefully as those of other medical technology.

Commercial Pressures and Professionalism

We've described how alluring commercial influences are, and how pervasive conflicts of interest have become in modern medicine. In most cases, these conflicts exist precisely because of the incentives created by new advances. And commercial pressures of various types have become a major obstacle to practicing evidence-based medicine.

Dr. Rennie believes that practicing evidence-based medicine is against human nature:

> It's against human nature to make decisions based on evidence, and I really believe that—even though no one could be more wedded than I am to the idea. Doctors form cozy relationships with nice people who respect them, or seem to respect them, and give them presents. It's why those doctors so willingly prescribe the latest brand name drug without ever looking into the evidence whatsoever . . . because it makes them happy, it makes the patient happy, it makes the drug rep happy.

He goes on to describe the pressures created by advertising aimed directly at patients:

> I think a doctor in a sense would be foolhardy or reckless with his own time and energy to spend time trying to go against the direct-to-consumer advertising. "I will lose this patient if I don't prescribe what she or he is demanding right now." I sympathize with people who make a cost benefit analysis in a flash and say "I just can't afford the time." So I'm just saying the system, irrespective of any transfer of money into my pocket, is working against evidence.

Can doctors and hospitals resist?

Medicine is one of the three traditional "learned professions": law, religion, and medicine. These professions acquired this stature because they worked with ubiquitous, profound human needs. Professionals in these fields had to be trusted with the intimate details of a client's mind, body, and personal life. A professional had to be trusted to use such intimate knowledge for the benefit of the client, not for exploitation. Self-governance, service, quality, autonomy, altruism, self-sacrifice, and a high level of learning are seen as defining characteristics of learned professions. These traits are the basis for the trust most patients still have in their own doctors.[8]

On the other hand, of course, medicine is a business. It's the way doctors, nurses, administrators, technicians, maintenance experts, manufacturers, and salespeople make a living. Without income, doctors and hospitals couldn't stay in business, nor could the drug and device makers. Business standards are different from professional standards, and they mainly focus on return on investment. Medical practice is always a balancing act between the professional and the business sides of practice.

Many leaders of American medicine, including prominent journal editors and leaders of professional societies, have become concerned that the balance between business and professional values has recently tilted dangerously toward the business side. As we have discussed, both doctors and hospitals today often seem to make choices based on a corporate mentality that focuses on financial return rather than on good evidence of benefit to patients. When the choices involve new treatments, the assumption is almost always that more and newer can only be better. Conveniently, this stance almost always coincides with financial self-interest.

Several professional organizations, including the American College of Physicians and the American Board of Internal Medicine Foundation, have issued recent calls for strengthening professional values among physicians.[9,10] Though the initiatives are short on specifics or sanctions, they may serve to refocus attention on this problem and to enhance the inculcation of professional values in medical school and specialty training. In some cases, it seems, we've become so preoccupied with technical training that we've forgotten to convey the ethical and social values on which the profession is built. Perhaps a combination of better training in evidence-based medicine and reinvigorated attention to true professionalism will help to counter the commercial pull against evidence-based practice.

Finally, more support for primary care medical practice may help deflect some of the pressures to use unproven treatments. Unlike the cardiologist or the orthopedist, primary physicians have little to gain from using new procedures or gadgets (although they may be susceptible to blandishments from the drug companies). They can therefore afford to be more dispassionate about them. The primary care doctor—typically a family doctor, general internist, or pediatrician—can serve the role of providing unbiased information and assisting patients with many difficult medical decisions.

Furthermore, such practitioners handle the majority of complaints as effectively as specialists, and usually in a lower-tech style. Their role shouldn't be that of gatekeeper—a role that they dislike, that patients distrust, and that's proved to be ineffective. Instead, they can serve the role of knowing the patient and his or her values best, handling most routine problems, and offering objective advice on more specialized, more technological care.

18

For Insurers and Researchers

Pay Now or Pay More Later

Without the data generated from clinical research, even expert opinions on novel medical treatments are not much better than a coin toss. —Jose A. Bufill, MD[1]

Modern medicine has left in the public mind the conviction that we know almost everything about everything. This is as good a time as any to amend the impression . . . biomedical science . . . good as it is, is perhaps not entitled to all the credit it gets from the general public. —Lewis Thomas, MD[2]

MAYBE THIS GOES without saying, but more and better scientific research will be the main source of better treatments for our common ailments. The problem is that good clinical research, and especially clinical trials, require lots of time, money, patience, and patients. There's no substitute for randomized trials to test the effectiveness and safety of most treatments in medicine. But as we've seen, the randomized trials we need are often delayed for years or decades.

If the ALLHAT study of drugs for high blood pressure had been done twenty years earlier—which it could have been—it would have saved countless dollars and complications from high blood pressure. If the Women's Health Initiative trial on hormone replacement therapy had been started fifteen years earlier—which it could have been—it, too, would have saved countless dollars and avoidable complications. If the randomized trial of encainide and flecainide had been done years earlier, it would have saved thousands of lives. If the trials of bone marrow transplant for advanced breast cancer had been completed faster, they would have saved billions of dollars and thousands of complications. Can't we speed up the process?

Part of the problem in each of these cases is that drug makers and doctors had little incentive to do the definitive trials: Their preferred treatments were already in wide use, and better evidence could only hurt market share. In most cases, doctors were wrongly convinced that they were doing the right thing, and patients were pleased to have the new treatments. But patients and the public had unrecognized incentives to learn more and learn faster: their safety and their pocketbooks.

Partnerships for Funding Clinical Research

The treatments described throughout this book were nearly all paid for by insurance. This sometimes makes them seem "free" to consumers because they don't see what's withheld from their paychecks, and their federal taxes seem abstract and unalterable. But the insurance payments literally came out of everyone's pockets, to the tune of billions and billions of dollars. And the rising cost of insurance is the reason fewer and fewer people can get it. Had the research been done earlier, it would have cost millions. But the payoff would have been a saving of billions of unnecessary expenditures and costs for unnecessary side effects. So even though good research is very expensive, we can pay for it now or we can pay for it later, with huge costs in the meantime. Cost-effectiveness studies suggest that medical research delivers good value for money.[3] All of us, through our insurance companies and Medicare, have a financial stake in getting better and faster research done.

Instead of just paying for unproven but popular treatments, what if insurers made this deal: "We'll pay for the treatment, but only if you participate in a clinical trial to find out how well it really works"? This is exactly what Medicare did when it was faced with the prospect of covering an expensive new treatment for emphysema.

In the early 1990s, surgeons developed a new technique for treating severe emphysema. Patients with severe emphysema develop big empty cavities in the lungs that fill space in the chest, but don't provide any oxygen exchange like that of normal lung tissue. Sometimes these cavities come to occupy so much space inside the chest that it's hard for the patient to breathe in and out with the remaining functioning lung. The new technique allowed surgeons to remove the most severely affected parts of the lungs, freeing up space in the chest so that the remaining lung tissue could expand and function more efficiently. The new operation was called lung volume reduction surgery.

The operation seemed to make perfect sense. And patients were too eager to wait for definitive studies of the effectiveness of this treatment. They wanted immediate access to the procedure, assuming that it worked because it was new and because some surgeons were vocal advocates of it. Insurance companies and Medicare were reluctant to cover an unproven and expensive operation that might apply to many people, but patients were clamoring to their congressional representatives, among others, for access to the new operation. Because the new treatment wasn't a drug and involved only a modest device, there was no company to fund a trial and little FDA authority over the procedure.

As with many new technologies, the first researchers pursued case reports and small series of patients, inductive reasoning, and theoretical justification for the operation. Encouraging initial reports led to the treatment's widespread use, but there remained no definitive data on its effectiveness or safety. There was also wide variability in how the operation was performed.

Medicare took a remarkable step that may be a model for future technology evaluations. The agency decided that it wouldn't pay for the procedure except for patients who agreed to enter a randomized trial. Medicare would fund the costs of medical care for patients in the trial, and the National Institutes of Health (NIH) would organize the trial and pay for the research costs. The NIH would be responsible for designing the study, choosing the researchers, collecting the data, and analyzing the results.[4] Yet another federal agency, the Agency for Healthcare Research and Quality, would fund an economic analysis of data from the trial. Researchers enrolled the first patients in the study in 1998 and published the main results in 2003.[5]

Without this collaborative funding, which was novel, the trial would probably never have been done, because of the expense. The patient care alone was expected to cost around $70 million.[4] Because of the NIH involvement and the expertise of its researchers, the trial was rigorously designed and executed, with adequate numbers of patients, uniform procedures, and appropriate safety and ethical safeguards. Although this model created challenges and problems, and may not be applicable for every new treatment, we think it's a model that should be expanded.

If you're curious about the results of the trial, they were complex—emphasizing the value of a large, carefully designed study. First, patients with the most severe emphysema had a higher risk of dying with surgery than with nonsurgical treatment.[6] Even among the survivors in this severe group, quality of life wasn't improved with surgery. So we quickly learned that some patients shouldn't have the operation at all.

Even after excluding this high-risk group, the risk of early death was still greater in the surgery group: over 2 percent after one month, compared to less than half a percent for the nonsurgery group. Long-term mortality was similar in the two groups. Even so, the researchers determined that there was a subgroup that had worse survival with surgery, and one that had better survival with surgery.[5] Overall, quality of life favored the surgery group. So, because of the study, we have a much better idea of which patients are likely to be helped by the new treatment and which ones are more likely to be hurt. The modest benefits of surgery came at a high price. (For aficionados of cost-effectiveness analysis, it cost an estimated $190,000 per year of "quality-adjusted" life gained, compared to the nonsurgical treatment.[7]) Medicare chose to cover the operation only for the carefully selected subgroup who stood to benefit.

This isn't the only example of an insurer getting involved with funding of research. When high-dose chemotherapy with bone marrow transplantation for late-stage breast cancer was gaining in popularity, some private insurers helped to fund the clinical trials that provided definitive results.[8] But these examples still aren't the norm. Because insurers are the ones who may have to pay for ineffective, unproven treatments, they have an incentive to help fund better and earlier research. And remember, of course, that the source of all insurance funds is our own pockets, so we all individually share the incentive.

We think private insurers should help to support the testing of novel treatments in clinical trials, just as Medicare did with lung volume reduction surgery. At the same time, they could resist paying for the treatments outside of rigorous studies designed to determine if the treatments work.[9] And Medicare should do more of the same.

Insurers resist paying for research because the routine medical care alone is so expensive, even without adding any research costs. Yet by avoiding paying for the research, they pay billions of dollars for useless or harmful therapy every year. If every medical insurance company and government payer—including Medicare, Medicaid, the VA, and the military—

set aside just 1 percent of its budget for research on treatment effectiveness, this would generate around $10 billion per year to help find better answers. An expert panel recently suggested that even one-quarter of one percent of the budgets of all the stakeholders would provide sufficient support for a new "National Clinical Research Enterprise."[10] This would complement the $27 billion budget of the NIH, which would continue to support both basic biological and clinical research.

Reporting *All* the Research Results

We've seen that drug and device makers sometimes suppress research results that are unfavorable to their products. Sometimes they publish favorable data from the same patients several times, creating redundant research reports that make it hard to know just how many studies were really done and how many patients were studied.

Companies provide some research results to the FDA in order to gain approval for new products, but they aren't required to publish these results where other scientists and doctors can evaluate them. For example, a recent systematic review on nonsteroidal anti-inflammatory drugs—ibuprofen, naproxen, Celebrex, Vioxx, and others—found that only one of thirty-seven studies reported in FDA reviews had been published.[11]

And the problem with unpublished research goes even farther. Many randomized trials get started but are never finished, for a variety of reasons. These rarely get reported, but they may offer important insights to doctors and patients.[12] Even when trials are completed, the ones that turn out negative—that is, showing no advantage for a new treatment—are less likely to get published than the ones that are positive.[13,14] Some clinical trials get reported only verbally at research meetings or in meeting abstracts; some never get published at all.[15]

The reasons are complex, but it appears likely that when the results of their research are negative, researchers often lose their enthusiasm and fail to write up the results and submit them for publication. Less often, journal editors or reviewers may be biased against publishing negative studies. Even if all the trials on a topic do get published, the ones with positive results tend to get published faster than the ones with negative results.[13] Therefore, the good news about a treatment often appears well before the bad news. The media coverage, in turn, tends to be unrealistically favorable.

The greater likelihood for favorable studies than for negative studies to get published has been labeled *publication bias*. The bias it creates in adopting medical advances may actually harm patients. As an example, one study of drugs for suppressing abnormal heart rhythms was completed in 1980, but was not published until 1993.[16] The study showed higher mortality in the group with the active drug than with placebo, consistent with the later studies of encainide and flecainide. Had these negative results been widely known, some experts believe that the use of dangerous drugs might have decreased sooner, saving many lives. Besides distorting the evidence for what works, failure to publish leads to waste and duplication in research efforts.

Consequently, many scientists, journal editors, expert panels, and even presidential committees have argued for a system that would register all clinical trials.[15] The NIH and some other groups have made steps in this direction, but they've been only partly successful. Even though the FDA has mandated registration of clinical trials evaluating new drugs for serious or life-threatening diseases, it has no mechanism for enforcement, and compliance appears to be poor. The barriers have been reluctance of the drug industry to participate, lack of funding, lack of any enforcement authority, and lack of publicity or awareness.[15]

In late 2004, this issue is coming to a head, after allegations that drug companies tried to suppress studies showing a higher risk of suicidal behavior among children taking antidepressants. In September, a group of twelve editors from prestigious medical journals announced they would refuse to publish results from drug companies' clinical trials unless they were listed at the outset on a national registry of clinical trials. Details of study design would have to be provided before patients were enrolled and before any results were known.

Congressional hearings also began in September, inquiring into possible suppression of data on antidepressants. Legislation was being formulated to require disclosure of all clinical trial results. PhRMA, the drug industry group, announced a proposal for a voluntary registry. This was criticized by journal editors, however, who argued that a voluntary registry wouldn't guard against suppression of unfavorable results. They felt an independent registry was essential. How far these efforts will be pursued, and how effective they will be, remains to be seen.

So we agree with recommendations from Kay Dickersin, director of the U.S. Cochrane Center in San Francisco, and Drummond Rennie, deputy editor of the *Journal of the American Medical Association.* They recommend several steps, including NIH leadership in developing a comprehensive registry, a requirement of ethical review that trials be registered, an agreement within the drug industry to register trials, a requirement by medical journals that trials be registered if they are to be published, and a change in federal law requiring that registration be part of the mandatory ethical review process.[15]

As Dickersin and Rennie argue, this may be an important issue for patient advocacy organizations to take up. Not only would registration of clinical trials guard against suppression of critical results or duplicate presentation of results, it would improve access to clinical trials by interested patients. In fact, one early impetus for creating a clinical trial registry came from a desire to make clinical trials known to cancer patients and their doctors. Before agreeing to participate in a clinical trial, patients should insist that the trial be listed in a central registry. This would help to assure adequate numbers of patients in clinical trials, and would allow patients who wish to contribute to new knowledge to do so. This, in turn, would speed the delivery of the best treatments to the medical community and to the public.

Increasing Participation in Research and Making Subjects Better Informed

Once patients understand how little is known about most medical problems and treatments, perhaps their interest in being participants in medical research will increase. Some experts believe that patients who are enrolled in clinical trials get better medical care than those outside clinical trials, regardless of whether they are receiving an experimental treatment or standard care.[17] And participating in research is the best way to get better answers about what really works.

It's disappointing that only about 3 percent of adult cancer patients participate in research studies. In contrast, over 70 percent of children with cancer are enrolled in clinical trials.[18] High participation in clinical trials among kids has made it possible to answer some important medical and scientific questions in a timely manner, even for rare diseases. If research participation among adults were as high, we'd have a much better chance of separating the lemons from the cherries among new treatments before we spend huge sums on the lemons. This is exactly the argument of retired

General Norman Schwartzkopf and chair of Paramount studios Sherry Lansing, who have written to encourage wider participation in research among cancer patients.[19]

We'll expand on this point when we talk about empowering patients, because we think this really is a form of empowerment. Of course, this assumes that patients are appropriately informed when they enter trials, and there's still room for improvement on this score. But then, patients who seek experimental treatments outside of clinical trials, convinced that they're getting the "newest treatment," are also often poorly informed about the true state of knowledge. They may be guinea pigs without realizing it at all.

One aspect of informed consent that should be assured is that patients understand the researchers' conflicts of interest. If the researchers hold stock in the company that makes the products they're testing, patients should know that. If the researchers have a grant from the manufacturer to do the research, patients should know that. If the researchers receive a special reimbursement for every subject they enroll, patients should know that. And if the researchers simply get consulting fees from the corporate sponsor of the research, patients should know that, too.

Surprisingly, this information, and even the identity of the research sponsor, isn't currently a required part of the informed consent process at many institutions. We think that such disclosures should be a routine aspect of the ethical review process and a part of every research consent form.

Evidence-Based Insurance Coverage

Making insurance coverage decisions is a hot potato—something no one really wants to do. As we'll see, several federal agencies have been driven out of existence because of a perception that their recommendations would hurt commercial interests. Policy makers effectively turned the decisions over to managed care in the 1990s, and it seriously wounded managed care. The decisions now are largely in the hands of Medicare and private insurers, who often follow Medicare's lead.

In the past, the insurance industry simply covered anything that was judged appropriate by expert opinion and "accepted" medical practice. Increasingly, it's trying to move toward decisions based on rigorous and systematic evaluation of the evidence.[20]

This sometimes means that there's a gap between FDA approval and coverage decisions. Remember that FDA approval doesn't mean that a product is the best or most efficient for a given purpose. Remember also that approval may come before major risks are recognized. Because the FDA can base its approval on surrogate outcomes, it may not even mean that a product has a net benefit in terms of quality or length of life. Finally, remember that once a product has been approved for any purpose, doctors can legally prescribe it for other purposes, whether or not there's evidence to support those uses. These are the reasons insurance companies are now trying to make their own decisions, and FDA approval alone isn't a deciding factor.

The idea of requiring good evidence for coverage decisions is embraced, in principle, by most stakeholders. But in practice, doctors, patients, manufacturers, and advocacy groups have often been unpleasantly surprised by, and vocally opposed to, some decisions that arose from evidence-based methods. In such cases, media tactics, lawsuits, and political influence are often used to override the best evidence.

The story of high-dose chemotherapy with bone marrow transplantation for late-stage breast cancer (presented in Chapter 11) offered one of the clearest examples, and illustrated a range of tactics. Many insurers resisted coverage for this procedure based on the lack of evidence for its safety and efficacy. Nonetheless, lawsuits, threatened lawsuits, and eventually even state laws forced them to cover it. Make no mistake—that requirement cost all of us in the form of higher insurance premiums and higher taxes. In the end, the insurance companies' skepticism was valid, but a host of nonscientific forces made an evidence-based coverage decision impossible.

Of course, insurance companies won't always be right. Sometimes well-intentioned people come to different conclusions, even when they are looking at the same evidence. And the evidence for or against a given treatment will change over time, reaching successively better approximations of the truth. Like science in general, evidence-based principles aren't infallible. Furthermore, insurers drag their feet when they perceive that it's in their best interest.

In part for these reasons, Harvard psychiatrist James Sabin and Tufts ethicist Norman Daniels argue that insurance coverage decisions should meet three key conditions. First, the rationale for a decision should be clear and publicly available. Second, the rationale should explain how the decision promotes "value for money" in meeting the varied health needs of a defined population within reasonable financial constraints. And third, there should be a mechanism for challenge, dispute resolution, and the introduction of new facts and arguments.[21]

Evidence-based clinical guidelines prepared by multidisciplinary groups with transparent methods can help insurers in making coverage decisions. Truly independent guidelines may help stakeholders to achieve some common understanding. But what about the problem of making decisions early in the life of a new treatment, often before definitive studies are available and while the treatment itself may be rapidly changing?

As Medicare official Steven Scheingold suggests, this is a situation in which simple yes-or-no decisions may not be consistent with evidence-based thinking. In contrast to the usual all-or-none approach, insurers should have the option of providing provisional coverage while more experience is gained. This leaves open the option of reversing or modifying the decision. Insurers should also have the option of giving partial coverage—say, for the use of a drug or device for one purpose, but not for others. Another important option, which we've already alluded to, is to provide coverage only in the context of clinical trials, so that we can acquire stronger evidence for or against a new treatment when little is available.[20]

Though they aren't the sole solution, evidence-based approaches to insurance coverage make good sense, and we'd argue for giving them a better chance to work. Of course, using them rigorously and in a timely manner will require expertise and money, but the investment would be a good one. Politicians, manufacturers, advocacy groups, and the media are less likely to produce valid decisions using their usual methods.

What Kind of Research?

Funding from the NIH has historically focused on basic biomedical research. This is the type of research that goes on in laboratories; it involves test tubes, centrifuges, cell cultures, and mice. It's focused on understanding the basic behavior of molecules, cells, and tissues. It doesn't generally involve human beings as subjects. Some people believe that more of this basic research will solve our health-care cost problems. The director of the NIH, Dr. Elias Zerhouni, reportedly has said, "Only a revolutionary understanding of disease process can put a brake on these costs." He went on to say that the solution might be both prevention and "molecular pre-emption of disease."[22]

The early promise of the human genome project was that we would understand The Cause of many diseases, and be able to develop true preventions and cures. Molecular biology, embodied in the genome project, has been the darling of NIH.

And yet, the insights of the human genome project so far have largely been to teach us that genes are rarely deterministic. Instead, multiple genes often interact with each other and with environmental factors to raise or lower the likelihood of a disease, rather than "causing" it in some absolute, highly predictable way. Those environmental factors include nutrition, exercise, smoking habits, chemical exposures, infections, and the like. In the words attributed to Judith Stern, a professor of nutrition at the University of California at Davis, "Genetics may load the gun, but environment pulls the trigger."[23]

In other words, the chronic diseases that most plague our society in the twenty-first century—diabetes, heart disease, strokes, cancer, AIDS—all have a great deal to do with lifestyle and behavior, not just bad luck in inheriting genes. Think of the roles of cigarette smoking, overeating, sedentariness, sexual practices, and drug use in these conditions.

Optimal care for or prevention of these problems is increasingly complex, and we're asking patients to take a more active role in their own care. This includes lifestyle changes, but also following complicated medication regimens, self-monitoring, rehabilitation, and the like. Taking advantage of medical advances increasingly requires that patients have literacy, computer skills, education, income, and the ability to follow complex instructions. We can't expect that smoking, overeating, sedentariness, sexual practices, or difficulty with medications will yield to a new pill, gene assay, implant, or surgical technique.[24] Hence the need for more "biobehavioral" research.

Also, as we've seen, changing a physiological measure, like extra heartbeats, doesn't necessarily translate into tangible benefits. There often are surprises between the laboratory and the medicine cabinet. Even promising biomedical research findings need to be tested as they'd actually be used in real life. Hence the need for more clinical research on treatment effectiveness, and especially clinical trials.

Research on prevention, epidemiology, treatment effectiveness, and delivery of health-care services is sometimes dismissed as boring and bureaucratic.[24] But we'd argue that the national research portfolio needs to include a substantial program in health behavior, helping to understand how individuals can make best use of new biological knowledge to prevent or treat disease. It needs to include a major commitment to clinical trials and posttreatment surveillance if we are to understand the effectiveness and safety of promising treatments that arise from basic biological research. And it needs to include the study of health-care quality and efficiency if we are to make the fruits of basic biomedical research widely available.

Ultimately, we all have an interest in getting better and faster research results when new technology emerges. The strategies of having insurers provide better support for research, registering all clinical trials, promoting wider participation in high-quality research, encouraging evidence-based insurance coverage, and broadening the research portfolio would serve us all well.

19

For All Decision Makers

Getting Value for Money

As a society, sooner or later we will have to determine whether there are some benefits that are just too small to justify the cost. —David Eddy, MD[1]

SO FAR, we've focused mainly on treatments that turned out to be useless, that did more harm than good, or that were both less effective and more expensive than alternatives. In cases like these, it's easy to decide against routinely using the new treatment. No sensible person wants ineffective or harmful treatment. No one wants a more expensive treatment if a less expensive one is just as good. If we were more discriminating in the use of these treatments, we'd save billions every year.

But more common, more challenging, and more painful is the situation where a new treatment has some very small advantage over alternative treatments, but at a very high price. The number of such treatments is enormous, and we're definitely paying for them. Most of us would agree that an expensive new treatment is worth the added cost if there's a big bang for the buck. We don't mind rising health-care costs when the benefits are substantial. We're not necessarily looking to save money on health care, just to get value for our money.

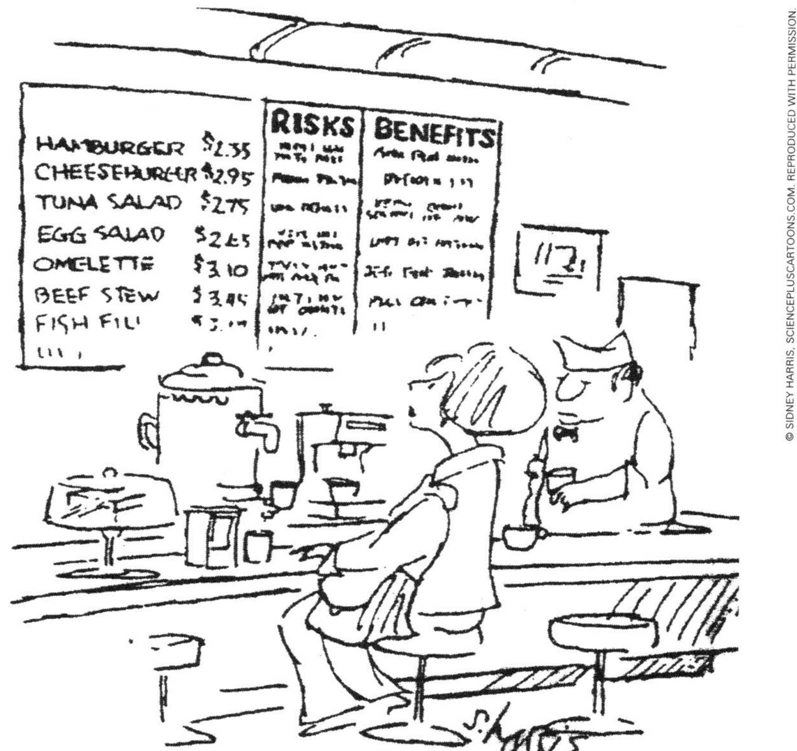

Unfortunately, as we all know, medical care is becoming unaffordable. Insurance covers more and more marginally useful new treatments, but fewer and fewer people have adequate insurance coverage for even the highly effective basics. We have to ask, are the benefits of some treatments so small and the costs so high that we shouldn't even make the treatments available?

There are no easy answers here. What looks like a trivial benefit to one person may look pretty important to another. When the patient is me or a member of my family, I may grasp at any straw. But some straws may not be worth grasping.

Some Cases to Ponder

CHEMOTHERAPY FOR LUNG CANCER

Consider different chemotherapy treatments for lung cancer. Recent studies compared five different treatment regimens and found that none of them resulted in better survival than the others.[2,3] The average survival was only eight months regardless of therapy. Side effects differed somewhat among the regimens, and it appeared that patients treated with carboplatin plus Taxol had somewhat less nausea than patients given the other treatments. As we noted in Chapter 13, the magnitude of this benefit remains a bit unclear, though, because patients in the Taxol group used more antinausea drugs. And, of course, drugs for nausea are an option with any of the treatments. Furthermore, overall quality of life measures were the same among the different groups. Nonetheless, the major cancer research groups in the United States adopted the carboplatin and Taxol treatment as the standard regimen for comparison in future studies.[3,4] So far, so good.

But consider the costs. Scott Ramsey, the doctor and economist at the University of Washington and the Fred Hutchinson Cancer Research Center, undertook a careful evaluation of the all the costs associated with the different treatment strategies. The new "standard regimen" costs up to $12,000 more per patient than the least expensive treatment. The more expensive treatment offered no savings in downstream costs like further hospitalization, emergency visits for treating side effects, other drugs, or blood transfusions. Given that almost 105,500 persons are diagnosed with this type of cancer each year, using the carboplatin and Taxol regimen as first-line therapy will cost about $1 billion more per year than the alternative treatments.[4]

Of course, what isn't clear from these studies is whether any of these chemotherapy treatments offer an improvement in quality or length of life compared to supportive care alone. And if so, how much?

Is $1 billion a year a reasonable price to pay for an uncertain reduction in nausea over an eight-month period for patients who are terminally ill? Before you answer, consider that insurers, who work within a budget, will have to cover these costs. To do so, they'll have to stop paying for other things, reduce the amount they pay for various services, or charge you higher premiums. Would you be happy to increase your insurance costs or your Medicare taxes to cover this particular treatment?

Medicare covers most patients with lung cancer, and there's little appetite for increasing Medicare taxes. Congress gives Medicare a fixed budget, and the agency is struggling to keep up with rapidly rising costs. In recent years, Medicare officials have sometimes decided to shrink payments to doctors rather than eliminate coverage for other services. Because of the cuts, some doctors have declared that they'll no longer care for new Medicare patients.[5] We have to consider this kind of trade-off if we want the more expensive new chemotherapy program.

NEW ANTI-INFLAMMATORY DRUGS FOR ARTHRITIS

Many people are familiar with the new arthritis drugs, Celebrex, Vioxx, and Bextra. They are so extensively advertised on TV that you could hardly miss them. Though the ads give the impression that these drugs offer a breakthrough in treatment effectiveness, all indications are that they're no more effective than older and cheaper drugs like ibuprofen and naproxen. What they may offer is a slightly reduced risk of stomach irritation and less risk of bleeding from the stomach. The cost of the newer medicines is five to ten times more than that of the older drugs.

To compare treatment costs and benefits for a nonfatal disease like arthritis, analysts often try to estimate the quality-of-life improvements from a new treatment. This makes it possible to give credit to a treatment that improves quality of life, but doesn't necessarily make people live longer. This is the situation for most medical treatments.

In the case of the new arthritis drugs, quality of life may be improved over the older drugs because the new drugs cause less belly pain and slightly less risk of bleeding. Because the new drugs reduce bleeding, using them may save some of the money used to treat the bleeding that occurs with the older drugs. Over a long period and many patients, the new drugs may even prevent a small number of deaths, though this is speculation. In fact, some may increase the risk of heart disease, so any benefit for survival is completely unclear.

Analysts try to calculate "quality-adjusted life years" as a way of giving credit to treatments that yield little or no benefit in terms of survival, but improve quality of life. There are some formal, but complicated, ways of trying to estimate how valuable an improvement is. For example, we might ask people how many days or weeks or months of life they'd be willing to give up in exchange for less belly pain and a lower risk of bleeding. That can give us an idea of how many quality-adjusted life years we gain from a treatment. These estimates are crude and controversial, but they give some ballpark figures of value for money.

Some expensive but widely accepted medical treatments cost in the range of $50,000 per quality-adjusted life year gained. Comparing the newer arthritis drugs with the older ones, one credible estimate is that it costs $250,000 plus for each quality-adjusted life year gained.[6]

Ponder for a moment some things we might do with that money. Would those other things improve your quality of life? Are these new arthritis drugs the best use of your dollars? Of our collective dollars?

LUNG VOLUME REDUCTION SURGERY

In the previous chapter, we described and admired a study of lung volume reduction surgery for patients with severe emphysema. The study found that some patients were made worse by the operation, but some were made better. Remember that overall, there was no improvement in survival, but there was a modest improvement in quality of life. Among patients who got the operation, medical bills in the first year averaged $63,000, compared with $13,000 for similar patients who got standard nonsurgical treatment.[7]

No one knows how many patients there are who might benefit from the operation, or how many would want it. But estimates are that offering the treatment will cost Medicare between $1 billion and $15 billion each year. Identifying the small group that benefits most certainly helps to improve cost-effectiveness, but costs are high even for this subgroup.

Medicare is also facing costs for expensive new coronary artery stents, implantable heart defibrillators, and special pumps to help failing hearts. All of these are likely to add billions in costs to a program that's already in financial straits.[8] The Medicare board of trustees recently estimated that under current conditions, the Medicare hospital insurance trust fund will be unable to cover its expenses by 2019.[9] Given the modest benefits of lung volume reduction surgery, we might reasonably ask if it's good value for money.

PEDICLE SCREWS FOR THE SPINE

We've already reviewed the evidence that the use of pedicle screws for spinal fusion surgery causes more complications than performing a fusion without the hardware. We've also seen that pedicle screws generally don't improve the results, in terms of pain relief and improved function.[10] Nonetheless, one group of researchers made the assumption that there was some small advantage in quality of life as a result of using the screws and tried to estimate the cost of adding the screws for each quality-adjusted year of life gained. Their best estimate was that adding pedicle screws to the procedure costs over $3 million per quality-adjusted year of life gained.[11] Are there ways to spend $3 million that would have more benefit for more people?

CHOLESTEROL DRUGS IN LOW-RISK PATIENTS

In many cases, new technology is a good value when doctors use it for certain types of patients, but not for others. The trick is to figure out who benefits most and use the new technology selectively. Cholesterol lowering offers a good example.

For people at high risk of having a heart attack, the use of cholesterol-lowering drugs seems to offer good value. In a man over age fifty-five with a cholesterol over three hundred and three other risk factors for heart disease (such as smoking, high blood pressure, and diabetes), treatment with a statin-type drug for lowering cholesterol probably costs about $20,000 per year of life saved.[12]

But in a low-risk person, the value of treatment is considerably less. For a forty-year-old woman with high cholesterol but no other risk factors, statin therapy would cost about $2 million per year of life saved.[12] Many people would therefore say, don't bother testing for cholesterol in such a low-risk person. But it happens routinely, and many such patients are treated.

So for many treatments, value for money isn't an all-or-nothing thing. For some kinds of patients the value may be excellent, and for others it may be terrible. If doctors aren't highly selective about whom they treat, even the value of effective treatments shrinks fast. Yet past history tells us doctors and patients both have difficulty saying no.

Economics and Decision Making

"But wait," you may protest, "all life is precious, and we can't attach a value to it." But we have to realize that the $2 million we would spend to save one year of life for a low-risk person might save many more lives if we used it instead for more efficient treatments. As Richard Lamm, former governor of Colorado, notes, "In public policy, everything we do prevents us from doing something else. Paying for treatment A to patient B, prevents us from delivering treatment Y to patient Z."[13]

Dr. David Eddy, an expert in clinical decision making and operations research, has offered some excellent examples of how this might work, for example, in a managed-care plan. We won't try to reproduce the math and the details here. But by focusing on treatment strategies that deliver high value for money, a health plan actually saves more lives than by paying for expensive services that provide only minor benefits.[14,15]

In other words, by paying high prices for small benefits, we actually may end up saving fewer lives than we might otherwise. We lose some patients who can't get more effective treatments that are less expensive. The treatments we've listed here don't appear to be useless, but the benefits seem small compared to the costs. Of course, if any savings were redistributed, we'd all need reassurance that it wasn't simply getting siphoned off to pay for ineffective treatments, to increase corporate profits, or to raise the CEO's salary.

So, are you willing to pay for these treatments? Whether you realize it or not, you *are* paying for them. You're paying in the form of higher insurance premiums, higher Medicare taxes, more out-of-pocket health-care costs, and higher prices for the consumer goods you buy. Employer-sponsored insurance premiums rose 14 percent in 2003, compared to an increase in gross domestic product of 2.7 percent. Experts forecast double-digit premium increases again for 2004.[16] One way or another, those costs get passed on to us.

The rapid growth of modestly effective, but very expensive treatments like those described here is the main reason why health insurance costs are rising so fast, with so little to show for it in terms of longevity or other public health statistics. It's also why fewer and fewer people can afford insurance at all. Are these treatments good value for money? We don't pretend to know the answer, but we do know that we can't afford every new test or treatment that will increase costs this much—and there are hundreds waiting for a coverage decision.

Richard Lamm, the former governor, argues that unless we address the questions of trade-offs and limits, we'll continue to move enormous amounts of resources into "marginal medicine." He believes that medical school culture, the legal system, and our insurance system are all programmed to maximize marginal medicine.[13]

Right now, we generally avoid deciding what's too expensive, and agree to cover nearly everything that offers even trivial benefits. This prices more and more people out of any health insurance and increases the amount you have to pay out of pocket. If health-care costs keep rising much faster than inflation, the logical extension is that at some point, our entire national wealth will go for health care. At some point, we may collectively decide that this isn't the best strategy.

Much as we may want to, we can't ignore the costs of new treatments. We'll have to decide if certain benefits are too small to justify the costs. In order to do so, we'll need better information on what new treatments will cost and what the real benefits will be. In other words, we need more good studies of effectiveness and of value for money. We'll also need to have that information communicated to consumers and doctors more clearly and completely. These needs are a legitimate—even essential—part of the research agenda.

Americans value autonomy and choice highly, so they may be unwilling to deny new treatments to those who want them, even when the value is modest relative to the cost. So we agree with those who argue for a solution that seems in keeping with American perspectives. Such a system might offer extensive information about the real clinical value of medical advances, and require higher out-of-pocket costs when these values are small.[16] This would force each of us to ask not just "Is this treatment worth it when someone else is subsidizing most of the cost," but "Is it worth it if I have to pay for a big chunk of it directly?"

Better data on clinical effectiveness and on value for money won't answer the tough questions for us. Decisions about what services to provide and pay for will never be based on economic analyses alone. But so-called cost-effectiveness studies may help to provide the information we need to inform both group and individual value judgments. Unfortunately, the value judgments can't be avoided.

20

For Government

Regulatory Approaches to Improve the Dissemination of Medical Innovations

A government, for protecting business only, is but a carcass, and soon fails by its own corruption and decay. —Amos Bronson Alcott, 1799–1888

There's no trick to being a humorist when you have the whole government working for you. —Will Rogers, 1879–1935

PITY YOUR poor senators and congressional Representatives. Many of them complain about the FDA's dragging its feet on approving new drugs and devices. They also want to promote business, so they favor policies that are good for drug and device manufacturers. They want jobs in their states and districts, so they eagerly promote the growing biotech industry and the jobs it creates. This leads them, in turn, to support rapid growth at the National Institutes of Health, which generates much of the basic scientific research leading to new products. They push Medicare to approve coverage of new gadgets and treatments more quickly. They want ever more medical innovations, and they want them disseminated ever more rapidly. Good for business, good for medicine, good for votes.

But while they argue for faster development, approval, and coverage of expensive new treatments, they complain that Medicare costs too much. The Medicare budget is rising too fast, and the aging population is rapidly increasing demand. Prescription drug coverage will add enormous expenses, and no one can figure out how to pay for it all. Furthermore, the number of uninsured Americans continues to rise as health insurance becomes more and more expensive. Do we raise taxes, cut benefits, tighten the eligibility criteria, or what?

We suspect that many lawmakers don't see a connection between the two issues: promoting rapid innovation and balancing the health-care budget. They frequently claim that the problems behind rising health-care costs are fraud and abuse, bureaucratic inefficiency, or insufficient market forces. But as we've seen, the major reason for rising health-care costs and shrinking insurance coverage is the rapid introduction of new medical treatments, often before they can be adequately evaluated for effectiveness, safety, or cost.

All the administrative reorganizing, exposing of fraud and abuse, and financial restructuring in the world aren't going to contain health-care costs unless new treatments can be more effectively managed. Our elected representatives can't have both: every promising but unproven or marginally effective medical innovation and affordable coverage.

In some cases, politicians are responding to constituents and advocacy groups, but often it's to lobbyists and campaign contributors. As we've seen, the drug industry is one of the greatest political benefactors in Washington (and the state legislatures), as well as a great benefactor to many advocacy groups. The device industry, organized medicine, and hospitals have powerful lobbies as well, often advocating for what is likely to be lucrative new technology.

So far, in their efforts to contain health-care costs, it seems that most politicians and administrators have tried to pass the buck on difficult individual decisions about which medical advances to support and which to let languish. It's easier to increase premiums, push more out-of-pocket costs, tweak financial incentives, seek out fraud and abuse, blame malpractice lawyers, or simply make fewer people eligible.

But we suspect that the tough job of slogging through scientific evidence—and often insisting on better evidence—for new devices, drugs, or operations can't be avoided. Blanket decisions won't work. Our current approach—simply denying any insurance coverage to more and more people—seems a risky course for both individuals and society. Simply paying for any innovation that any company, inventor, doctor, politician, or patient can think of is also a strategy that won't work.

The FDA approval process is critically important and valuable, but as we've seen, the FDA has no mandate or budget for many of the evaluations we need. Individual insurance carriers can continue to make decisions about coverage, but this strategy results in widely variable decisions and enormous duplication of effort. Some of those decisions are capricious, the process is rarely visible, and many decisions end up being challenged in court. Are there regulatory approaches to improving the dissemination of medical innovations that would be acceptable to Americans and more effective than the current process?

Changes in Marketing

Marketing of new drugs and devices clearly has its place. But its place shouldn't be to sell doctors and patients on products they don't need, products that barely work, or products that are more expensive but no better than readily available alternatives. Despite the ads, the "latest and greatest" is often only the most expensive. We can't afford the cost in dollars or in adverse effects.

Except among drug and device manufacturers, tighter controls on certain aspects of drug marketing would be welcome. For example, recent changes in the drug industry have reduced some gifts to doctors, but others persist, and the changes are voluntary. Some states, like Vermont, have proposed that drug companies be required to report any gifts to doctors that are over $25 in value.[1] Though the definition of a gift may sometimes be ambiguous, this seems like a good start.

The Bush administration has proposed guidelines that would also address switching arrangements, in which doctors receive gifts for switching patients from one drug to another or for getting new drugs added to hospital or organizational formularies. Not surprisingly, drug companies and the American Medical Association have opposed the guidelines, although consumer groups like the AARP have supported them.[2] We think they're a good idea.

A related practice that seems to escape the gift-giving guidelines is the use of payments to physicians for attending meetings of "advisory committees." An example recently cited in the press was a meeting of psychiatrists for dinner at the Omni Berkshire Place Hotel in Manhattan. The doctors were paid $300 for participating in the dinner, where they discussed using the drug Carbatrol for bipolar disorder (also known as manic-depressive illness). The FDA had not even approved the medicine for this purpose.[1] We think that such payments, like gifts, should be outlawed or be reported. Similar restrictions need to be placed on device manufacturers, some of whose "consulting" or "advising" fees look suspiciously like kickbacks for using their products.[3] Reducing the exposure of medical students and residents to drug reps is another strategy to consider.[4]

The accuracy of drug ads directed toward both doctors and the public should be routinely assured before the ads are printed or broadcast, not in hit-or-miss fashion afterwards. Some medical editors have suggested creating a drug "advertising advisory board," with representation from health professionals, consumers, institutions, drug manufacturers, government, and the media. This board would provide an independent review of advertisements before they become public. Professional organizations in both medicine and public health have endorsed the idea of mandatory pre-broadcast approval of drug ads.[5,6]

Another promising approach has been proposed by Senator Debbie Stabenow of Michigan. Stabenow suggests limiting the amount of a drug company's marketing expenses that can be claimed as a tax deduction. As things currently stand, drug companies can deduct both marketing and research costs from their taxable income. Stabenow would still allow deductions for both, but would limit the deduction for advertising to the amount deducted for research. So if a company spends more on marketing than on research, its marketing tax deduction couldn't exceed the amount deducted for research. Stabenow noted, "Our concern is that market research not be more important than medical research."[7,8]

Others in Congress and the Bush administration have proposed various types of legislation that would encourage faster emergence of generic drugs, with lower prices than brand-name drugs. For example, the seemingly limitless ability of drug companies to extend their patents on drugs might be curtailed by appropriate legislation. Such efforts would help to make drugs more affordable and would at least limit the period of the most aggressive advertising of new drugs.[9,10]

The drug industry generally argues that such measures stifle lifesaving research, their mantra for opposing all controls on the industry. But given the magnitude of their profits, the actual allocation of their resources, their proclivity for spending research dollars on lucrative "me too" drugs, and their already drying pipeline of new drugs, we're skeptical of the claim. Furthermore, the National Institutes of Health, which sponsors most of the basic science that leads to true breakthroughs, is still going strong. Even further measures to speed the introduction of generic drugs and curb patent abuses would be welcome.

Approval and Monitoring of Drugs and Devices

Drug approval requires the most rigorous form of testing: randomized controlled trials. Yes, there are some problems and shortfalls with the information from these studies, but certain biases are reduced or eliminated when the trials are well conducted. Knowing whether a new heart valve, artificial hip, or spine screw is safe and effective seems just as important as knowing whether drugs are safe and effective. Maybe more so, since implants can't be easily reversed, like stopping a drug.

Yet in many cases, the strength of evidence required for approving medical devices falls far short of that required for drugs. The strategy of gaining regulatory approval by claiming that nearly all new devices are equivalent to something used prior to 1976 is silly and inadequate. Let's do away with the double standard and require the same rigor of evidence for devices that we ask of drugs—at least for more of the devices that carry the greatest costs or risks.

Performing randomized trials of devices is in some ways more challenging than performing randomized trials of drugs, but it's certainly not impossible. There would need to be careful methodological development in this area, but the issues are too important to ignore.

An important reform that is needed for both drugs and devices is more rigorous surveillance of safety after the products are marketed. This is often when rare but serious complications first become apparent, but current monitoring depends heavily on haphazard reporting by doctors. One drug expert has suggested that only 1 percent of adverse effects of new drugs get reported.[11] Experts have outlined the need for a more proactive system for monitoring safety and have suggested new research approaches to identifying adverse effects.[12,13]

Better surveillance would require more resources; the number of people and the FDA budget for surveillance are almost laughably small for the task of monitoring the over five thousand drugs that are currently on the market.[12,14] Also, as we've seen, relying on user fees to pay the bills at the FDA makes the agency beholden to the drug and device companies. The companies become, in essence, sponsors of the agency. It makes sense for the industry to support the related regulatory functions, but perhaps a tax mechanism rather than a user fee would help to weaken the tie between agency support and approval of individual products.

Some experts suggest that an agency charged with monitoring drug safety should be independent of the FDA.[14] This would be analogous to

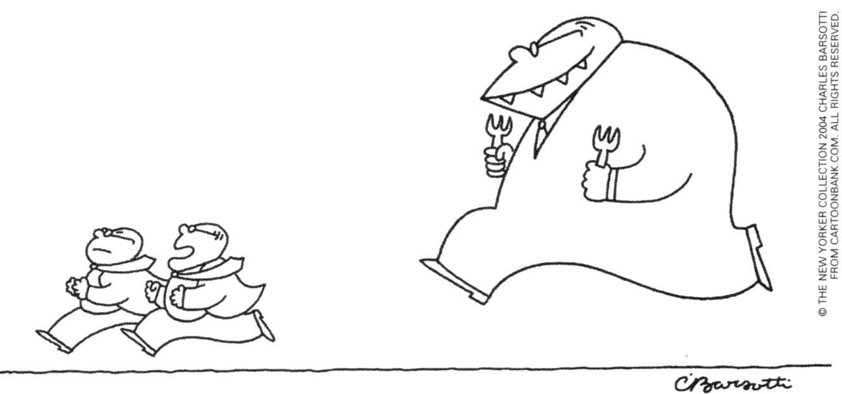

"No, I didn't. I never said there should be no government regulation."

the National Transportation Safety Board, which investigates plane crashes. It is separate from the Federal Aviation Administration and can therefore criticize both the airline industry and FAA standards, when appropriate. Such an agency might be asked to investigate all drug recalls, just as the NTSB investigates all plane crashes. The organization could ask whether warning signs were missed and whether other drugs may pose similar risks.

Advocates point out that a drug safety board might also help to protect manufacturers, to some degree. The antinausea drug Bendectin was forced off the market by lawsuits, for example, despite the absence of persuasive evidence that it was harmful. Similarly, many of the putative hazards of breast implants seem to have been overblown.

The tension between rapid approval of new products and thorough evaluation of safety and efficacy isn't going to go away. This suggests the value of more formal mechanisms for provisional approval of drugs and devices. That is, a drug or device might be given approval only for a limited period of time or in certain pilot markets, with thorough reevaluation required for full approval. This would limit the number of patients exposed to possible unknown risks prior to widespread marketing. It would also allow the FDA to impose rigorous criteria for further data collection and analysis (these tasks are now sometimes requested by the FDA, but the request is often ignored after a drug is approved). It would allow a new drug or device to be tested as it would actually be used in practice. This would include a wider range of patient ages and medical conditions than are typically included among the fastidiously selected patients who enter the clinical trials required for initial drug approval.

Similarly, insurers may wish to experiment with conditional and flexible coverage decisions, rather than simple yes-or-no decisions. The impact and cost of new treatments could then be evaluated in actual practice before making firm decisions. This approach might also encourage coverage for a drug or device for certain medical conditions, but not others. The notion of ongoing review through all stages of a product's life cycle should become routine. Both acceptances and refusals of coverage need to be continuously reevaluated in the light of new scientific research. Medicare has experimented with such flexible coverage decisions, and this approach should be encouraged.[15]

The changes we propose would be moderately expensive. The FDA would need a bigger budget. We think that's a good idea.

Comparing Drugs

In 2003, Representatives Tom Allen (D-Maine) and Jo Ann Emerson (R-Missouri) introduced a bill that would earmark funds specifically for comparing the cost and effectiveness of prescription drugs.[16] This is exactly the type of comparison that the FDA assiduously avoids. Lawmakers on both sides of the aisle have declared such comparisons to be key to reducing the cost of drugs. As Representative Nancy Johnson (R-Connecticut) said, "There are many expensive products on the market that are no better than aspirin. We need to be able to demonstrate that and provide senior citizens and all Americans with that information so they can choose the most cost-effective, medically effective pharmaceutical for their particular needs."[17]

The story of diuretic therapy versus expensive new blood pressure medications made the point dramatically. The ALLHAT study that showed diuretics to be equally or more effective was funded by the National Institutes of Health.[18] Ditto for the trial that demonstrated the dangers of encainide and flecainide for abnormal heart rhythms.[19] Ditto for the study showing that aspirin was as effective as ticlopidine for preventing strokes in African Americans.[20] These studies weren't required by the FDA and weren't carried out by the drug companies, which had no incentive to do them. Cost is obviously an issue, but it's not the only one. We'd all be willing to pay for drugs that are more effective or safer. These examples suggest that we need the comparisons for our own health, as well as for our pocketbooks.

Researchers suggest that direct drug comparisons might address, for example, whether cholesterol drugs that are now available inexpensively as generics are just as good as the expensive new ones, whether the newly generic version of Prilosec is just as good as newer medicines for heartburn and ulcers, and whether new anti-inflammatory drugs like Celebrex and Vioxx have any advantage over older drugs like ibuprofen and naproxen. There are plenty of other examples, and the agenda would be large.[17]

Not surprisingly, the pharmaceutical industry opposes such legislation. On the other hand, the AARP, some unions, companies like General Motors, and professional groups like the American Academy of Family Physicians support the efforts.[17] We think these comparisons would fill a critical need. Funding for the work might go to the NIH, to Medicare, to designated centers, or to a new agency. A strategy for prioritization would be critical.

Efforts to Provide Centralized Assessments

At this point, some people may logically be thinking, "Why not have a national clearinghouse to evaluate new drugs and technologies before they get widely disseminated and cost us all a fortune? The clearinghouse could define what works, what doesn't, what's safe, and how much it'll cost. Then insurance companies and Medicare would have a clearer idea of what's 'experimental' and what's 'standard care,' and coverage could be more consistent." Not a bad idea! But there's some history behind this idea that we have to consider.

Even in the 1960s and 1970s, many observers thought that it would be unreasonable for Medicare to pay for just anything and everything. According to Norm Weissman, PhD, who spent many years with the Public Health Service, the question people were asking about new treatments was, "Does this make a difference? Is it better? Is it going to make a difference in health care somehow?" The result was the creation of a Peer Review Office in the Public Health Service to help advise Medicare about coverage decisions. Weissman doesn't know the motivation, but he recalls that the office was killed by Senator Warren Magnuson from Washington state. It became the first of several now-defunct agencies intended to evaluate new medical technology.

In 1978, the Carter administration created the National Center for Health Care Technology, with a similar goal in mind. Norm Weissman became part of that center, but only briefly—because in January 1980, in one of his first acts as president, Ronald Reagan eliminated the agency. It actually ended its operations in December 1981.[21] Weissman says he later learned, informally, that the organizations representing the drug and device industries—PhRMA and AdvaMed under their earlier names—had brought pressure to eliminate the agency. AdvaMed, representing the medical device manufacturers, was then known as HIMA, the Health Industry Manufacturers Association.

The late Seymour Perry headed the center and wrote about the opposition of HIMA and also of the American Medical Association.[21] He concluded that the "unalterable bottom line for the Health Industry Manufacturer's Association in its opposition was the fear that the Center's activities had the potential ability to constrain industry's freedom in the marketplace." For the AMA, the fear seemed to be that doctors would lose the autonomy to make any decisions they wanted about new treatments. Perry noted that many other organizations, including the American College of Physicians, the Association of American Medical Colleges, and several insurance companies, urged the continuation of the agency, but Congress nonetheless ended its funding. Make that two government agencies for evaluating medical technology to die under political pressure.

That development left another government agency still in a position to evaluate new medical technology: the congressional Office of Technology Assessment. This office had been created in 1972, and it provided Congress with summaries on many scientific issues, not just those related to health care. It had three divisions, dealing with defense, transportation and energy, and health and life sciences. The office sometimes made recommendations regarding coverage of expensive new medical advances and was sometimes heavily lobbied by drug makers. But the office had bipartisan support for much of its life, and a bipartisan board endorsed nearly all its assessments. One exception, however, may have been important.

In the mid-1980's, the OTA issued a critique of Ronald Reagan's "Star Wars" Strategic Defense Initiative. This report was seen by some conservative Republicans—including Newt Gingrich—as biased and ideological.[22,23] When Gingrich became Speaker of the House in 1995, in a time of budget-cutting fervor, OTA got the hatchet. There were other criticisms of the agency, and other political factors may have been important, but a third agency that performed medical technology assessments came to a halt.

In 1989, yet another agency assumed some of the responsibility for evaluating medical technology—the Agency for Health Care Policy and Research. Congress gave the agency a mandate to produce clinical guidelines to try to make medical care more consistent. The agency also created Patient Outcome Research Teams to study what works and what doesn't work in each of several common disease areas.

We described in Chapter 14 how, again in 1995, this agency had a "near death" experience caused by the emergence of the new congressional leadership. Some members of Congress saw the director of the agency as a partisan for the Clinton health plan, and spine surgeons, aroused by research and guidelines that they opposed, had become committed enemies of the agency. Though the agency survived, it ended its guideline work, ended the Patient Outcome Research Teams, and suffered a substantial budget cut. Spine surgeons, who were concerned about reimbursement, and spine implant manufacturers had become some of the strongest opponents of the agency's work.[24]

Some of the work of assessing new treatments is still being done by the Agency for Health Care Policy and Research (under a new name), some is being done by the National Academy of Science, some is being done by Medicare itself, and some is being done by private insurance companies like Blue Cross/Blue Shield. But the work is fragmented and of variable quality. Furthermore, some highly desirable original research, like direct comparisons between competing drugs, isn't being consistently done by any of these groups. In its defense, the current approach is fairly low profile and diffused, so it's been tolerated by industry and politicians.

A Health Care "Fed"?

Some observers think there's a need for greater medical technology assessment capacity at a national level.[14, 25–27] Proposals to fund direct comparisons between drugs look smart to us, but what about comparisons of competing devices? What about comparing surgical treatments with drug treatments for the same condition? Important past studies have compared surgery versus drugs for heartburn, for angina, and for preventing strokes. The agenda clearly goes beyond drugs alone. If such comparative information were available to doctors, patients, employers, and insurers, it would go a long way toward helping all of us decide how to spend our healthcare dollars.

The demise of the National Center for Health Care Technology and the Office of Technology Assessment has to some degree left a void. If a new agency were to fill the void, it would need to be protected from both political and corporate pressures, like the U.S. Federal Reserve Board. Like the Federal Reserve Board, the new agency would need to be well respected, powerful, and independent. Unlike the Federal Reserve Board, though, a new health technology assessment center need not be regulatory. Instead, it would provide doctors, consumers, and insurers with the information they now lack for making the most effective and efficient medical decisions.[27]

Such a center would assume the painful role of assessing new tests and treatments one by one and helping us all make better-informed decisions. As some advocates have suggested, there may be no other way to assure that medical care is affordable and accessible to all Americans, whatever health-care financing structure you favor.

Princeton's highly regarded health economist, Uwe Reinhardt, envisions an organization that would set standards for measuring and reporting health-care quality as well as evaluate alternative treatment approaches. Reinhardt says, "Given what is at stake, would asking a 'Health Care Fed' to be funded with, say, one percent of total health care spending be that outrageous?"[28] That 1 percent of health-care spending would amount to several billion dollars—a good start for such a monumental task.

Most other developed countries now have medical technology assessment agencies. Some have argued that these agencies might provide models from which to create an American agency. There's an irony here: Most of the agencies in other countries were modeled after our own now-defunct Office of Technology Assessment.[29]

If the United States were to fund a major effort in this area, its success would depend on several commitments. While there are many advocates of such an effort, some realists fear that a new agency would be dead on arrival, given our past history. As Dartmouth's Dr. Jack Wennberg argues, such an effort requires:

> The long view: stable funding; strong peer review to assure good science and freedom from conflicts of interest that affect judgments; policies that sustain the careers of leading scientists over a professional lifetime (keeping them free of dependency on funding

from the drug and device companies whose products they evaluate); and deep commitment on the part of the scientific establishment, sufficient to withstand the wrath of practitioners and others with vested interests who find their favorite theories slain by evidence or demands for their services reduced because informed patients want less.[30]

21

For Consumers

Shared Decision Making

I know of no safe depository of the ultimate power of the society but the people themselves; and if we think them not enlightened enough to exercise their control with a wholesome discretion, the remedy is not to take it from them, but to inform their discretion. —Thomas Jefferson[1]

CONSUMERS HAVE a critically important role in helping to restrain the use of ineffective, marginal, or harmful new medical treatments. They create the demand for new treatments, and they ultimately pay for those treatments. They deserve their money's worth for these treatments, and their health may depend on them. Consumers have become more wary and more knowledgeable about many consumer products, like cars and stereos. But they typically have little experience on which to base their judgments about new medical technology. In an unfamiliar arena, they often have to trust expert advice.

And yet, as we've seen, medical technology includes some lemons, just like the car lots do. And sometimes even experts have sold lemons. Consumers may have faced buying a car or a house dozens of times, and gotten smarter about it each time. But when they are faced with a decision about treatment for breast cancer, whether or not to have back surgery, or which treatment is best for coronary heart disease, they're likely to be facing the decision for the first time, and the stakes are high.

In this situation, many people now turn to the Internet for information. Unfortunately, the accuracy of the medical information on the Internet is highly variable.[2,3] Many sites are designed to market a product, service, or facility. As we've seen, industry is a poor source of balanced or complete information. Worse, the average consumer finds it difficult to sort the wheat from the chaff and risks inadvertently fixing on information that really isn't relevant to his or her particular situation. Doctors should be able to help in this situation. Often, though, it's impossible to find the particular piece of information that we want most.

There may be several remedies for this situation, all of which require some cultural shifts by doctors, consumers, and even regulatory agencies. One is the evolution of patient decision aids that focus on particular medical decisions and summarize in an engaging fashion the benefits and risks of competing approaches. Another is open access by patients to their medical records. In an age when more and more medical records are electronic, this is increasingly feasible, and it is being pilot-tested in some cutting-edge health-care facilities. Some doctors at Dartmouth suggest requiring drug labels that mimic the nutritional labels now required on everything at the grocery store. Patients should support clinical trials, recognizing that the fact that something is "experimental" doesn't mean that it's cutting-edge therapy; it means that we don't know if it works. Consumers should become skeptics about medical treatments, rather than jumping on bandwagons or accepting authoritarian pronouncements.

In other words, patients and the public (all of whom are probably future patients), need to become resourceful and more involved in their own care. As chronic diseases like diabetes, high blood pressure, breast cancer, and heart disease become the dominant problems in medical care, patients will need to be more involved than ever in planning and arranging for their own care. Let's investigate some promising approaches in more detail.

Shared Decision Making

Some medical decisions are clear-cut. There's strong agreement on the effectiveness of treatment, and also on the desirability of treatment. Thyroid hormone replacement in patients who clearly have symptoms that are due to an underactive thyroid is an example. The treatment is effective, affordable, and safe, and it can make a big difference. Untreated, the condition can become serious. Having an appendectomy for appendicitis fits the same description. Setting broken bones and deciding whether to prescribe antibiotics for pneumonia are usually easy decisions.

In other situations, we have a good idea of what treatments can accomplish, but different patients may prefer different approaches. In some cases, different treatments have only small differences in their results. In yet other situations, we just don't know as much about the results of different approaches as we'd like. Many medical decisions aren't black and white, but various shades of gray. In the face of these uncertainties, informed patient preferences should play a big role in decision making.

As just one example, consider a sixty-five-year-old man with newly diagnosed prostate cancer that hasn't spread. Having a prostatectomy, or removal of the prostate gland, can reduce his risk of dying from prostate cancer by 50 percent.[4] Sounds like surgery is the way to go. But wait.

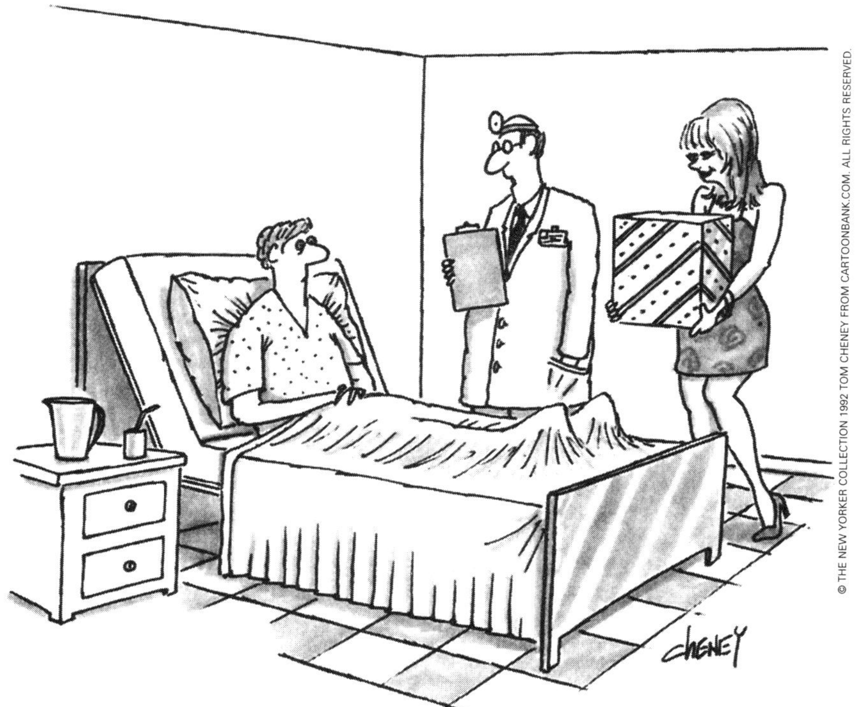

"In your case, Dave, there's a choice—elective surgery, outpatient medicinal therapy, or whatever's in the box that our lovely Carol is holding."

That 50 percent *relative* reduction in the risk of dying from prostate cancer is an *absolute* reduction from about 9 percent to about 4½ percent. The 9 percent risk is cut in half, hence the "50 percent" figure. But the absolute drop of 4½ percent in the risk of dying from prostate cancer seems more modest. Furthermore, older men are susceptible to dying from other causes as well. It turns out that the *overall* mortality, regardless of cause, is nearly the same with or without a prostatectomy. In other words, the 4½ percent drop in prostate cancer mortality is balanced by more deaths from other things, including postoperative death and deaths from other cancers.[4,5]

Furthermore, the operation may leave our sixty-five-year-old man impotent or incontinent, wearing adult diapers. His chance of dying in the next six years is about the same with or without surgery, but with surgery he's more likely to be impotent or incontinent. Maybe the choice of surgery isn't a slam dunk.

Making a decision in this situation is complex, and reasonable people may come to different conclusions for themselves. We think that this kind of information needs to be routinely available to patients, and that they should become more engaged in the decision-making process.

Doctors often argue that patients are already involved in decision making and that we inform patients of their choices. After all, we have people sign "informed consent" forms before any invasive test or procedure, right? And the consent forms list the dire things that occasionally go wrong, right?

But when researchers tape-recorded the conversations in doctors' offices (with everyone's consent), they found that doctors may describe the nature of such decisions to their patients, but they discuss the risks or benefits less often, and they rarely check to see how well the patient understands.[6] Getting "informed consent" usually consists of soliciting patient agreement with a recommendation, rather than providing the best information on the benefits and risks of several alternative choices.

The educational materials in a doctor's office—from commercial publishers, consumer groups, professional societies, and drug companies—are often inadequate. When asked, patients say that these materials are too simple or too technical; omit treatments that they're interested in; and offer too little information on treatment effectiveness, alternative treatments, uncertainties, self-care, or prevention. When specialists have reviewed such materials, they report that many offer false impressions of treatment effectiveness, emphasizing benefits and minimizing risks.[7] The same criticisms apply to most Web-based materials and (as we've seen) many media reports on medical treatments.

As we've seen, in many cases, biased patient information results from conflicts of interest. Drug and device manufacturers, insurance companies, and medical specialty societies may all have preferred treatments. They often prepare literature that's designed subtly to persuade rather than to provide complete and objective information.

So a new generation of decision aids is called for, and is being developed. These are most helpful for the many "gray areas" of medicine, where no one choice is always right, where reasonable doctors make different recommendations, and where reasonable patients make different choices for themselves. And help with decision making may be especially important for patients who have little knowledge about the condition or treatments, who have unrealistic expectations, or whose preferences are unclear. Common medical situations of this sort include surgical procedures like most back surgery or the choice of treatments for prostate enlargement. Many drug treatments also fit the description: whether or not to use hormone replacement for menopausal symptoms or to take blood thinners for certain abnormal heart rhythms.

The new decision aids differ substantially from the older generation of educational materials. They make the choices explicit, rather than implying a preferred course. They use the best available evidence, usually from randomized trials, to quantify the benefits and risks of competing treatments. Most of them are interactive, allowing a patient to obtain information specific to his or her age, disease severity, and other medical problems. The programs are usually multimedia, incorporating charts, pictures, diagrams, and audio narration in addition to written materials. Most of them include examples of other patients who have faced the problem, and how they came to different decisions. Often they include exercises to help you clarify your own values regarding the personal importance of various benefits or harms. Many are computer- or video-based, allowing animated graphics and patient interviews, though these don't seem to be essential.

Since we've advocated evidence-based medicine, you should be thinking, "Sounds cool, but do these things really work? Do they make any difference?" Although this is a new area of inquiry, there are some thirty-four randomized trials comparing what happens when patients do or don't use these decision aids. In general, the aids improve patient knowledge, enhance realistic expectations, reduce their uncertainty, and stimulate a more active role in decision making. The aids have little effect on patient satisfaction, but they sometimes modify the decisions that patients make.[8]

In comparison to patients without the aids, those who see such aids tend to make different decisions from those they might have made if they had simply talked with their doctors. In many cases, patients using the aids have chosen less aggressive therapy, whether it was surgical or drug therapy.[8] It seems that when they understand the real magnitude of benefit (often less than they imagined) and the real magnitude of risk (often more than they imagined), patients often choose less technologically intensive treatments. And yet in every trial so far, those who saw the decision aids had treatment results at least as good as those who didn't.

These results suggest that at least in some cases, less aggressive and less expensive care can result in equally good outcomes and patient satisfaction. On a larger scale, treatment complications may be reduced. And perhaps "informed consent" will become a more meaningful term.

Here are some examples:

- With a decision aid for back problems, patients with herniated discs were less likely to choose surgical treatments.[9]
- An informational package combined with a pretreatment interview resulted in fewer hysterectomies than standard care for women with excessive menstrual bleeding.[10]
- Among patients with atrial fibrillation (an abnormal heart rhythm), those who used a decision aid were less likely to undergo treatment with powerful blood thinners.[11]
- Men who viewed a decision aid regarding screening blood tests for prostate cancer chose the screening less often.[12]
- Among patients with coronary artery narrowing but stable symptoms, those who viewed a decision aid chose less bypass surgery or angioplasty, and more medication therapy.[13]

So, it seems that when they're well informed, some patients are less enchanted with high-tech solutions than they would be otherwise. When patients are provided with realistic expectations, preferences sometimes change. Despite the apparent effect on patient choices, these studies found the process to be highly acceptable to both patients and doctors, and found that patients didn't feel that they were making unilateral decisions. The doctor-patient relationship wasn't hurt, and patients generally became more active in the decision making.

There are some formidable barriers to making these decision aids more widely available. It takes plenty of time, money, and expertise to assemble the best scientific evidence, identify patients' key concerns, get the perspectives of relevant specialists, pilot-test the programs, and package them in an attractive way. Keeping decision aids up-to-date is another challenge, but newer resources like the Cochrane Collaboration should help. Using video presentations may require office space and staff, though it's easy to imagine greater use of the Internet for this purpose, making the presentations accessible at home. So far, only a few insurance companies have been willing to reimburse doctors for using programs of this sort. But producing and updating such programs needs more consistent funding support than from research grants—the source of most of this work to date.[14]

Perhaps the greatest concern is maintaining the integrity of such programs. It would be easy to persuade patients to make certain choices, and, of course, this is the purpose of marketing. Sometimes only minor changes in framing a problem or the manner in which information is presented can have important effects on consumer choices. People without a vested interest in a particular treatment approach should do the production work, to avoid steering people toward certain products, toward less expensive care, or toward one's favored approach.

Another problem is that some oxen may be gored by well-constructed decision aids. If they result in less surgery or less use of certain drugs, vested interests may attack the process. And it remains to be seen whether such decision aids can meet the challenge of direct-to-consumer advertising by manufacturers and health-care providers, whose well-funded ads offer highly persuasive messages urging one particular approach.[15] In the past, technology assessment efforts have sometimes been doomed by industry opposition, and these educational efforts may risk the same fate. Protecting the sources of decision aids may be necessary.

Open Access to Medical Records

At first blush, open access to medical records may seem to have little to do with reducing the use of ineffective technology. But it may be an important part of giving patients a more realistic understanding of their health problems. Open access to medical records may allow patients to better understand the uncertainties in their care and the decisions that their doctors face. They almost certainly would become better informed about tests or treatments that they've already had, and better able to avoid duplicating them. Those with chronic diseases would be able to track their own progress, and could in some cases become the best repositories of information about their own conditions.

And patients would be better positioned to participate in their own care. With access to details about their own test results and doctors' findings, they'd be better prepared to find and interpret information about their own conditions.

Until now, the paper medical record posed a barrier to this vision. It couldn't be in both the patient's hands and the doctor's hands. It often was handwritten, illegible, and poorly organized. New information was sometimes slow in reaching the chart, so keeping it current was challenging.

Electronic medical records are changing this scene. Indeed, we think information technology is one form of new technology that's been underused in medicine. Though they're not yet part of most medical practices, electronic records are becoming more and more commonplace in large hospitals and large medical practices.

In places where patient access is being tested, patients can access their records by computer from home. Notes and reports are no longer handwritten, and lab data are perfectly tabulated. New data are in the record almost immediately. The innovators are beginning to link patient educational aids to certain parts of the record, so that patients can get easily understood online explanations of lab results, medical terms, recommended screening tests, and the like. Patients can point out errors in the record, and it becomes a much more interactive tool. Though medical records are currently designed mainly for doctors' use, greater patient access might well prompt redesign of the records to make them more understandable and useful to patients. We can even imagine different presentations of the same electronic information for different purposes.

Of course, there's some resistance to this vision. Some doctors are afraid that the assessments and comments in the record may become less candid. Perhaps some information will be alarming to patients. Perhaps it will generate more questions and require more time explaining things, with little hope for better reimbursement. There are probably some valid concerns, but the benefits of routine patient access may come to outweigh any drawbacks. And it may be one small piece that helps patients to understand when and why high-tech interventions may not be their best bet.

"Nutritional" Labels for Drugs

Another idea for providing better information to patients is to improve the labeling of medicines. Drs. Steve Woloshin, Lisa Schwartz, and Gil Welch, internists at Dartmouth Medical School and the White River Junction VA Medical Center, have suggested labels similar to the nutrition labels that are now required on all food packaging.

Rather than the confusing language of "indications," "mechanism of action," and "contraindications" that appears on many drug package inserts, Woloshin, Schwartz, and Welch propose the simpler and more informative format shown in Figure 21-1. This approach clearly identifies what the drug is for, who should consider using it, alternative treatments that may be available, how long the drug has been approved, and details of the research study that led to the drug's approval. Information on the research might include the type of patients who were studied, the number of patients who participated, and how many improved or had certain results among those taking the drug and among those taking a placebo (or alternative treatment). It might list the incidence of the three or four most common side effects and the three or four most serious side effects.

In fact, it's not too hard to imagine providing similar patient-oriented evidence summaries for medical devices and surgical procedures. These might be very similar in design to the summary that Woloshin and colleagues propose for drugs. Trying to develop such summaries might spotlight the lower level of evidence required to unleash devices and operations on the public, compared to that required for drugs. Summaries might have to be developed to deal with off-label uses of drugs and devices as well.

An advantage of this approach is that patients could see at a glance the real magnitude of any benefits and harms, and exactly who is most likely to benefit. Instead of being told, for example, "this drug will reduce your risk of stroke by 50 percent" patients could see whether that meant from 40 percent to 20 percent or from 1 percent to 0.5 percent—both of which could be called 50 percent reductions. Similarly, rather than an exhaustive list of rare or uncertain side effects, without any indication of their frequency, patients could see at a glance what problems are most common, how often they occur, and what the most serious possibilities might be.

FIGURE 21-1

DRUG FACTS: NOLVADEX (TAMOXIFEN) FOR *PREVENTING* BREAST CANCER

What is this drug for? Reduce the chance of getting breast cancer.

Who might consider taking it? Women at high risk of getting breast cancer based on strong family history, age, and other risk factors. You can calculate your breast cancer risk at http://bcra.nci.nih.gov/brc/.

Other treatments to consider: No other medicines have been shown to reduce the chance of getting breast cancer.

Drug's track record: Year FDA approved drug for this use, 1999 (first approved for *treating* breast cancer, 1982)

What you need to do when taking tamoxifen:

1. Have a yearly gynecologic examination (with a Pap smear).
2. Check up yearly blood tests.
3. Use birth control (do not get pregnant).

TAMOXIFEN STUDY FACTS

Who was in the study? 13,175 women age 35 and older who previously had lobular carcinoma in situ OR whose 5 year risk of breast cancer was calculated to be 1.7% or greater

Length of study	**6 Years**	
	Women NOT TAKING Tamoxifen	**Women TAKING Tamoxifen**
How drug might help?		
Getting invasive breast cancer	2.70%	1.40%
Dying from breast cancer* (difference may be due to chance)	0.09%	0.05%
How drug might harm?		
Life-threatening side effects		
Blood clot	0.4%	0.8%
Stroke	0.4%	0.6%
Invasive uterine cancer	0.2%	0.5%
Less serious side effects		
Cataracts requiring surgery	1.1%	1.7%
Hot flashes	69%	81%
Vaginal discharge	35%	55%
Died for any reason	1.1%	0.9%
Average monthly price	$103.85 (at 20 mg. a day dose)	

* To learn more about Nolvadex (tamoxifen), the study (Journal of the National Cancer Institute: 1998:90: 1371–1388), and the box, go to http://www.drugfactsbox.gov.

Source: This example provided by Dr. Steven Woloshin.

Getting Experimental Treatment Outside Research Trials: Something to Avoid

The examples of bone marrow transplantation for breast cancer, AZT for AIDS, lung volume reduction surgery for emphysema, and encainide for abnormal heart rhythms should make everyone wary of jumping on the bandwagon of an experimental treatment too soon. "Experimental" really doesn't mean "cutting-edge new therapy that's just not widely available yet." It means "we don't know if it's better, worse, or the same as standard treatments." When faced with life-threatening illness, of course, a natural instinct is to try anything that may offer any hope. It may seem like there's nothing to lose.

But some people have had regrets about trying experimental treatments. We previously described James Quinn, who survived nine months with an artificial heart, seven of them in the hospital. After suffering two strokes, Quinn said, "This is nothing like I thought it would be. If I had to do it over again, I wouldn't do it."[16] In response to a newspaper article on the ineffectiveness of bone marrow transplant for breast cancer, a doctor wrote, "My late sister-in-law's bone marrow transplant resulted in two anguished months of recovery that might have been spent with her family."[17] Unexpected deaths and complications in gene therapy trials have affected young patients and shortened their lives. Even terminally ill patients may discover that they really do have something to lose.

A recent study suggests that just knowing that a clinical trial of a new treatment is underway makes the treatment more attractive to doctors and patients. When they learn about a clinical trial, many seem to assume that the experimental treatment works and rush to get it. They're unwilling to wait for the trial results that will show whether the experimental treatment is safe and effective. Many such patients aren't inclined to enter the research study, seemingly because they're convinced that the treatment is worth trying. So if the experimental treatment is available outside the research study, they seek it out.

This study focused on the use of apheresis, a technique that separates the components of blood. The hope was that this technique could be used to remove circulating immune substances or proteins that might cause disease. The technique was known to work for some conditions, so it was already available in some centers. But it was being tested for three new conditions. The researchers found that when apheresis was being tested as treatment for the new diseases, there was a sudden increase in use of the treatment outside the clinical trials. In fact, more people got treated outside the trials than in them.[18]

This was analogous to the situation for bone marrow transplantation for widespread breast cancer. The researchers labeled this phenomenon "jumping the gun." A result of jumping the gun was that many patients may have received experimental treatment without appropriate consent. That's because the treatment was simply provided as if it weren't experimental—as if we knew the answer. Furthermore, the trials that would help define the optimal treatment approach were delayed, because recruitment of subjects was slower than it might otherwise have been. As it turned out, apheresis was effective for one of the problems, but not for a second. The third trial is still ongoing.

Rather than stampeding to gain access to experimental treatments, patients should consider enrolling in clinical trials that will determine whether the treatments really work. Avoiding clinical trials can only delay getting valid answers about a new treatment's effectiveness. When you go into an ethically designed trial, it's impossible for you to know whether you'll be better off with the new treatment or the standard one. Furthermore, there's every indication that patients in many clinical trials get a better quality of care—regardless of which treatment they get—than patients in routine care. This is because the treatments, the visits, the follow-up tests, and the number of people devoted to their care are often optimized in a research study, thanks to research funds that aren't available for routine care.

If we want to reduce the amount of useless technology we pay for, we should all support high-quality clinical trials. Advocacy groups should support this type of research as strongly as they support increased research funding and increased access to experimental treatments. As patients and advocacy groups assume more authority, they also assume this responsibility. If the concept of evidence-based medicine is to succeed, this will be a key element.

Becoming a Skeptic

Becoming a skeptic about medical advances doesn't mean becoming a nihilist. We shouldn't assume that everything new is bad, any more than we should assume that everything new is good. Certainly, some advances offer major advantages over older treatments, even if they aren't miracle cures. But everyone should be aware of the spin machine that accompanies nearly all new medical technology.

In their book titled *Trust Us, We're Experts,* journalists John Stauber and Sheldon Rampton offer advice about recognizing overblown claims and propaganda.[19] They led us to the Jefferson quote that starts this chapter. We've adapted some of their suggestions to the problem of analyzing claims for new medical technology.

Exaggeration and fear-mongering are hallmarks of propaganda. When I (Rick) studied a type of electrical stimulator for the skin that's sometimes used to treat back pain (transcutaneous electrical nerve stimulation, or TENS), I found that it was no more effective than a sham stimulator.[20] In a subsequent radio interview, a representative of the manufacturer disputed the results and suggested that without TENS, patients would be "condemned" to the "living hell" of chronic pain or narcotic addiction. He didn't point out the many other treatments that are available to patients with chronic pain. Furthermore, a recent review of TENS in the Cochrane Collaboration concluded, "The evidence from randomized controlled trials does not support the use of TENS alone in the treatment of chronic low back pain."[21]

"Glittering generalities" are a second tactic.[19] Think of phrases like "proven effective," which don't tell you how much better one treatment is than another. At least for drugs, if a product is FDA approved, it's probably at least slightly better than nothing, and that's all "proven effective" really means. Likewise, beware of "lifesaving" technologies or "miracle cures," which rarely are. Even "high-tech" should raise a red flag: It's often offered as a lure before credible evidence is available. It also helps to justify high prices.

Testimonials should also make you wary. As an example, expert guidelines from the U.S. Preventive Services Task Force haven't recommended for or against routine PSA screening for prostate cancer. This is because there are many uncertainties about the test, the treatments, and the relative advantages and disadvantages.[22] But when celebrities endorse PSA testing, consumers listen. Said one man, even after enduring a prostate biopsy for a false-positive PSA test, "If Joe Torre [the Yankees' manager] and Bob Dole recommend screening, then screening must be a good thing. With all their money, you know they are getting the best care in the world."[23] That's exactly the assumption the drug companies are banking on.

The tactic of celebrity endorsements for prescription drugs began in 1998 with Joan Lunden, the former *Good Morning America* anchor, plugging

Claritin. Supermodel Cheryl Tiegs was busily promoting postmenopausal estrogen therapy before new research disclosed its hazards and lack of benefits for the heart. Baseball hero Cal Ripken figured prominently in ads for a drug he doesn't use (Prinvil) that treats a condition he doesn't have (high blood pressure).[24] So a critical consumer might ask, why should I regard this person as a trustworthy source of information on this subject? And what are the merits of the idea without the endorsement?

Bandwagons are another useful tool of propaganda. Remember the organizing efforts of "Astroturf" organizations funded mainly by drug companies. Requests to join a bandwagon are usually a clue that you should look at who's funding the effort.

Rampton and Stauber point out that when you hire a contractor or an attorney, that person is working for you, because you are paying for her or his services. But generally, the visible experts who appear on the public stage to "educate" you about new medical treatments aren't working for you; they're working for a client whose interests and values may be very different from yours. This is especially true of corporate sponsors, because they have a clear and almost explicit bias—the desire to maximize profits. And the money that corporations put into influencing public policy or public opinion far exceeds that from nonprofit organizations. Money doesn't always create bias, but it's a leading indicator. So follow the money.

It's wise to ask, "What's in a name?" Rampton and Stauber point out that industry front groups try to portray themselves as moderate, representing the "middle ground." So they use names like "Citizens for Better Medicare" or the "Center for Patient Advocacy," which make them sound like benign, neutral organizations. The names don't reveal that one was founded by the drug industry to help lobby for keeping drug prices high, or that the other was founded by orthopedic surgeons who were angry at government-sponsored research and guidelines. Words like *sensible, responsible,* and *sound* often appear in the titles of industry-sponsored groups.[19]

Finally, Rampton and Stauber urge caution regarding the pronouncements of "think tanks." They point out that think tanks virtually always have a decided political leaning, and that there are twice as many conservative think tanks as liberal ones. Think tanks are often well funded by big business, and they supply experts to testify for Congress, write op-ed pieces, and appear as TV commentators. Rampton and Stauber argue that they're often more like PR fronts than sources of genuine scholarship.[19]

Avoiding the Risks of New Medical Treatments

Part of shared and informed decision making is simply being judicious about the use of any new treatment. None of us wants to forgo the benefits of the major advances—the cherries—that come along in the medical world, but we sure don't want the lemons. Some practical advice may be in order here.

The examples discussed in this book suggest that consumers should be cautious, rather than jumping on the new drug bandwagon. When your doctor prescribes a drug, ask how long it's been on the market. Also ask if there are older drugs that are substantially similar. Ask about generic drugs. If the first drug of a class has lost its patent and become generic, it may be very similar to a new drug, but at a much lower price. Many new drugs, including some that are heavily marketed, are simply "me too" drugs—chemically similar to older drugs, and often similar in effectiveness. Many drugs that have been recalled for serious side effects were simply "me too" drugs, and exposure to them could have been easily avoided. Go with the older drug unless you've tried it and it's failed already. This may mean resisting the siren call of direct-to-consumer ads that saturate the airways. Similar considerations apply to new medical devices.

If a drug or device has been on the market for less than a year, be especially wary. Many problems show up only with time. Many recalled drugs get pulled within a year of hitting the market, so this seems like a prudent delay. Asked if patients should take a new medicine that has been sold for less than a year, Dr. Raymond Woosley, a drug-safety expert and cardiologist now at the University of Arizona, said, "I sure wouldn't. I don't personally, and I don't usually prescribe it unless I have to."[25]

Don't complain if the FDA seems to take its sweet time with new drugs and devices. It may be saving you from snake oil or worse. And live by an old aphorism to doctors: Don't be either the first or the last to adopt a new drug.

With new surgical operations, how can you avoid being an inadvertent guinea pig? Or at least avoid preventable complications, if you must have surgery? Surgeon David Flum says, "First of all, there's no such thing as a small procedure. 'Minimally invasive' surgery just means that the incision is minimal. It doesn't mean that what we're doing inside or the complications are minimal. So the rush to get elective surgery should be tempered—should really be tempered—by asking yourself 'How am I going to feel if I have to get re-operated for bleeding or if I have a wound infection?'"

If you're having elective (not emergency) surgery, don't rush in. Be sure you know what the nonsurgical treatment options and results may be. Find out how long the operation you're considering has been done in general, and how many your surgeon has performed in particular. Says Flum, "Every patient should ask his doctor, how many of these have you done, Doc? Patients should understand that we don't really think there's a magic number of operations required to prevent bad results. But if the doctor doesn't give a satisfactory answer, then it may be time to move on to a second opinion. Sometimes patients choose a less-experienced surgeon because of proximity, better rapport, or hospital preferences. But surgeons should be willing to disclose this important piece of information to allow for a more informed decision."

Also, remember that the best surgeon in the world needs the support of superb nurses, operating room technicians, x-ray technicians, laboratory personnel, and pathologists. Modern medicine is a team sport. So find out whether the hospital where your operation will take place has done lots of the same operation. For most types of surgery, there's a clear connection between the number of operations done in a hospital and that hospital's success rate. This is why a group of major corporations (like IBM and General Motors), called the Leapfrog Group, recommend that their employees have surgery only in so-called high-volume hospitals. If IBM and GM want to play that way, you can too.

Aficionados of 1960s rock music recall Jimi Hendrix, who wasn't afraid of being blunt. For both your doctor and your hospital, just remember Jimi's first hit album, *Are You Experienced?* Jimi may have had something else on his mind, but this is also the key question to ask anyone who proposes to "open you up."

Conclusions

Medical technology is here to stay, and it's a good thing. But it's the primary reason for rising health-care costs, which threaten to leave more and more people uninsured. Rapid medical advances, coupled with a financing system that pays most of the costs and few mechanisms to evaluate the clinical effectiveness of new advances, create a recipe for inefficient care. Relatively low out-of-pocket costs to patients make price seem irrelevant. Payment systems generally encourage doctors and hospitals to do ever more, and to concentrate on specific lucrative services. And patients have too little information about treatment effectiveness to make well-informed decisions. This is a perfect storm.

But don't be duped into thinking that everything new is good, or at least better than the alternatives. Consumers can help to improve their own care and help to restrain medical costs at the same time by being careful shoppers. This is more challenging than looking for the best department store bargains, but it beats the heck out of being sold a bill of goods.

Information on comparative effectiveness is hard to find, because those who create products and services have little to gain by providing it. The developers and providers of medical treatments have been more politically effective than those who seek to evaluate these treatments. Better public funding for evaluating medical advances seems highly appropriate, as it would serve the interests of public payers, private payers, and taxpayers.[26]

Consumers and patients should ask for the best possible information on their medical choices, preferably from unbiased decision aids. They should be vocal about wanting access to their own medical records, because they can become more expert on their own problems and choices with this information in hand. They can advocate for better information, not only in the form of decision aids and better access to records, but also in the form of more informative drug labeling. They should support clinical trials rather than decry them, because this is the ultimate source of good information. And they should arm themselves with better "crap detectors" when they are confronted with glowing pronouncements about new medical treatments.

Finally, those who are concerned about the quality and cost of medical care may want to become activists for changes in clinical and public policy. Improved access to generic drugs, better surveillance of new drugs and devices after they're marketed, minimizing conflicts of interest in the approval process, greater use of evidence-based medicine, and access to better information should be nonpartisan issues that nearly everyone can support. They will require action by doctors, hospitals, the media, and the government. And they will happen only if we insist.

REFERENCES

CHAPTER 1

1. Szasz T. *The Second Sin.* London: Routledge Kegan and Paul, 1974.

2. Bufill JA. Patients need patience rather than the latest technology. *St. Louis Post-Dispatch,* March 20, 2000, p. D17.

3. Stolberg SG. On Medicine's frontier: The last journey of James Quinn. *The New York Times,* October 8, 2002, p. D1.

4. How a new policy led to seven deadly drugs; Medicine: Once a wary watchdog, the U.S. Food and Drug Administration set out to become a "partner" of the pharmaceutical industry; today, the American public has more remedies, but some are proving lethal. *Los Angeles Times,* December 20, 2000, p. A1.

5. Writing Group for the Women's Health Initiative Investigators. Risks and benefits of estrogen plus progestin in healthy postmenopausal women. *JAMA* 2002; 288: 321–333.

6. Moseley JB, O'Malley K, Petersen NJ, Menke TJ, Brody BA, Kuykendall DH, et al. A controlled trial of arthroscopic surgery for osteoarthritis of the knee. *N Engl J Med* 2002; 347: 81–88.

7. Bartley N. Cancer mistake ravages a life. *Seattle Times,* April 25, 2001, p. B1.

8. Stadtmauer EA, O'Neill A, Goldstein LJ, Crilley PA, Mangan KF, Ingle JN, et al. Conventional-dose chemotherapy compared with high-dose chemotherapy plus autologous hematopoietic stem-cell transplantation for metastatic breast cancer. Philadelphia Bone Marrow Transplant Group. *N Engl J Med* 2000; 342: 1069–1076.

9. Mello MM, Brennan TA. The controversy over high-dose chemotherapy with autologous bone marrow transplant for breast cancer. *Health Affairs* 2001; 20(5): 101–117.

10. The ALLHAT Officers and Coordinators for the ALLHAT Collaborative Research Group. Major outcomes in high-risk hypertensive patients randomized to angiotensin-converting enzyme inhibitor or calcium channel blocker vs diuretic: The Antihypertensive and Lipid-Lowering treatment to prevent Heart Attack Trial (ALLHAT). *JAMA* 2002; 288: 2981–2997.

11. Petersen M. Diuretics' value drowned out by trumpeting of newer drugs. *The New York Times,* December 18, 2002, p. A32.

12. Kleinke JD. *Oxymorons: The Myth of a U.S. Health Care System.* San Francisco: Jossey-Bass, 2001, p. 79.

13. Callahan D. *False Hopes: Why America's Quest for Perfect Health Is a Recipe for Failure.* New York: Simon and Schuster, 1998.

14. Kolata G. New heart studies question the value of opening arteries. *The New York Times*, March 21, 2004, sec. 1, p. 1.

15. Steinberg EP, Tunis S, Shapiro D. Insurance coverage for experimental technologies. *Health Affairs* 1995; 14: 143–158.

CHAPTER 2

1. Boden WE, O'Rourke RA, Crawford MH, et al. Outcomes in patients with acute non-Q-wave myocardial infarction randomly assigned to an invasive as compared with a conservative management strategy. *N Engl J Med* 1998; 338: 1785–1792.

2. Lange RA, Hillis LD. Use and overuse of angiography and revascularization for acute coronary syndromes. *N Engl J Med* 1998; 338: 1838–1839.

3. Leape LL. Unnecessary surgery. *Annu Rev Public Health* 1992; 13: 363–383.

4. Woloshin S, Schwartz LM, Byram SJ, Sox HC, Fischhoff B, Welch HG. Women's understanding of the mammography screening debate. *Arch Intern Med* 2000; 160: 1434–1440.

5. Kim M, Blendon RJ, Benson JM. How interested are Americans in new medical technologies? A multicountry comparison. *Health Affairs* 2001; 20: 194–201.

6. Segal HP. *Technological Utopianism in American Culture.* Chicago: University of Chicago Press, 1985.

7. Illich I. *Medical Nemesis: The Expropriation of Health.* New York: Pantheon Books, 1976.

8. Fuchs VR. *Who Shall Live? Health Economics and Social Choice.* New York: Basic Books, 1974.

9. Priester R. A values framework for health system reform. *Health Affairs* 1992 11(1), 84–108.

10. Lamm R. Marginal medicine. *JAMA* 1998; 280: 931–933.

11. Blendon RJ, Donelan K, Leitman R, Epstein A, Cantor JC, Cohen AB, et al. Physicians' perspectives on caring for patients in the United States, Canada, and West Germany. *N Engl J Med* 1993; 328 (14), 1011–1016.

12. Lasch C. *Culture of Narcissicism: American Life in an Age of Diminishing Expectations.* New York: Norton, 1978.

13. Delbanco T, Sands DZ. Electrons in flight—e-mail between doctors and patients. *N Engl J Med* 2004; 350: 1705–1708

14. Beard SM, Wall L, Gaffney L, Sampson F. Aggressive non-Hodgkin's lymphoma: economics of high-dose therapy. *Pharmacoeconomics,* 2004; 22 (4), 207–224.

15. McVie JG, Dalesio O, Smith IE. *Autologous Bone Marrow Transplantation and Solid Tumors.* New York: Raven Press, 1984.

16. Rogers EM. *Diffusion of Innovations,* 4th ed. New York: The Free Press, 1995, p. 11.

17. Groopman, J. *Anatomy of Hope: How People Prevail in the Face of Illness.* New York: Random House, 2004.

18. Callahan D. Death and the research imperative. *N Engl J Med* 2000; 342: 654–656.

19. Fisher LM. The race to cash in on the genetic code. *The New York Times*, August 29, 1999, sec. 3, p. 1.

20. Last acts. A coalition to improve care and caring near the end of life. Available at: www.lastacts.org. Accessed May 4, 2004.

21. Preston TA. The artificial heart, in Dutton D, *Worse Than the Disease: Pitfalls of Medical Progress*. New York: Cambridge University Press, 1988, pp. 91–126.

22. Koenig BA. The technological imperative in medical practice: The social creation of a "routine" treatment, in Lock M, Gordon DR (eds.), *Biomedicine Examined*. Boston: Kluwer Academic Publishers, 1988, pp. 465–496.

23. Hogness JR, VanAntwerp M (eds.). *The Artificial Heart, Prototypes, Policies, and Patients*. Washington, D.C.: Institute of Medicine, National Academy Press, 1991.

CHAPTER 3

1. Lister J. By the *London Post:* Christmas books. *N Engl J Med* 1975; 292: 467–469.

2. Cousins N. *Anatomy of an Illness*. New York: W.W. Norton, 1979, p. 28.

3. Newhouse JP and the Insurance Experiment Group. *Free for all? Lessons from the RAND Health Insurance Experiment*. Cambridge, Mass.: Harvard University Press, 1993.

4. Keeler EB, Rolph JE. How cost sharing reduced medical spending of participants in the health insurance experiment. *JAMA* 1983; 249: 2220–2222.

5. Rogers WH, O'Rourke TW, Ware JE, Brook RH, Newhouse JP. Effects of cost sharing in health insurance on disability days. *Health Policy* 1991; 18: 131–139.

6. Goodman DC, Fisher ES, Little GA, Stukel TA, Chang C-H, Schoendorf KS. The relation between the availability of neonatal intensive care and neonatal mortality. *N Engl J Med* 2002; 346: 1538–1544.

7. Grumbach K. Specialists, technology, and newborns—too much of a good thing. *N Engl J Med* 2002; 346: 1574–1575.

8. Hirschmann JV. Antibiotics for common respiratory tract infections in adults. *Arch Intern Med* 2002; 162: 256–264.

9. Geyman JP. Evidence-based medicine in primary care: An overview. *J Am Board Fam Pract* 1998; 11: 46–56.

10. Center for the Evaluative Clinical Sciences at Dartmouth Medical School. The Dartmouth Atlas of Health Care. Variations in the use of discretionary surgery. Available at www.dartmouthatlas.org/reports/quickreport_surgery.php. Accessed May 12, 2004.

11. Volinn E, Mayer J, Diehr P, Van Koevering D, Connell FA, Loeser JD. Small area analysis of surgery for low-back pain. *Spine* 1992; 17: 575–581.

12. Keller RB, Atlas SJ, Soule DN, Singer DE, Deyo RA. Relationship between rates and outcomes of operative treatment for lumbar disc herniation and spinal stenosis. *J Bone Joint Surg* 1999; 81-A: 752–762.

13. Cherkin DC, Deyo RA, Loeser JD, Bush T, Waddell G. An international comparison of back surgery rates. *Spine* 1994; 19: 1201–1206.

14. Leape LL. Unnecessary surgery. *Annu Rev Public Health* 1992; 13: 363–383.

15. HCUPnet, Healthcare Cost and Utilization Project. Statistics for U.S. hospital stays, the national bill for conditions treated in the hospital. Agency for Healthcare Research and Quality, Rockville, MD. Available at: http://www.ahrq.gov/data/hcup/

hcupnet.htm. Accessed June 9, 2002.

16. Somogyi-Zalud E, Zhong Z, Hamel MB, Lynn J. The use of life-sustaining treatments in hospitalized persons aged 80 and older. *J Am Geriatr Soc* 2002; 50: 930–934.

17. Fisher ES, Wennberg DE, Stukel TA, Gottlieb DJ, Lucas FL, Pinder EL. The implications of regional variations in Medicare spending. Part 1: The content, quality, and accessibility of care. *Ann Intern Med* 2003; 138: 273–287.

18. Fisher ES, Wennberg DE, Stukel TA, Gottlieb DJ, Lucas FL, Pinder EL. The implications of regional variations in Medicare spending. Part 2: Health outcomes and satisfaction with care. *Ann Intern Med* 2003; 138: 288–298.

19. Weinberger M, Oddone EZ, Henderson WG, et al. Does increased access to primary care reduce hospital readmissions? *N Engl J Med* 1996; 334: 1441–1447.

20. Kendrick D, Fielding K, Bentley E, et al. Radiography of the lumbar spine in primary care patients with low back pain: Randomised controlled trial. *Br Med J* 2001; 322: 400–405.

21. Potosky AL, Reeve BB, Clegg LX, et al. Quality of life following localized prostate cancer treated initially with androgen deprivation therapy or no therapy. *J Natl Cancer Inst* 2002; 94: 430–437.

22. Deyo RA. Cascade effects of medical technology. *Annu Rev Public Health* 2002; 23: 23-–44.

23. Deyo RA, Weinstein JN. Low back pain. *N Engl J Med* 2001; 344: 363–370.

24. Lurie JD, Birkmeyer NJ, Weinstein JN. Rates of advanced spinal imaging and spine surgery. *Spine* 2003; 28: 616–620.

25. Jarvik JG, Hollingworth W, Martin B, Emerson SS, Gray DT, Overman S, et al. Rapid magnetic resonance imaging vs radiographs for patients with low back pain: A randomized controlled trial. *JAMA* 2003; 289 (21): 2810–2818.

26. Black WC, Welch HG. Advances in diagnostic imaging and overestimations of disease prevalence and the benefits of therapy. *N Engl J Med* 1993; 328 (17): 1237–1243.

27. Bartley N. Cancer mistake ravages a life. *Seattle Times,* April 25, 2001, p. B1.

28. Bartley N. Couple retell anguish of false cancer diagnosis. *Seattle Times*, May 19, 2001, p. B1.

29. Bartley N. Trial unraveling misdiagnosis. *Seattle Times*, May 24, 2001, p. B1.

30. Skolnik S, Sunde S. UW and drug company share blame. *Seattle Post-Intelligencer*, June 30, 2001, p. A-1.

31. Rice TH. The impact of changing Medicare reimbursement rates on physician-induced demand. *Med Care* 1983; 21: 803–815.

32. Ginsburg PB, Koretz DM. Bed availability and hospital utilization: Estimates of the "Roemer effect." *Health Care Financ Rev* 1983; 5(1): 87–92.

33. Wennberg JE, Fisher ES, Skinner JS. Geography and the debate over Medicare reform. *Health Affairs* 2002 (supp Web exclusive) W96–W114.

34. Fisher ES, Wennberg JE, Stukel TA, Skinner JS, Sharp SM, Freeman JL, Gittelsohn AM. Associations among hospital capacity, utilization, and mortality of U.S. Medicare beneficiaries, controlling for sociodemographic factors. *Health Serv Res* 2000; 34: 1351–1362.

35. Vandenburgh H. *Feeding Frenzy: Organizational Deviance in the Texas Psychiatric Hospital Industry.* Lanham, Md.: University Press of America, 1999.

36. American Health Line. Health Care Costs: Employers waste $390B annually. June 11, 2002. Available at: www.nationaljournal.com.

37. Schuster MA, McGlynn EA, Brook RH. How good is the quality of health care in the United States? *Milbank Q* 1998; 76: 517–563.

38. Landefeld CS. Medical marvels and muda. *SGIM Forum*, 2000.

CHAPTER 4

1. Braun ML. *DES Stories: Faces and Voices of People Exposed to Diethylstilbestrol.* Rochester, N.Y.: Visual Studies Workshop Press, 2001.

2. Smith L. The DES legacy; children of women given the hormone DES decades ago now cope with their own—and even their children's—health problems. *The Washington Post*, September 23, 2003, p. F1.

3. Centers for Disease Control. DES update: Health care providers. Available at: www.cdc.gov/DES. Accessed May 8, 2004..

4. Palmer JR, Hatch EE, Rosenberg CL, et al. Risk of breast cancer in women exposed to diethylstilbestrol in utero: Preliminary results (United States). *Cancer Causes Control* 2002; 13: 753–758.

5. Dutton DB. *Worse Than the Disease: Pitfalls of Medical Progress.* New York: Cambridge University Press, 1988, pp. 31–90.

6. Stadtmauer EA, O'Neill A, Goldstein LJ, Crilley PA, Mangan KF, Ingle JN, et al. Conventional-dose chemotherapy compared with high-dose chemotherapy plus autologous hematopoietic stem-cell transplantation for metastatic breast cancer. Philadelphia Bone Marrow Transplant Group. *N Engl J Med* 2000; 342: 1069–1076.

7. Mello MM, Brennan TA. The controversy over high-dose chemotherapy with autologous bone marrow transplant for breast cancer. *Health Affairs* 2001; 20(5): 101–117.

8. The ALLHAT Officers and Coordinators for the ALLHAT Collaborative Research Group. Major outcomes in high-risk hypertensive patients randomized to angiotensin-converting enzyme inhibitor or calcium channel blocker vs diuretic: the Antihypertensive and Lipid-Lowering treatment to prevent Heart Attack Trial (ALLHAT). *JAMA* 2002; 288: 2981–2997.

9. Petersen M. Diuretics' value drowned out by trumpeting of newer drugs. *New York Times*, December 18, 2002, p. A32.

10. How a new policy led to seven deadly drugs; Medicine: Once a wary watchdog, the U.S. Food and Drug Administration set out to become a "partner" of the pharmaceutical industry; today, the American public has more remedies, but some are proving lethal. *Los Angeles Times,* December 20, 2000, p. A1.

11. Petersen M, Berenson A. Papers indicate that Bayer knew of dangers of its cholesterol drug. *The New York Times*, February 22, 2003, p. A1.

12. Misocky MA. Letter to Carol Sever, Bayer Corporation, October 25, 1999. FDA Center for Drug Evaluation and Research, Warning letters and untitled letters to Pharmaceutical Companies, 1999. Available at: www.fda.gov/cder/warn/oct99/wl102599.pdf. Accessed July 23, 2004.

13. Maisel WH, Sweeney MO, Stevenson WG, Ellison KE, Epstein LM. Recalls and safety alerts involving pacemakers and implantable cardioverter-defibrillator devices. *JAMA* 2001; 286: 793–799.

14. Bell R. *Impure Science*. New York: John Wiley and Sons, 1992, pp. 162–176.

15. FDA Capsules. *Newsday*, April 22, 2003, p. A35.

16. FDA: Suspends sale of gel used in gynecological operations. *American Health Line*, April 17, 2003. Available at www.nationaljournal.com. Accessed April 17, 2003.

17. Lasser KE, Allen PD, Woolhandler SJ, Himmelstein DU, Wolfe SM, Bor DH. Timing of new black box warnings and withdrawals for prescription medications. *JAMA* 2002; 287: 2215–2220.

18. Wood AJJ. The safety of new medicines: The importance of asking the right questions. *JAMA* 1999: 281; 1753–1754.

19. Moore TJ, Psaty BM, Furberg CD. Time to act on drug safety. *JAMA* 1998; 279: 1571–1573.

20. Ernst FR, Grizzle AJ. Drug-related morbidity and mortality: Updating the cost-of-illness model. *J Am Pharm Assoc* (Wash) 2001; 41 (2): 192–199.

21. Johnson JA, Bootman JL. Drug-related morbidity and mortality: A cost-of-illness model. *Arch Intern Med* 1995; 155: 1949–1956.

22. Nesi T. False hope in a bottle. *The New York Times*, June 5, 2003, p. A-35.

23. Writing Group for the Women's Health Initiative Investigators. Risks and benefits of estrogen plus progestin in healthy postmenopausal women. *JAMA* 2002; 288: 321–333.

24. Grady D, Herrington D, Bittner V, et al. Cardiovascular disease outcomes during 68 years of hormone therapy: Heart and Estrogen/progestin Replacement Study Follow-up (HERS II). *JAMA* 2002; 288: 49–57.

25. Jacobson RM, Feinstein AR. Oxygen as a cause of blindness in premature infants: "Autopsy" of a decade of errors in clinical epidemiologic research. *J Clin Epidemiol* 1992; 45: 1265–1287.

26. Silverman WA. Medical inflation. *Perspect Biol Med* 1980 (Summer): 617–637.

27. Grady D. Operation for obesity leaves some in misery. *The New York Times*, May 4, 2004, p. F1.

28. Moseley JB, O'Malley K, Petersen NJ, Menke TJ, Brody BA, Kuykendall DH, et al. A controlled trial of arthroscopic surgery for osteoarthritis of the knee. *N Engl J Med* 2002; 347: 81–88.

29. Flum DR, Koepsell T, Heagerty P, Sinanan M, Dellinger EP. Common bile duct injury during laparoscopic cholecystectomy and the use of intraoperative cholangiography: Adverse outcome or preventable error? *Arch Surg* 2001; 136: 1287–1292.

30. Flum DR, Koepsell T, Heagerty P, Pellegrini CA. The nationwide frequency of major adverse outcomes in antireflux surgery and the role of surgeon experience, 1992–1997. *J Am Coll Surg* 2002; 195: 611–618.

31. Levin AA, Geiger E. 2001 reported volume for selected procedures performed in New York state licensed hospitals and ambulatory surgery centers. Available at: Center for Medical Consumers web site, www.medicalconsumers.org. Accessed August 9, 2003.

CHAPTER 5

1. Toner R, Stolberg SG. Decade after health care crisis, soaring costs bring new strains. *The New York Times*, August 11, 2002, sec. 1, p. 1.

2. Geyman JP. *Health Care in America: Can Our Ailing System Be Healed?* Boston: Butterworth-Heinemann, 2002, p.15

3. Organ Procurement and Transplantation Network. Transplants in the U.S. by recipient age. Available at: www.optn.org/latestData/rptData.asp. Accessed August 9, 2003.

4. Huizenga HF, Ramsey SD, Albert RK. Estimated growth of lung volume reduction surgery among Medicare enrollees, 1994–1996. *Chest* 1998; 114: 1583–1587.

5. Newhouse JP. An iconoclastic view of health cost containment. *Health Affairs* 1993 (Suppl): 153–171.

6. Chernew ME, Hirth RA, Sonnad SS, et al. Managed care, medical technology, and health care growth: A review of the evidence. *Med Care* Res Rev 1998; 55: 259–288.

7. Fuchs VR. Health care for the elderly: How much? Who will pay for it? *Health Affairs* 1999; 18: 11–21.

8. Broder JM, Pear R, Freudenheim M. Problem of lost health benefits is reaching into the middle class. *The New York Times*, November 25, 2002, p. A1

9. Kellerman AL. Physician support for covering the uninsured: Is the cup half empty or half full? *Ann Intern Med* 2003; 139: 858–859.

10. Cunningham PJ. Prescription drug access: Not just a Medicare problem. Center for Studying Health System change, Issue Brief No. 51, April 2002.

11. McCormack LA, Gabel JR, Whitmore H, Anderson WL, Pickreign J. Trends in retiree health benefits: Health benefits for retirees are eroding even in the best of times. *Health Affairs* 2002; 21(6): 169–176.

12. Kaiser Family Foundation. Eighteen percent of California seniors and 26 percent of those in poor health report skipping prescription doses or foregoing medications due to cost, new survey finds. Press release Oct. 31, 2002. Available at: www.kff.org/content/2002/6058/. Accessed October 5, 2003.

13. Kaiser Daily Health Policy Report. High cost of insurance leading some health people to opt out of employer-sponsored coverage. August 8, 2002. Available at: www.kaisernetwork.org/daily_reports. Accessed May 10, 2004.

14. Robinson JC. Reinvention of health insurance in the consumer era. *JAMA* 2004; 291: 1880–1886.

15. Kronick R, Gilmer T. Explaining the decline in health insurance coverage, 1979–1995. *Health Affairs* 1999; 18(2): 30–47.

16. Snow JW, Chao EL, Thompson TG, Barnhart JAB, Palmer JL, Saving TR, Smith DG. 2004 annual report of the boards of trustees of the federal hospital insurance and federal supplementary medical insurance trust funds. Available at: www.cms.hhs.gov/publications/trusteesreport/. Accessed July 23, 2004.

17. Mello MM, Brennan TA. The controversy over high-dose chemotherapy with autologous bone marrow transplant for breast cancer. *Health Affairs* 2001; 20: 101–117.

18. Heffler S, Smith S, Keehan S, Clemens MK, Zezza M, Truffer C. Health spending projections through 2013. *Health Affairs*, February 11, 2004 (Web Exclusive), W4-79–W4-93.

19. Schwartz WB. In the pipeline: A wave of valuable medical technology. *Health Affairs*, v. 13, no. 3, Summer 1994, 70–79.

20. Thomas L. *The Fragile Species*. New York: Macmillan, 1992, pp. 10–15.

21. Cohen L, Rothschild H. The bandwagons of medicine. *Perspect Biol Med* 1979; 22: 531.

22. Deyo RA. Cascade effects of medical technology. *Annu Rev Public Health* 2002; 23: 23–44.

23. Sackett DL, Haynes RB, Tugwell P. *Clinical Epidemiology: A Basic Science for Clinical Medicine*. Boston: Little Brown, 1985, pp. 176–178.

24. Echt DS, Liebson PR, Mitchell LB, et al. Mortality and morbidity in patients receiving encainide, flecainide, or placebo. The Cardiac Arrhythmia Suppression Trial. *N Engl J Med* 1991; 324: 781–788.

25. Thacker SB, Stroup D, Chang M. Continuous electronic heart rate monitoring for fetal assessment during labor (Cochrane Review): The Cochrane Library, Issue 4. Chichester, UK: John Wiley & Sons, Ltd., 2003.

26. Rogers EM. *Diffusion of Innovations*, 4th ed. New York: Free Press, 1995.

27. Dixon AS. The evolution of clinical policies. *Med Care* 1990; 28: 201–220.

28. Schwartz WB. The inevitable failure of current cost-containment strategies: Why they can provide only temporary relief. *JAMA* 1987; 257: 220–224.

29. Altman DE, Levitt L. The sad history of health care cost containment as told in one chart. *Health Affairs*, January 23, 2002 (Web exclusive), W83–W84.

CHAPTER 6

1. Osler W. Quoted in Cushing H. *Life of Sir William Osler*, Oxford: Clarendon Press, 1925.

2. Navarro J. *Health*. Washington, D.C.: Pan American Health Organization, 2002, p. 181.

3. Crovo D, Bajwa ZH, Warfield CA. Pain associated with herpes zoster infection. UpToDate version 11.3. Available at: www.uptodate.com. Accessed May 10, 2004.

4. Soumerai SB, Ross-Degnan D, Avorn J, et al. Effects of Medicaid drug-payment limits on admission to hospitals and nursing homes. *N Engl J Med* 1991; 325: 1072–1077.

5. Soumerai SB, McLaughlin TJ, Ross-Degnan D, Casteris CS, Bollini P. Effects of limiting Medicaid drug-reimbursement benefits on the use of psychotropic agents and acute mental health services by patients with schizophrenia. *N Engl J Med* 1994; 331: 650–655.

6. Vermont Congressman Bernard Sanders's web site. Comparison of drug prices between the U.S. and Canada. Available at: http://bernie.house.gov/prescriptions/drugsheet.asp. Accessed May 10, 2004.

7. Sager A. Americans would save $38 billion in 2001 if we paid Canadian prices for brand name prescription drugs. Testimony before the Subcommittee on Consumer Affairs, Foreign Commerce, and Tourism, Committee on Commerce, Science, and Transportation, U.S. Senate, September 5, 2001. Available at: http://dcc2.bumc.bu.edu/hs/ushealthreform.htm. Accessed July 23, 2004.

8. National Institute for Health Care Management. Prescription drug expenditures in 2001: Another year of escalating costs. May 2002. Available at: www.nihcm.org. Accessed July 23, 2004.

9. Angell M. The pharmaceutical industry—to whom is it accountable? *N Engl J Med* 2000; 342: 1902–1904.

10. Levitt L. Prescription drug trends. The Henry J. Kaiser Foundation, November 2001.

11. Socolar D, Sager A. Pharmaceutical marketing and research spending: The evidence does not support PhRMA's claims. Presented at Annual Meeting of the American Public Health Association, Atlanta, Georgia, October 21, 2001. Available at: http://dcc2.bumc.bu.edu/hs/ushealthreform.htm. Accessed July 23, 2004.

12. General Accounting Office. *Prescription drugs: FDA oversight of direct-to-consumer advertising has limitations.* Publication GAO-03-177, October 2002.

13. National Institute for Health Care Management. Changing patterns of pharmaceutical innovation. May 2002. Available at: www.nihcm.org. Accessed July 23, 2004.

14. Kaufman M. Decline in new drugs raises concerns; FDA approvals are lowest in a decade. *The Washington Post*, November 18, 2002, p. A1.

15. Relman AS, Angell M. America's other drug problem. *New Republic,* December 16, 2002, pp. 27–41.

16. National Institute for Health Care Management Research and Educational Foundation. Prescription drugs and mass media advertising, 2000. November 2001, pp. 1–17. Available at: www.nichm.org. Accessed July 23, 2004.

17. Wilkes MS, Bell RA, Kravitz RL. Direct-to-consumer prescription drug advertising: Trends, impact, and implications. *Health Affairs* 2000; 19(2): 110–128.

18. Burton B. New Zealand moves to ban direct advertising of drugs. *Br Med J* 2004; 328: 68.

19. Watson R. EU ministers reject proposal for limited direct to consumer advertising. *Br Med J* 2003; 326: 1284.

20. Rosenthal MB, Berndt ER, Donohue JM, Frank RG, Epstein AM. Promotion of prescription drugs to consumers. *N Engl J Med* 2002; 346: 498–505.

21. The Henry J. Kaiser Family Foundation. Survey: Nearly one in three adults has talked to a doctor and one in eight has received a prescription in response to a drug ad. Publication 3197, November 2001. Available at: www.kff.org/marketplace. Accessed July 23, 2004.

22. Holmer AF. Direct-to-consumer prescription drug advertising builds bridges between patients and physicians. *JAMA* 1999; 281: 380–384.

23. Kelly P. DTC advertising's benefits far outweigh its imperfections. A drug industry executive supports this growing practice. *Health Affairs*, April 28, 2004 (Web exclusive), W4-246–W4-248.

24. Bero LA. "Educational" advertisements—I haven't seen one yet!" *West J Med* 2001; 174: 395.

25. Woloshin S, Schwartz LM, Tremmel J, Welch HG. Direct-to-consumer advertisements for prescription drugs: What are Americans being sold? *Lancet* 2001; 358: 1141–1146.

26. Bell RA, Wilkes MS, Kravitz RL. The educational value of consumer-targeted prescription drug print advertising. *J Fam Pract* 2000; 49: 1092–1098.

27. Woloshin S, Schwartz LM, Welch HG. The value of benefit data in direct-to-consumer drug ads. *Health Affairs*, April 28, 2004 (Web exclusive), W4-234–W4-245.

28. Hall SS. Claritin and Schering-Plough: A prescription for profit. *The New York*

Times, March 11, 2001, Section 6, p. 40.

29. Del Carpio J, Kabbash L, Turenne Y, et al. Efficacy and safety of loratadine (10 mg once daily), terfenadine (60 mg twice daily), and placebo in the treatment of seasonal allergic rhinitis. *J Allergy Clin Immunol* 1989; 84(5 Pt 1): 741–746.

30. Schoenwetter W, Lim J. Comparison of intranasal triamcinolone acetonide with oral loratidine for the treatment of patients with seasonal allergic rhinitis. *Clin Ther* 1995; 17: 479–492.

31. Jordana G, Dolovich J, Briscoe MP, et al. Intranasal fluticasone propionate versus loratadine in the treatment of adolescent patients with seasonal allergic rhinitis. *J Allergy Clin Immunol* 1996; 97: 588–595.

32. Gawchik SM, Lim J. Comparison of intranasal triamcinolone acetonide with oral loratidine in the treatment of seasonal ragweed-induced allergic rhinitis. *Am J Manag Care* 1997; 3: 1052–1058.

33. National Center for Health Statistics. Fast stats A to Z. Number, percent distribution and therapeutic classification for the 20 drugs most frequently prescribed at physician offices. Available at: www.cdc.gov/nchs/fastats/drugs.htm. Accessed December 4, 2001.

34. Freeman L. Aggressive strategy helps propel Claritin to top slot. *Advertising Age*, 1998; 69 (11): S6–S7.

35. Gahart MT, Duhamel LM, Dievier A, Price R. Examining the FDA's oversight of direct-to-consumer advertising. *Health Affairs*, February 26, 2003 (Web exclusive), W3-120–W3-123.

36. Petersen M. Who's minding the drug store? *The New York Times*, June 29, 2003, sec. 3, p. 1.

37. Adams C. FDA scrambles to police drug ads truthfulness. *The Wall Street Journal*, January 2, 2001, p. A24.

38. Bell RA, Kravitz RL, Wilkes MS. Direct-to-consumer prescription drug advertising and the public. *J Gen Intern Med* 1999; 14: 651–657.

39. Lipsky MS, Taylor CA. The opinions and experiences of family physicians regarding direct-to-consumer advertising. *J Fam Pract* 1997; 45: 495–459.

40. Moore TJ, Psaty BM, Furberg CD. Time to act on drug safety. *JAMA* 1998; 279: 1571–1573.

41. Lasser KE, Allen PD, Woolhandler SJ, Himmelstein DU, Wolfe SM, Bor DH. Timing of new black box warnings and withdrawals for prescription medications. *JAMA* 2002; 287; 2215–2220.

42. Mintzes B, Barer ML, Kravitz RL, et al. Influence of direct to consumer pharmaceutical advertising and patients' requests on prescribing decisions: Two site cross sectional survey. *Br Med J* 2002; 324: 278–279.

43. Mintzes B, Barer ML, Kravitz RL, et al. How does direct-to-consumer advertising (DTCA) affect prescribing? A survey in primary care environments with and without legal DTCA. *Can Med Assoc J* 2003; 169: 405–412.

44. Schwartz RK, Soumerai SB, Avorn J. Physician motivations for nonscientific drug prescribing. *Soc Sci Med* 1989; 28: 1989.

45. Bell RA, Wilkes MS, Kravitz RL. Advertisement-induced prescription drug requests: Patients' anticipated reactions to a physician who refuses. *J Fam Pract* 1999; 48: 446–452.

46. Terzian TV. Direct-to-consumer prescription drug advertising. *Am J Law Med* 1999; 25(1): 149–167.

47. Hamilton DP. Celebrities help "educate" public on new drugs. *The Wall Street Journal*, April 22, 2002, p. B1.

48. Petersen M. Heartfelt advice, hefty fees. *The New York Times*, August 11, 2002, sec. 3, p.1.

49. Moore TJ. *Deadly Medicine*. New York: Simon and Schuster, 1995, pp. 163–176.

50. Adams C. Doctors on the run can "dine'n'dash" in style in New Orleans: Drug companies pick up tabs and make sales pitches; free Christmas trees, too. *The Wall Street Journal*, May 14, 2001, p. A-1.

51. Zoellner T. America's other drug problem. *Men's Health,* October 2001, pp. 118–123.

52. Gammage J, Stark K. Under the influence: Drug companies spend billions, showering gifts on doctors, to persuade them to prescribe new medicine. Critics say it's bad for patients' wallets—and maybe their bodies. *Philadelphia Inquirer Magazine*, March 9, 2002.

53. PBS broadcast of *Now with Bill Moyers*. Science for sale? Transcript available at: www.pbs.org/now/printable/transcript_scienceforsale_print.html. Accessed November 22, 2002.

54. Dana J, Loewenstein G. A social science perspective on gifts to physicians from industry. *JAMA* 2003; 290: 252–255.

55. Scott-Levin. Rx's and RSVP's: Pharmaceutical companies holding more meetings and events. Press release, July 9, 2001.

56. Wazana A. Physicians and the pharmaceutical industry: Is a gift ever just a gift? *JAMA* 2000; 283: 373–380.

57. Gibbone RV, Landry FJ, Blouch DL, Jones DL, Williams FK, Lucey CR, Kroenke K. A comparison of physicians' and patients' attitudes toward pharmaceutical industry gifts. *J Gen Intern Med* 1998; 13: 151–154.

58. Zuger A. Fever pitch: Getting doctors to prescribe is big business. *The New York Times*, January 11, 1999, p. A1.

59. Anonymous. Desloratidine (Clarinex). *Med Let* 2002; 44: 27–28.

60. Scott-Levin. Doctors prefer to see specialty pharmaceutical reps. Press release, February 20, 2001.

61. Ferguson RP, Rhim E, Belizaire W, Egede L, Carter K, Lansdale T. Encounters with pharmaceutical sales representatives among practicing internists. *Am J Med* 1999; 107: 149–152.

62. Ziegler MG, Lew P, Singer BC. The accuracy of drug information from pharmaceutical sales representatives. *JAMA* 1995; 273: 1296–1298.

63. Huang E, Stafford RS. National patterns in the treatment of urinary tract infections in women by ambulatory care physicians. *Arch Intern Med* 2002; 162: 41–47.

64. American Health Line. Antibiotics: Doctors not following UTI guidelines. www.nationaljournal.com. Accessed January 14, 2002.

65. Orlowski JP, Wateska L. The effects of pharmaceutical firm enticements on physician prescribing patterns. There's no such thing as a free lunch. *Chest* 1992; 102: 270–273.

66. Wilkes MS, Doblin BKH, Shapiro MF. Pharmaceutical advertisements in leading medical journals: Experts' assessments. *Ann Intern Med* 1992; 116: 912–919.

67. Moore T. *Deadly Medicine*. New York: Simon and Schuster, 1995, p. 174.

68. Westfall JM, McCabe J, Nicholas RA. Personal use of drug samples by physicians and office staff. *JAMA* 1997; 278: 141–143.

69. Chew LD, O'Young TS, Hazlet TK, Bradley KA, Maynard C, Lessler DS. A physician survey of the effect of drug sample availability on physicians' behavior. *J Gen Intern Med* 2000; 15: 478–483.

70. Hollon MF. Direct-to-consumer marketing of prescription drugs: Creating consumer demand. *JAMA* 1999; 281: 382–384.

CHAPTER 7

1. Kaufman M. Deal to boost drug approval, oversight; industries agree to higher fees so FDA can hire more employees. *The Washington Post*, March 7, 2002, p. A2.

2. Pear R. Drug companies increase spending on efforts to lobby Congress and governments. *The New York Times*, June 1, 2003, sec. 1, p. 33.

3. The Center for Responsive Politics, Washington, D.C. Data on campaign contributions and lobbying activities collected from government sources. Available at: www.opensecrets.org. Accessed February 26, 2002.

4. Mintz M. What's new about prescription… *The Washington Post*, February 11, 2001, p. B1.

5. Gordon G, Gustafson K. Drug firms flex their political muscles: Industry has many weapons this election year, including strong ties with Lieberman. *Minneapolis Star Tribune*, August 27, 2000, p. 1-A.

6. American Health Line. Rx drug costs II: Senators under fire for industry ties. July 19, 2000. Available at: www.nationaljournal.com. Accessed July 19, 2000.

7. Noble HB. E-medicine—a special report; Hailed as a Surgeon General, Koop is faulted on web ethics. *The New York Times*, September 5, 1999, sec. 1, p. 1.

8. Hamburger T, McGinley L, Cloud DS. Influence market: Industries that backed Bush are now seeking return on investment. *The Wall Street Journal*, March 6, 2001, p. A1.

9. Aaron C, Lincoln T, Pattison N, Link D, Clemente F, Peck B. The other drug war 2003: Drug companies deploy an army of 675 lobbyists to protect profits. Public Citizen Congress Watch, available at www.citizen.org. Accessed May 13, 2004.

10. Gerth J, Stolberg SG. Medicine merchants: Cultivating alliances. With quiet, unseen ties, drug makers sway debate. *The New York Times*, October 5, 2000, p. A-1.

11. Burbach C. Drug lobbying group buys Terry ads. *Omaha World-Herald*, November 4, 2000, NEWS p. 54.

12. Public Citizen. New report documents how Citizens for Better Medicare is a drug industry sham group designed to mislead America's seniors. June 20, 2000. Available at: www.citizen.org/pressroom/print_release.cfm?ID=269. Accessed July 23, 2004.

13. The Center for Responsive Politics. Preventive Medicine. Citizens for Better Medicare and prescription drug coverage. Available at www.opensecrets.org. Accessed February 26, 2002.

14. Hamburger T. Drug-industry ads aid GOP—"educational grant" funds seniors' prescription-benefit campaign. *The Wall Street Journal*, June 18, 2002, p. A4.

15. Hamburger T. Drug industry moves to boost image before vote. *The Wall Street Journal*, September 16, 2002, p. A6.

16. Anonymous. Generic drugs: The stalling game. *Consumer Reports*, July 2001, pp. 36–40.

17. Hall SS. Claritin and Schering-Plough: A prescription for profit. *The New York Times*, March 11, 2001, Section 6, p. 40.

18. News Release. Tufts Center for the Study of Drug Development pegs cost of a new prescription medicine at $802 million. November 30, 2001. Available at: http://csdd.tufts.edu/newsevents/recentnews.asp?newsid=6. Accessed July 23, 2004.

19. Public Citizen. Tufts drug study sample is skewed; true figure of R&D costs likely is 75 percent lower. December 4, 2001. Available at: www.citizen.org. Accessed December 21, 2003.

20. IMS Health. Lipitor leads the way in 2003. IMS World Review, March 18, 2004. Available at: www.ims-global.com/insight/news_story_040316.htm. Accessed May 12, 2004.

21. Petersen M. Consumer groups sue in generic drug dispute. *The New York Times*, April 8, 2001, sec. 1, p. 34.

22. Abate T. Lawsuit alleges illegal delay of generic drug introduction; group attacks Squibb's 11th-hour patent extension. *San Francisco Chronicle*, April 16, 2001, p. B1.

23. Petersen M. Bristol-Myers held culpable in patent move against rivals. *The New York Times*, February 20, 2002, p. C1.

24. Rowley J, Decker S. Bristol-Myers settles: Misused patent laws to block generics. Most of the FTC charges concern alleged manipulation of FDA's registry of patents. *The Gazette (Montreal)*, March 8, 2003, p. B14.

25. National Institute for Health Care Management. A primer: Generic drugs, patents, and the pharmaceutical marketplace. June 2002. Available at: www.nihcm.org. Accessed July 23, 2004.

26. Carey J, Barrett A. Drug prices: What's fair? *Business Week*, December 10, 2001, pp. 61–70.

27. Relman AS, Angell M. America's other drug problem. *New Republic*, December 16, 2002, pp. 27–41.

28. Zimmerman R. Child play: Pharmaceutical firms win big on plan to test adult drugs on kids—by doing inexpensive trials, they gain 6 more months free from generic rivals—FDA: Law does some good. *The Wall Street Journal*, February 5, 2001, p. A1.

29. Bloomberg News. Merck gains extension for sales of cholesterol drug. *The New York Times*, July 19, 2001, p. C4.

30. Stolberg SG. Children test new medicines despite doubts. *The New York Times*, February 11, 2001, Section 1, p. 1.

31. Connolly C. Coalition seeks to curb drug patent extensions. *The Washington Post*, March 25, 2002, p. A1. McGinley L, Hensley S. Leading the news: Drug makers aim to protect patents; pharmaceuticals industry exhorts companies to avoid coalition favoring generics. *The Wall Street Journal*, May 3, 2002, p. A3.

32. Abbott K. Drug firm took bribes, suit says; pharmaceutical maker in Broomfield accused of keeping meds off market. *Rocky Mountain News (Denver)*, September 28, 2001, p. 4A.

33. Anonymous. Cipro saga exposes how drugmakers protect profits. *USA Today*, October 29, 2001, p. 14A.

34. FTC web site. FTC Health Care Antitrust Report—conduct involving health care services and products. Available at: www.ftc.gov/bc/hcindex/conduct.htm. Accessed February 26, 2002.

35. Petersen M. Whistle-blower says marketers broke the rules to push a drug. *The New York Times*, March 14, 2002, p. C1.

36. Petersen M. Doctor explains why he blew the whistle. *The New York Times*, March 13, 2003, p. C1.

37. Petersen M. Suit says company promoted drug in exam rooms. *The New York Times*, May 15, 2002, p. C1.

38. Reuters. Company news; FDA approves Alpharma's generic epilepsy drug. *The New York Times*, September 13, 2003, p. C4.

39. Kowalczyk L. Drug company push on doctors disclosed. *The Boston Globe*, May 19, 2002, p. A1.

40. Petersen M. Court papers suggest scale of drug's use. *The New York Times*, May 30, 2003, p. C1.

41. Harris G. Pfizer to pay $430 million over promoting drug to doctors. *The New York Times*, May 14, 2004, p. C1.

42. American Health Line. Johnson & Johnson: Bribe MDs to prescribe drug, suit says. June 26, 2002. Available at: www.nationaljournal.com. Accessed June 26, 2002.

43. Peterson M. Methods used for marketing arthritis drug are under fire. *The New York Times*, April 11, 2002, p. C1.

44. Dembner A. $840M penalty is expected for drug company. *The Boston Globe*, May 28, 2001, p. A1.

45. Haddad C, Barrett A. A whistle-blower rocks an industry. *Business Week*, June 24, 2002, p. 126.

46. Gaul GM, Flaherty MP. Drugmaker discusses deal to end free-sample case. *The Washington Post*, September 20, 2002, p. E3.

47. Partlow J, Kaufman M. U.S., drug company settles scam charges; AstraZeneca admits free-sample scheme. *The Washington Post*, June 21, 2003, p. E1.

48. Appleby J. Pfizer to pay $49M over drug discount. *USA Today*, October 29, 2002, p. 3B.

49. Harris G. Drug makers settled 7 suits by whistle-blowers, group says. *The New York Times*, November 6, 2003, p. C8.

50. American Health Line. Eli Lilly: Employees disciplined over free Prozac mailing. July 24, 2002. Available at: www.nationaljournal.com. Accessed July 24, 2002.

51. Liptak A. Free Prozac in the junk mail draws a lawsuit. *The New York Times*, July 6, 2002, p. A1.

52. Lo B, Alpers A. Uses and abuses of prescription drug information in pharmacy benefits management programs. *JAMA* 2000; 283: 801–806.

53. O'Harrow R. Prescription sales, privacy fears; CVS, Giant share customer records with drug marketing firm. *The Washington Post*, February 15, 1998, p. A1.

54. O'Harrow R. Giant Food stops sharing customer data; prescription-marketing plan drew complaints. *The Washington Post*, February 18, 1998, p. A1.

55. American Health Line. Rx drugs: Schumer asks FTC to probe promotional tactics. May 6, 2002. Available at: www.nationaljournal.com. Accessed May 6, 2002.

56. Choudhry NK, Stelfox HT, Detsky AS. Relationships between authors of clinical practice guidelines and the pharmaceutical industry. *JAMA* 2002; 287: 612–617.

57. Lenzer J. Alteplase for stroke: Money and optimistic claims buttress the "brain attack" campaign. *Br Med J* 2002; 324: 723–726.

58. Wardlaw JM, Warlow CP, Counsell C. Systematic review of evidence on thrombolytic therapy for acute ischaemic stroke. *Lancet* 1997; 350: 607–614.

59. Katzan IL, Furlan AJ, Lloyd LE, et al. Use of tissue-type plasminogen activator for acute ischemic stroke: The Cleveland area experience. *JAMA* 2000; 283: 1151–1158.

60. Bravata DM, Kim H, Concato J, Krumholz HM, Brass LM. Thrombolysis for acute stroke in routine clinical practice. *Arch Intern Med* 2002; 162: 1994–2001.

61. Jorgensen HS, Nakayama H, Kammersgaard LP, Raaschou HO, Olsen TS. Predicted impact of intravenous thrombolysis on prognosis of general population of stroke patients: Simulation model. *Br Med J* 1999; 319: 288–289.

62. Kleindorfer D, Kissela B, Schneider A, et al. Eligibility for recombinant tissue plasminogen activator in acute ischemic stroke. A population-based study. *Stroke* 2004, vol. 35, no. 2: e27-9.

63. Adams JG, Chisholm CD, on behalf of the SAEM Board of Directors. The Society of Academic Emergency Medicine position on optimizing care of the stroke patient. *Acad Emerg Med* 2003; 10: 805.

64. Lenzer J. Prescription for Controversy. MotherJones.com, May/June 2001 issue. Available at: www.motherjones.com/news/outfront/2001/05/prescription.html, Accessed January 25, 2004.

65. Warlow C. Commentary: Who pays the guideline writers? *Br Med J* 2002; 324: 726–727.

66. Wardlaw JM, Del Zoppo G, Yamaguchi T, Berge E. Thrombolysis for acute ischemic stroke (Cochrane Review). In: The Cochrane Library. Issue 3, 2004. Chichester, UK: John Wiley and Sons, Ltd.

CHAPTER 8

1. Petrella RJ, DiSilvestro MD, Hildebrand C. Effects of hyaluronate sodium on pain and physical functioning in osteoarthritis of the knee. *Arch Intern Med* 2002; 162: 292–298.

2. Felson DT, Anderson JJ. Hyaluronate sodium injections for osteoarthritis: Hope, hype, and hard truths. *Arch Intern Med* 2002; 162: 245–247.

3. InfoPOEMS web site: Hyaluronate ineffective for treating osteoarthritis of the knee. Available at: http://www.infopoems.com/clients/epocrates/index.cfm?client=epocrates&ID=40555. Accessed July 10, 2002.

4. Lo GH, LaValley M, McAlindon T, Felson DT. Intra-articular hyaluronic acid in treatment of knee osteoarthritis: A meta-analysis. *JAMA* 2003; 290: 3115–3121.

5. Friedman LS, Richter ED. Relationship between conflicts of interest and research results. *J Gen Intern Med* 2004; 19: 51–56.

6. Lexchin J, Bero LA, Kjulbegovic B, Clark O. Pharmaceutical industry sponsorship and research outcome and quality: Systematic review. *Br Med J* 2003; 326: 1167–1170.

7. Kjaergard LL, Als-Nielson B. Association between competing interests and authors' conclusions: Epidemiological study of randomized clinical trails published in the BMJ. *Br Med J* 2002; 325: 249.

8. Als-Nielson B, Chen W, Gluud C, Kjaergard LL. Association of funding and conclusions in randomized drug trials: A reflection of treatment effect or adverse events? *JAMA* 2003; 290: 921–928.

9. Silverstein FE, Faich G, Goldstein JL, et al. Gastrointestinal toxicity with celecoxib vs nonsteroidal anti-inflammatory drugs for osteoarthritis and rheumatoid arthritis. The CLASS study: A randomized controlled trial. *JAMA* 2000; 284: 1247–1255.

10. Gottlieb S. Researchers deny any attempt to mislead the public over *JAMA* article on arthritis drug. *Br Med J* 2001; 323: 301.

11. Hrachovec JB, Mora M, Wright JM, Perry TL, Bassett KL, and Chambers GK. Reporting of 6-month vs 12-month data in a clinical trial of celecoxib. *JAMA* 2001; 286: 2398–2400.

12. Okie S. Missing data on Celebrex; full study altered picture of drug. *The Washington Post*, August 5, 2001, p. A11.

13. Dong BJ, Hauck WW, Gambertoglio JG, et al. Bioequivalence of generic and brand-name levothyroxine products in the treatment of hypothyroidism. *JAMA* 1997; 277: 1205–1213.

14. Rennie D. Thyroid storm. *JAMA* 1997; 277: 1238–1243.

15. King RT. How a drug firm paid for university study, then undermined it. *The Wall Street Journal*, April 25, 1996, p. A1.

16. Bodenheimer T. Uneasy alliance: Clinical investigators and the pharmaceutical industry. *N Engl J Med* 2000; 342: 1539–1544.

17. Davidoff F, DeAngelis CD, Drazen JM, et al. Sponsorship, authorship, and accountability. *Ann Intern Med* 2001; 135: 463–466.

18. Schulman KA, Seils DM, Timbie JW, et al. A national survey of provisions in clinical-trial agreements between medical schools and industry sponsors. *N Engl J Med* 2002; 347: 1335–1341.

19. Blumenthal D, Campbell EG, Anderson MS, Causino H, Louis KS. Withholding research results in academic life science. Evidence from a national survey of faculty. *JAMA* 1997; 277: 1224–1228.

20. Schultz S. True, false, whatever. Physicians are putting a stop to the publication of misleading drug data. *U.S. News & World Report*, September 17, 2001, pp. 72–73.

21. Stern JM, Simes RJ. Publication bias: Evidence of delayed publication in a cohort study of clinical research projects. *Br Med J* 1997: 315: 640–645.

22. Krzyzanowska MK, Pintilie M, Tannock IF. Factors associated with failure to publish large randomized trials presented at an oncology meeting. *JAMA* 2003; 290: 495–501.

23. Melander H, Ahlqvist-Rastad J, Meijer G, Beermann B. Evidence b(i)ased medicine—selective reporting from studies sponsored by pharmaceutical industry: review of studies in new drug applications. *Br Med J* 2003; 326: 1171–1175.

24. Kolata G. Ideas and Trends; Science needs a healthy negative outlook. *The New York Times*, July 7, 2002, sec. 4, p.10.

25. Huston P, Moher D. Redundancy, disaggregation, and the integrity of medical research. *Lancet* 1996; 347: 1024–1026.

26. Tramer MR, Reynolds DJM, Moore RA, McQuay HJ. Impact of covert duplicate publication on meta-analysis: A case study. *Br Med J* 1997; 315: 635–640.

27. Johansen HK, Gotzsche PC. Problems in the design and reporting of trials of antifungal agents encountered during meta-analysis. *JAMA* 1999; 282: 1752–1759.

28. Rennie D. Fair conduct and fair reporting of clinical trials. *JAMA* 1999; 282: 1766–1768.

29. Bero LA, Rennie D. Influences on the quality of published drug studies. *Int J Technol Assess Health Care*. 1996; 12: 209–237.

30. Ray WA, Griffin MR, Avorn J. Evaluating drugs after their approval for clinical use. *N Engl J Med* 1993; 329: 2029–2032.

31. Pynchon T. *Gravity's Rainbow*. New York: Penguin Books, 1973, p. 251.

32. Kessler DA, Rose JL, Temple RJ, Schapiro R, Griffin JP. Therapeutic-class wars—drug promotion in a competitive marketplace. *N Engl J Med* 1994; 331: 1350–1353.

33. Oxman AD, Chalmers I, Sackett DL. Publish and be damned: A practical guide to informed consent to treatment. *Br Med J* 2001; 323: 1464–1466.

34. Bekelman JE, Li Y, Gross CP. Scope and impact of financial conflicts of interest in biomedical research; a systematic review. *JAMA* 2003; 289: 454–465.

35. Brennan TA. Buying editorials. *N Engl J Med* 1994; 331: 673–675.

36. Larkin M. Whose article is it anyway? *Lancet* 1999; 354: 136.

37. Flanagin A, Carey LA, Fontanorosa PB, Phillips SG, Pace BP, Lundberg GD, Rennie D. Prevalence of articles with honorary authors and ghost authors in peer-reviewed medical journals. *JAMA* 1998; 280: 222–224.

38. Elliott, C. Pharma buys a conscience. *The American Prospect*, September 24–October 8, 2001, 16–20.

CHAPTER 9

1. Johnson T. Shattuck Lecture: Medicine and the media. *N Engl J Med* 1998; 339: 87–92.

2. Shaw D. Medical miracles or misguided media? *Los Angeles Times*, February 13, 2000, p. A1.

3. Winsten JA. Science and the media: The boundaries of truth. *Health Affairs* 1985; 4(1): 5–23.

4. Entwistle V. Reporting research in medical journals and newspapers. *Br Med J* 1995; 310: 920–923.

5. Woloshin S, Schwartz LM. Press releases: Translating research into news. *JAMA* 2002; 287: 2856–2858.

6. Steinbrook R. Medical journals and medical reporting. *N Engl J Med* 2000; 342: 1668–1671.

7. Shell ER. The Hippocratic wars. *The New York Times Magazine*, June 28, 1998, pp. 34–38.

8. Moynihan R, Bero L, Ross-Degnan D, Henry D, et al. Coverage by the news media of the benefits and risks of medications. *N Engl J Med* 2000; 342: 1645–1650.

9. Shaw D. Overdose of optimism? Stories on what you eat, drink reflect lack of context, appetite for conflict. *Los Angeles Times*, February 14, 2000, p. A11.

10. Psaty BM, Weiss NS, Furberg CD, et al. Surrogate end points, health outcomes, and the drug-approval process for the treatment of risk factors for cardiovascular disease. *JAMA* 1999; 282: 786–790.

11. Echt DS, Liebson PR, Mitchell LB, et al. Mortality and morbidity in patients receiving encainide, flecainide, or placebo. The Cardiac Arrhythmia Suppression Trial. *N Engl J Med* 1991; 324: 781–788.

12. Loo LK, Byrne JM, Hardin SB, Castro D, Fisher FP. Reporting medical information: Does the lay press get it right? *J Gen Intern Med* 1998; 13: Suppl 1, abstract.

13. Burke W, Olsen AH, Pinsky LE, Reynolds SE, Press NA. Misleading presentation of breast cancer in popular magazines. *Effective Clinical Practice* 2001; 4: 58–64.

14. Rossouw JE, Anderson GL, Prentice RL, et al. Risks and benefits of estrogen plus progestin in health postmenopausal women: Principal results from the Women's Health Initiative randomized controlled trial. *JAMA* 2002; 288: 321–333.

15. Moynihan R. Alosetron: A case study in regulatory capture, or a victory for patients' rights? *Br Med J* 2002; 325: 592–595.

16. Moynihan R, Heath I, Henry D. Selling sickness: The pharmaceutical industry and disease mongering. *Br Med J* 2002; 324: 886–891.

17. Schoene ML. Media coverage of unproven spine treatments: Are patients getting an accurate view of the evidence? *The Back Letter* 2002; 17(6): 61–69.

18. Schoene M. A biologic cure for arthritis—or a tiny inconclusive study and a lot of media hype? *The Back Letter* 2001; 16: 40–41.

19. Mello MM, Brennan TA. The controversy over high-dose chemotherapy with autologous bone marrow transplant for breast cancer. *Health Affairs* 2001; 20(5): 101–117.

20. Stadtmauer EA, O'Neill A, Goldstein LJ, Crilley PA, Mangan KF, Ingle JN, et al. Conventional-dose chemotherapy compared with high-dose chemotherapy plus autologous hematopoietic stem-cell transplantation for metastatic breast cancer. Philadelphia Bone Marrow Transplant Group. *N Engl J Med* 2000; 342: 1069–1076.

21. Mills JL. Reporting provocative results: Can we publish "hot" papers without getting burned? *JAMA* 1987; 258: 3428–3429.

CHAPTER 10

1. Mello MM, Brennan TA. The controversy over high-dose chemotherapy with autologous bone marrow transplant for breast cancer. *Health Affairs* 2001; 20: 101–117.

2. Writing Group for the Women's Health Initiative Investigators. Risks and benefits of estrogen plus progestin in healthy postmenopausal women. *JAMA* 2002; 288: 321–333.

3. Fenton JJ, Deyo RA. Patient self-referral for radiologic screening tests: Clinical and ethical concerns. *J Am Board Fam Pract* 2003; 16: 494–501.

4. Napoli M. PSA screening test for prostate cancer: An interview with Otis Brawley, MD. Available at: Center for Medical Consumers web site, www.medicalconsumers.org. Accessed August 9, 2003.

5. Bartley N. Cancer mistake ravages a life. *Seattle Times*, April 25, 2001, p. B1.

6. Anderson RE. Billions for defense; the pervasive nature of defensive medicine. *Arch Intern Med* 1999; 159: 2399–2402.

7. DeKay ML, Asch DA. Is the defensive use of diagnostic tests good for patients, or bad? *Med Decis Making* 1998; 18: 19–28.

8. Eichenwald K. Operating profits: Mining Medicare; How one hospital benefited from questionable surgery. *The New York Times*, August 12, 2003, p. A1.

9. Eichenwald K. Tenet Healthcare paying $54 million in fraud settlement. *The New York Times*, August 7, 2003, p. A1.

10. Fuhrmans V. FBI raids surgery clinics in probe; investigators say patients were paid to have surgery in a $300 million scam. *The Wall Street Journal*, March 19, 2004, p. A7.

11. Swedlow A, Johnson G, Smithline N, Milstein A. Increased costs and rates of use in the California workers' compensation system as a result of self-referral by physicians. *N Engl J Med* 1992; 327: 1502–1506.

12. Hillman BJ, Olson GT, Griffith PE, et al. Physicians' utilization and charges for outpatient diagnostic imaging in a Medicare population. *JAMA* 1992; 268: 2050–2054.

13. Kouri BE, Parsons RG, Alpert HR. Physician self-referral for diagnostic imaging: Review of the empiric literature. *AJR* 2002; 179: 843–850.

14. Mitchell JM, Sunshine JH. Consequences of physicians' ownership of health care facilities—joint ventures in radiation therapy. *N Engl J Med* 1992; 327: 1497–1501.

15. Lipper MH, Hillman BJ, Pates RD, Simpson PM, Mitchell JM, Ballard DJ. Ownership and utilization of MR imagers in the Commonwealth of Virginia. *Radiology* 1995; 195: 217–221.

16. Mitchell JM, Scott E. Physician ownership of physical therapy services. Effects on charges, utilization, profits, and service characteristics. *JAMA* 1992; 268: 2055–2059.

17. Abelson R. An M.R.I. machine for every doctor? Someone has to pay. *The New York Times*, March 13, 2004, p. A1.

18. Pham HH, Devers KJ, May JH, Berenson R. Financial pressures spur physician entrepreneurialism. *Health Affairs* 2004; 23: 70–81.

19. Kowalczyk L. Doctors feeling pinched seen seeking ways to hike incomes. *The Boston Globe*, March 9, 2004, p. D1.

20. Eichenwald K, Kolata G. Hidden interest—a special report; when physicians double as entrepreneurs. *The New York Times*. Nov. 30, 1999, p. A1.

21. Maulitz RC. That was the century that was: Historical perspectives on medical life at the fin de siecle. *Ann Intern Med* 1999; 131: 75–78.

22. Napoli M. The selling of heart scans to people without symptoms [interview with TB Graboys]. Available at: Center for Medical Consumers web site, www.medicalconsumers.org. Accessed August 9, 2003.

23. Graboys TB. Coronary angiography: A long look at a short queue. *JAMA* 1999; 281: 184–185.

24. Kowalczyk L. Surgeries on web find favor with hospitals. *The Boston Globe*, July 16, 2003, p. A1.

25. Rogers M. Battle ready. *Health Leaders* 2002; V (no. 12): 45–54.

26. Devers K, Brewster LR, Ginsburg PB. Specialty hospitals: Focused factories or cream skimmers? Center for Studying Health System Change Issue Brief No. 62, April 2003.

27. General Accounting Office. Specialty hospitals. Information on national market share, physician ownership, and patients served. GAO-03-683R, April 18, 2003.

28. Clinton HR. Now can we talk about health care? *The New York Times Magazine*, April 18, 2004, p. 26.

CHAPTER 11

1. Dresser R. *When Science Offers Salvation: Patient Advocacy and Research Ethics*. New York: Oxford University Press, 2001.

2. Stolberg SG. Patients lobby for cash for research into illness. *The New York Times*, April 14, 1999, p. A18.

3. Kolata G. FDA debate on speedy access to AIDS drugs is reopening. *The New York Times*, September 12, 1994, p. A13.

4. Belkin L. Charity begins at . . . the marketing meeting, the gala event, the product tie-in. *The New York Times Magazine*, December 22, 1996, p. 40.

5. Mello MM, Brennan TA. The controversy over high-dose chemotherapy with autologous bone marrow transplant for breast cancer. *Health Affairs* 2001; 20(5): 101–117.

6. Aaron LA, Buchwald D. A review of the evidence for overlap among unexplained clinical conditions. *Ann Intern Med* 2001; 134 (9 pt. 2): 868–881.

7. Barsky AJ, Borus FJ. Functional somatic syndromes. *Ann Intern Med* 1999; 130: 910–921.

8. Wessely S. Chronic fatigue syndrome—trials and tribulations. *JAMA* 2001; 286: 1378–1379.

9. Fitzpatrick M. Health: The making of a new disease: Michael Fitzpatrick on why the medical profession's latest ruling on ME (or chronic fatigue syndrome) is nothing short of disastrous. *The Guardian (London)*, February 7, 2002, G2, p. 14.

10. Townsel LJ. Symptoms are "all over the map." *St. Louis Post-Dispatch*, July 24, 1999, Lifestyle, p. 35.

11. Deyo RA, Psaty BM, Simon G, Wagner EH, Omenn GS. The messenger under attack—intimidation of researchers by special-interest groups. *N Engl J Med* 1997; 336: 1176–1180.

12. Steere AC. Lyme disease. *N Engl J Med* 2001; 345: 115–125.

13. Klempner MS, Hu LT, Evans J, et al. Two controlled trials of antibiotic treatment in patients with persistent symptoms and a history of Lyme disease. *N Engl J Med* 2001; 345: 85–92.

14. Barnard A. Ticked off long-term sufferers of Lyme disease fight for help. *The Boston Globe*, July 10, 2001, p. B1.

15. Gross J. In Lyme disease debate, some patients feel lost. *The New York Times*, July 7, 2001, p. B1.

16. Gerth J, Stolberg SG. Medicine merchants: Cultivating alliances; with quiet, unseen ties, drug makers sway debate. *The New York Times*, October 5, 2000, p. A1.

17. Lenzer J. Lay campaigners for prostate screening are funded by industry. *Br Med J* 2003; 326: 680.

18. Lenzer J. The grassroots are greener. Praxis Post: the webzine of medicine and culture, March 21, 2001. Available at: http://praxis.md/post/trends/032101. Accessed August 21, 2002.

19. O'Harrow R Jr. Grass roots seeded by drugmaker; Schering-Plough uses "coalitions" to sell costly treatment. *The Washington Post*, September 12, 2000, p. A1.

20. California Attorney General's Office. What's in a nonprofit's name? Public trust, profit and the potential for public deception. April 1999. Available at: http://caag.state.ca.us/publications/nonprofit/index.html. Accessed December 14, 2002.

CHAPTER 12

1. Horton R. Lotronex and the FDA: A fatal erosion of integrity. *Lancet* 2001; 357: 1544–1545.

2. Deyo RA. Gaps, tensions, and conflicts in the FDA approval process: Implications for clinical practice. *J Am Board Fam Pract* 2004; 17: 142–149.

3. Lipsky MS, Sharp LK. From idea to market: The drug approval process. *J Am Board Fam Pract* 2001; 14: 362–367.

4. Lasser KE, Allen PD, Woolhandler SJ, Himmelstein DU, Wolfe SM, Bor DH. Timing of new black box warnings and withdrawals for prescription medications. *JAMA* 2002; 287: 2215–2220.

5. Friedman MA, Woodcock J, Lumpkin MM, Shuren JE, Hass AE, Thompson LJ. The safety of newly approved medicines: Do recent market removals mean there is a problem? *JAMA* 1999; 281: 1728–1734.

6. Maisel WH, Sweeney MO, Stevenson WG, Ellison KE, Epstein LM. Recalls and safety alerts involving pacemakers and implantable cardioverter-defibrillator devices. *JAMA* 2001; 286: 793–799.

7. Writing Group for the Women's Health Initiative Investigators. Risks and benefits of estrogen plus progestin in healthy postmenopausal women. *JAMA* 2002; 288: 321–333.

8. Grady D, Herrington D, Bittner V, et al. Cardiovascular disease outcomes during 68 years of hormone therapy: Heart and Estrogen/progestin Replacement Study Follow-up (HERS II). *JAMA* 2002; 288: 49–57.

9. The ALLHAT officers and Coordinators for the ALLHAT Collaborative Research Group. Major outcomes in high-risk hypertensive patients randomized to angiotensin-converting enzyme inhibitor or calcium channel blocker vs diuretic: The Antihypertensive and Lipid-Lowering treatment to prevent Heart Attack Trial (ALLHAT). *JAMA* 2002; 288: 2981–2997.

10. Echt DS, Liebson PR, Mitchell LB, et al. Mortality and morbidity in patients receiving encainide, flecainide, or placebo. The Cardiac Arrhythmia Suppression Trial. *N Engl J Med* 1991; 324: 781–788.

11. Moore TJ. *Deadly Medicine: Why Tens of Thousands of Heart Patients Died in America's Worst Drug Disaster*. New York, Simon and Schuster, 1995.

12. Petersen M. Diuretics' value drowned out by trumpeting of newer drugs. *The New York Times*, December 18, 2002, p. A32.

13. Gorelick PB, Richardson D, Kelly M, Ruland S, Hung E, Harris Y, et al. Aspirin and ticlopidine for prevention of recurrent stroke in black patients: A randomized trial. *JAMA* 2003; 289: 2947–2957.

14. Anonymous. Montelukast (Singulair) for allergic rhinitis. *Med Lett*, March 17, 2003: 45: 21–22.

15. Gilpin KN. Pfizer pays large fine to settle drug suit. *International Herald Tribune*, May 14, 2004, sec. 1, p. 11.

16. Gahart MT, Duhamel LM, Dievier A, Price R. Examining the FDA's oversight of direct-to-consumer advertising. *Health Affairs*, February 26, 2003 (Web exclusive), W3-120–W3-123.

17. Ramsey SD, Luce BR, Deyo R, Franklin G. The limited state of technology assessment for medical devices: Facing the issues. *Am J Managed Care* 1998; 4(special issue): SP188–SP199.

18. Merrill RA. Modernizing the FDA: An incremental revolution. *Health Affairs* 1999; 18(2): 96–111.

19. Food and Drug Administration web site. Available at: http://www.fda.gov. Accessed August 19, 2002.

20. Handelsman H. Intermittent positive pressure breathing (IPPB) therapy. *Health Technol Assess Rep* 1991; 1: 1–9. U.S. Department of Health and Human Services, Agency for Health Care Policy and Research, December 1991, AHCPR Pub. No. 92-0013.

21. FDA Center for Devices and Radiological Health, Office of Device Evaluation Annual Report 2002. Available at: http://www.fda.gov/cdrh/annual/fy2002/ode/index.html. Accessed April 11, 2003.

22. Lundblad J, Kaplan S, et al. How a new policy led to seven deadly drugs; Medicine: Once a wary watchdog, the U.S. Food and Drug Administration set out to become a "partner" of the pharmaceutical industry; today, the American public has more remedies, but some are proving lethal. *Los Angeles Times*, December 20, 2000. p. A1.

23. Adams C, Hensley S. Health & Technology: Drug makers want FDA to move quicker. *The Wall Street Journal*, January 29, 2002, p. B12.

24. Adams C. FDA may start assessing fees on makers of medical devices. *The Wall Street Journal*, May 21, 2002. p. D6.

25. Angell M, Relman AS. Prescription for profit. *The Washington Post*, June 20, 2001, p. A27.

26. Adams C. FDA looks to cure its high attrition rate. Agency's efficiency may suffer as workers defect, quit or retire. *The Wall Street Journal*, August 19, 2002, p. A4.

27. Goldberg R. FDA needs a dose of reform. *The Wall Street Journal*, September 30, 2002.

28. Moore TJ, Psaty BM, Furberg CD. Time to act on drug safety. *JAMA* 1998; 279: 1571–1573.

29. Adams C. Test data for some drugs are long overdue at the FDA. *The Wall Street Journal*, January 28, 2003, p. B1.

30. Ahmad SR. Adverse drug event monitoring at the Food and Drug

Administration: Your report can make a difference. *J Gen Intern Med* 2003; 18: 57–60.

31. Wood AJJ. The safety of new medicines: The importance of asking the right questions. *JAMA* 1999: 281; 1753–1754.

32. Cauchon D. FDA advisers tied to industry. *USA Today*, September 25, 2000, p. 1A.

33. Cauchon D. Number of drug experts available is limited. Many waivers granted for those who have conflicts of interest. *USA Today*, September 25, 2000, p. 10A.

34. Gribbin A. House investigates panels involved with drug safety. Mismanagement claims spur action. *The Washington Times*, June 18, 2001, p. A1.

35. Pear R. Drug makers' generic tactics criticized. *The New York Times*, April 24, 2002, p. C6.

36. Anonymous. Doctor groups settle FTC charges. *USA Today*, August 21, 2002, p. 1B.

37. Gugliotta G. FTC says six firms used false online ads; medical, diet claims targeted by crackdown. *The Washington Post*, June 15, 2001, p. E1.

CHAPTER 13

1. Anonymous. The therapeutics of the cacodylates. *JAMA* 1903; 40: 651–652.

2. Much of this section was previously published and is reproduced here with modest revision and with permission from Deyo RA. Bruce Psaty and the risks of calcium channel blockers. *Qual Saf Health Care* 2002; 11: 294–296.

3. Psaty BM, Heckbert SR, Koepsell TD, et al. The risk of myocardial infarction associated with antihypertensive drug therapies. *JAMA* 1995; 274: 620–625.

4. Joint National Committee on Detection, Evaluation, and Treatment of High Blood Pressure. The Fifth Report of the Joint National Committee on Detection, Evaluation, and Treatment of High Blood Pressure (JNC V). *Arch Intern Med* 1993; 153: 154–183.

5. Deyo RA, Psaty BM, Simon G, Wagner EH, Omenn GS. The messenger under attack—intimidation of researchers by special-interest groups. *N Engl J Med* 1997; 336: 1176–1180.

6. Stryer DB, Lurie P, Bero LA. Dear Doctor . . . regarding calcium channel blockers. *JAMA* 1996; 275: 517.

7. Horton R. Bayer accused of disinformation. *Lancet* 1995; 346: 891–892.

8. Borhani NO, Mercuri M, Borhani PA, et al. Final outcome results of the Multicenter Isradipine Diuretic Atherosclerosis Study (MIDAS). A randomized controlled trial. *JAMA* 1996; 276: 785–791.

9. Pahor M, Psaty BM, Alderman MH, et al. Health outcomes associated with calcium antagonists compared with other first-line antihypertensive therapies: A meta-analysis of randomized controlled trials. *Lancet* 2000; 356: 1949–1954.

10. Neal B, MacMahon S, Chapman N. Effects of ACE inhibitors, calcium antagonists, and other blood-pressure lowering drugs: Results of prospectively designed overviews of randomized trials. Blood Pressure Lowering Treatment Trialists Collaboration. *Lancet* 2000; 356: 1955–1964.

11. Pahor M, Psaty BM, Alderman MH, et al. Blood pressure-lowering treatment (letter). *Lancet* 2001; 358: 152–153.

12. The ALLHAT officers and coordinators for the ALLHAT Collaborative Research Group. Major outcomes in high-risk hypertensive patients randomized to angiotensin-converting enzyme inhibitor or calcium channel blocker vs. diuretic. The Antihypertensive and Lipid-Lowering treatment to prevent Heart Attack Trial (ALLHAT). *JAMA* 2002; 288: 2981–2997.

13. Furberg CD, Psaty BM, Pahor M, Alderman MH. Clinical implications of recent findings from the Antihypertensive and Lipid-Lowering treatment to prevent Heart Attack Trial (ALLHAT) and other studies of hypertension. *Ann Intern Med* 2001; 135: 1074–1078.

14. Kizer JR, Kimmel SE. Epidemiologic review of the calcium channel blocker drugs: An up-to-date perspective on the proposed hazards. *Arch Intern Med* 2001; 161: 1145–1158.

15. Trend of the Month. Global pharmaceutical sales up 11%. *Drug Benefit Trends* 2001; 13(11): 8

16. Langreth R. The new drug war. *Forbes* March 31, 2003, p. 84a.

17. Fischer MA, Avorn J. Economic implications of evidence-based prescribing for hypertension. Can better care cost less? *JAMA* 2004; 291: 1850–1856.

18. Agodoa LY, Appel L, Bakris GL, et al. Effect of ramipril vs amlodipine on renal outcomes in hypertensive nephrosclerosis: a randomized controlled trial. *JAMA* 2001; 285: 2719–2728.

19. Lewis EF, Hunsicker LG, Clarke WR, et al. Renoprotective effect of angiotensin-receptor antagonist irbesartan in patients with nephropathy due to type 2 diabetes. *N Engl J Med* 2001; 345: 851–860.

20. Joint National Committee on Prevention Detection, Evaluation, and Treatment of High Blood Pressure. The Sixth Report of the Joint National Committee on Prevention, Detection, Evaluation, and Treatment of High Blood Pressure. *Arch Intern Med* 1997; 157: 2413–2446.

21. Maclure M, Dormuth C, Naumann T, et al. Influences of educational interventions and adverse news about calcium-channel blockers on first line prescribing of antihypertensive drugs to elderly people in British Columbia. *Lancet* 1998; 352: 943–948.

22. Stelfox HT, Chua G, O'Rourke K, Detsky AS. Conflict of interest in the debate over calcium-channel antagonists. *N Engl J Med* 1998; 338: 101–106.

23. Rennie D. Thyroid storm. *JAMA* 1997; 277: 1238–1243.

24. King RT. Bitter pill: How a drug firm paid for university study, then undermined it. *The Wall Street Journal*, April 25, 1996, p. A1.

25. Dong BJ, Hauck WW, Gambertoglio JG, et al. Bioequivalence of generic and brand-name levothyroxine products in the treatment of hypothyroidism. *JAMA* 1997; 227: 1205–1213.

26. American Health Line. Rx Industry: "60 Minutes" uncovers Synthroid controversy. December 20, 1999. Available at: www.nationaljournal.com. Accessed December 20, 1999.

27. Kelly K, Crowley J, Bunn PA, et al. Randomized phase III trial of paclitaxel plus carboplatin versus vinorelbine plus cisplatin in the treatment of patients with advanced non-small-cell lung cancer: A Southwest Oncology Group trial. *J Clin Oncol* 2001; 19: 3210–3218.

28. Cloud DS, McGinley L. How drug makers influence Medicare reimbursements to doctors. *The Wall Street Journal*, September 27, 2000, p. B1.

29. Dembner A. $840M penalty is expected for drug company. *The Boston Globe*, May 28, 2001, p. A1.

30. Rybak DC. Drugmaker sued; Attorney General Mike Hatch says government insurers are being charged huge markups on drugs—a practice he intends to stop. *Star Tribune (Minneapolis)*, June 19, 2002, p. 1D.

31. Abelson R. Drug sales bring huge profits, and scrutiny, to cancer doctors. *The New York Times*, January 26, 2003, sec. 1, p.1.

32. Iglehart JK. Medicare and drug pricing. *N Engl J Med* 2003; 348: 1590–1597.

33. Powell JH. Drug firm sued for alleged overcharges. *Boston Herald*, January 4, 2002, p. 29.

34. Williamson T. Abbott reduces some prices for agencies, hospitals. *Chicago Sun-Times*, June 15, 2001, p. 62.

35. Emanuel EJ, Young-Xu Y, Levinsky NG, Gazelle G, Saynina O, Ash AS. Chemotherapy use among Medicare beneficiaries at the end of life. *Ann Intern Med* 2003; 138: 639–643.

36. Ramsey SD, Moinpour CM, Lovato LC, et al. Economic analysis of vinorelbine plus cisplatin versus paclitaxel plus carboplatin for advanced non-small-cell lung cancer. *J Nat Cancer Inst* 2002; 94: 291–297.

37. Moore TJ. *Deadly Medicine: Why Tens of Thousands of Heart Patients Died in America's Worst Drug Disaster.* New York: Simon and Schuster, 1995.

38. Echt DS, Liebson PR, Mitchell LB, et al. Mortality and morbidity in patients receiving encainide, flecainide, or placebo. The Cardiac Arrhythmia Suppression Trial. *N Engl J Med* 1991; 324: 781–788.

39. The Cardiac Arrhythmia Suppression Trial Investigators. Effect of the antiarrhythmic agent moricizine on survival after myocardial infarction. *N Engl J Med* 1992; 327: 227–233.

40. Alderson P, Bunn F, Lefebvre C, et al. Human albumin solution for resuscitation and volume expansion in critically ill patients. Cochrane Database syst Rev 2002; (1): CD001208.

41. Saltus R. AIDS drug researchers say firm pressured them. Findings published, but fight goes to court. *The Boston Globe*, November 1, 2000, p. A3.

42. Kellum JA, Decker JM. Use of dopamine in acute renal failure: A meta-analysis. *Crit Care Med* 2001; 29: 1526–1531.

43. Snow V, Weiss KB, LeFevre M, et al. Management of newly detected atrial fibrillation: A clinical practice guideline from the American Academy of Family Physicians and the American College of Physicians. *Ann Intern Med* 2003; 139: 1009–1017.

44. Writing Group for the Women's Health Initiative Investigators. Risks and benefits of estrogen plus progestin in healthy postmenopausal women. *JAMA* 2002; 288: 321–333.

45. Grady D. Minimal benefit is seen in drugs for Alzheimer's. *The New York Times*, April 7, 2004.

CHAPTER 14

1. Groopman J. A knife in the back. Is surgery the best approach to chronic back pain? *The New Yorker*, April 8, 2002, pp. 66–73.

2. Salkever A. How high tech is operating on medicine. *Business Week* online, October 15, 2002. Available at: www.businessweek.com. Accessed October 15, 2002.

3. Centers for Medicare and Medicaid Services. Health care industry market update: Medical devices and supplies. October 10, 2002. Available at: www.cms.hhs.gov/marketupdate. Accessed July 23, 2004.

4. Bell R. *Impure Science*. New York: John Wiley and Sons, 1992, pp. 162–176.

5. Camp JP, Smith M, Szurgot MA. Lessons of the Bjork-Shiley heart valve failure. University of Texas at Austin, December 3, 1997. Available at: www.me.utexas.edu/~uer/heartvalves/index.html. Accessed April 27, 2003.

6. Fielder JH. Ethical issues in biomedical engineering: The Bjork-Shiley heart valve. *IEEE Engineering in Medicine and Biology*, March 1991, pp. 76–78.

7. Lilliston B: Settling with Shiley. Available at: http://multinationalmonitor.org/hyper/issues/1994/08/mm0894_14.html. Accessed April 27, 2003.

8. Palast G. *The Best Democracy Money Can Buy*. New York: Plume Books, 2002, pp. 231–235.

9. Cherkin DC, Deyo RA, Wheeler K, Ciol MA. Physician variation in diagnostic testing for low back pain. Who you see is what you get. *Arthritis Rheum* 1994; 37: 15–22.

10. Turner JA, Ersek M, Herron L, Haselkorn J, Kent D, Ciol MA, Deyo R. Patient outcomes after lumbar spinal fusions. *JAMA* 1992; 268: 907–911.

11. Deyo RA, Ciol MA, Cherkin DC, Loeser JD, Bigos SJ. Lumbar spinal fusion. A cohort study of complications, reoperations, and resource use in the Medicare population. *Spine* 1993; 18: 1463–1470.

12. Bigos S, Bowyer O, Braen G, et al. Acute Low Back Problems in Adults. Clinical Practice Guideline No. 14. AHCPR Publication No. 95-0642. Rockville, MD: U.S. Department of Health and Human Services, Agency for Health Care Policy and Research, Public Health Service, December 1994.

13. Deyo RA, Psaty BM, Simon G, Wagner EH, Omenn GS. The messenger under attack—intimidation of researchers by special-interest groups. *N Engl J Med* 1997; 336: 1176–1180.

14. Stryker J. A scalpel in the back. National Public Radio, Marketplace, air date October 3, 1995.

15. Borzo G. Societies caught in fraud cases: Product-liability lawsuits raise questions about CME vs. promotion. *American Medical News,* May 12, 1997; 1: 24–25.

16. Weiser B. Settlement of medical device lawsuits stirs new dispute; rival firm calls deal "travesty of justice." *The Washington Post*, December 12, 1996, p. D3.

17. Deyo RA, Nachemson A, Mirza SK. Spinal fusion surgery: The case for restraint. *N Engl J Med* 2004; 350: 722–726.

18. Bono CM, Lee CK. Critical analysis of trends in fusion for degenerative disc disease over the last twenty years: Influence of technique on fusion rate and clinical outcome. Presented at the annual meeting of the International Society for the Study of the Lumbar Spine, Vancouver, B.C., Canada, May 13–17, 2003.

19. Abelson R, Petersen M. An operation to ease back pain bolsters the bottom line, too. *The New York Times*, December 31, 2003, p. A1.

20. Anonymous. Pedicle screws are at center of controversy. *The Washington Post*, April 18, 1995, p. Z12.

21. Dalen JE. The pulmonary artery catheter—friend, foe, or accomplice? *JAMA* 2001; 286: 348–350.

22. Parsons PE. Progress in research on pulmonary-artery catheters. *N Engl J Med* 2003; 348: 66–68.

23. Gore JM, Goldberg FJ, Spodick DH, et al. A community wide assessment of the use of pulmonary artery catheters in patients with acute myocardial infarction. *Chest* 1987; 92: 721–727.

24. Zion MM, Balkin J, Rosenmann D, et al. Use of pulmonary artery catheters in patients with acute myocardial infarction: analysis of experience in 5,841 patients in the SPRINT registry. *Chest* 1990; 98: 1331–1335.

25. Connors AF, Speroff T, Dawson NR, et al. The effectiveness of right heart catheterization in the initial care of critically ill patients. *JAMA* 1996; 276: 889–897.

26. Polanczyk CA, Rohde LE, Goldman L, et al. Right heart catheterization and cardiac complications in patients undergoing noncardiac surgery: an observational study. *JAMA* 2001; 286: 309–314.

27. Sandham JD, Hull RD, Brant RF, et al. A randomized, controlled trial of the use of pulmonary-artery catheters in high-risk surgical patients. *N Engl J Med* 2003; 348: 5–14.

28. Richard C, Warszawski J, Anguel N, et al, for the French Pulmonary Artery Catheter Study Group. Early use of the pulmonary artery catheter and outcomes in patients with shock and acute respiratory distress syndrome. A randomized controlled trial. *JAMA* 2003; 290: 2713–2720.

29. Powell JT, Greenhalgh RM. Small abdominal aortic aneurysms. *N Engl J Med* 2003; 348: 1895–1901.

30. Finz S. Guilty plea in medical fraud—12 patients die; Bay area branch of Guidant fined $92 million over malfunctions. *San Francisco Chronicle*, June 13, 2003, p. A1.

31. Eichenwald, K. Maker admits it hid problems in artery device. *The New York Times*, June 13, 2003, p. A1.

32. Feigal DW. FDA Public Health Notification: Problems with endovascular grafts for treatment of abdominal aortic aneurysm (AAA). Letter dated April 27, 2001. Available at: www.fda.gov/cdrh/safety/aaa.html. Accessed July 23, 2004.

33. Pauza K, Howell S, Dreyfuss P, Peloza J, Park K. A randomized, double-blind placebo controlled trial evaluating intradiscal electrothermal anuloplasty (IDET). Presented at Annual Meeting of the International Society for the Study of the Lumbar Spine, Vancouver, BC, 2003.

34. Freeman BJC, Fraser R, Cain CMJ, Hall DJ. A randomized, double-blind controlled efficacy study—intradiscal electrothermal therapy (IDET) versus placebo. Presented at Annual Meeting of the International Society for the Study of the Lumbar Spine, Vancouver, BC, May 13–17, 2003.

35. Anonymous. Maker recalls new type of heart valve. *The Washington Post*, January 25, 2000, p. A2.

36. Saririan M, Eisenberg MJ. Myocardial laser revascularization for the treatment of end-stage coronary artery disease. *J Am Coll Cardiol* 2003; 41: 173–183.

37. Anderson RE. Billions for defense; the pervasive nature of defensive medicine. *Arch Intern Med* 1999; 159: 2399–2402.

38. Feigal DW, Gardner SN, McClellan M. Ensuring safe and effective medical devices. *N Engl J Med* 2003; 348: 191–192.

CHAPTER 15

1. Navarro J (ed.). *Health*. Washington DC: Pan American Health Organization, 2002, p. 151.

2. Finlayson EVA, Birkmeyer JD. Operative mortality with elective surgery in older adults. *Eff Clin Pract* 2001; 4: 172–177.

3. Groopman J. A knife in the back. Is surgery the best approach to chronic back pain? *The New Yorker*, April 8, 2002, pp. 66–73.

4. Aiken LH, Clarke SP, Sloane DM, Sochalski J, Silber JH. Hospital nurse staffing and patient mortality, nurse burnout, and job dissatisfaction. *JAMA* 2002; 288: 1987–1993.

5. Lerner BH. *Breast Cancer Wars: Hope, Fear, and the Pursuit of a Cure in Twentieth-Century America*. New York: Oxford University Press, 2001.

6. Fisher B, Anderson S, Bryant J, et al. Twenty-year follow-up of a randomized trial comparing total mastectomy, lumpectomy, and lumpectomy plus irradiation for the treatment of invasive breast cancer. *N Engl J Med* 2002; 347: 1233–1241.

7. Veronesi U, Cascinelli N, Mariani L, et al. Twenty-year follow-up of a randomized study comparing breast-conserving surgery with radical mastectomy for early breast cancer. *N Engl J Med* 2002; 347: 1227–1232.

8. Mohler ER. Lymphedema. UpToDate Online 10.3, 2003, www.update.com. Accessed January 18, 2003.

9. Rutkow IM. William Stewart Halsted. *Arch Surg* 2000; 135: 1478.

10. Kolata G. Lumpectomies seen as equal in benefit to breast removals. *The New York Times*, October 17, 2002, p. A1.

11. Rubin R. Lumpectomy as safe a choice as mastectomy, studies say. *USA Today*, October 17, 2002, p. 13D.

12. Morrow M. Rational local therapy for breast cancer. *N Engl J Med* 2002; 347: 1270–1271.

13. Benson H, McCallie DP. Angina pectoris and the placebo effect. *N Engl J Med* 1979; 300: 1424–1429.

14. Beecher HK. Surgery as placebo. A quantitative study of bias. *JAMA* 1961; 176: 1102–1107.

15. Cobb LA, Thomas GI, Dillard DH, Merendino KA, Bruce RA. An evaluation of internal-mammary-artery ligation by a double blind technic. *N Engl J Med* 1959; 260: 1115–1118.

16. Dimond EG, Kittle CF, Crockett JE. Comparison of internal mammary artery ligation and sham operation for angina pectoris. *Am J Cardiol* 1960; 5: 483–486.

17. Kaptchuk TJ, Goldman P, Stone DA, Stason WB. Do medical devices have enhanced placebo effects? *J Clin Epidemiol* 2000; 53: 786–792.

18. Moseley JB, O'Malley K, Petersen NJ, Menke TJ, Brody BA, Kuykendall DH, et al. A controlled trial of arthroscopic surgery for osteoarthritis of the knee. *N Engl J Med* 2002; 347: 81–88.

19. Talbot M. The placebo prescription. *The New York Times Magazine*, January 9, 2000, p. 6-34.

20. Kolata G. Study casts doubt on value of popular knee surgery. *The New York Times*, July 10, 2002.

21. Felson DT, Buckwalter J. Debridement and lavage for osteoarthritis of the knee. *N Engl J Med* 2002; 347: 132–133.

22. The EC/IC Bypass Study Group. Failure of extracranial-intracranial arterial bypass to reduce the risk of ischemic stroke. Results of an international randomized trial. *N Engl J Med* 1985; 313: 1191–1200.

23. Haynes RB, Mukherjee J, Sackett DL, Taylor DW, Barnett HJ, Peerless SJ. Functional status changes following medical or surgical treatment for cerebral ischemia. Results of the extracranial-intracranial bypass study. *JAMA* 1987; 257: 2043–2046.

24. Okie S. Stroke operation deemed ineffective; popular surgery to redirect blood flow may be abandoned in light of new study. *The Washington Post*, July 17, 1985, *Health*, p. 7.

25. Grubb RL, Derdeyn CP, Fritsch SM et al. Importance of hemodynamic factors in the prognosis of symptomatic carotid occlusion. *JAMA* 1998; 280: 1055–1060.

26. Adams HP. Occlusion of the internal carotid artery: Reopening a closed door? *JAMA* 1998; 280: 1093–1094.

27. Kolata G. Parkinson's research is set back by failure of fetal cell implants. *The New York Times*, March 8, 2001, p. A1.

28. Freed CR, Greene PE, Breeze RE, et al. Transplantation of embryonic dopamine neurons for severe Parkinson's disease. *N Engl J Med* 2001; 344: 710–719.

29. Tarkan L. In many delivery rooms, a routine becomes less routine. *The New York Times*, February 26, 2002, p. F6.

30. Weber AM, Meyn L. Episiotomy use in the United States, 1979–1997. *Obstet Gynecol* 2002; 100: 1177–1182.

31. Carroli G, Belizan J. Episiotomy for vaginal birth (Cochrane Review). In: The Cochrane Library, Issue 4. Oxford: Update Software, 2002.

32. Marcus AD. Saying no to the knife—new research questions need for some common surgeries; antibiotics instead of scars. *The Wall Street Journal*, April 22, 2003, p. D1.

33. Venstrom JM, McBride MA, Tother KI, Hirshberg B, Orchard TH, Harlan DM. Survival after pancreas transplantation in patients with diabetes and preserved kidney function. *JAMA* 2003; 290: 2817–2823.

34. Neumayer L, Giobbie-Hurder A, Jonasson O, et al. Open mesh versus laparoscopic mesh repair of inguinal hernia. *N Engl J Med* 2004; 350: 1819–1827.

CHAPTER 16

1. Federal Trade Commission Consumer Alert. Paunch lines: Weight loss claims are no joke for dieters. Available at: www.ftc.gov/bcp/conline/pubs/alerts/paunch.htm. Accessed March 25, 2004.

2. O'Keefe M. O's pitcher dies after workout; heatstroke is cause; docs test for ephedra. *Daily News (New York)*, February 18, 2003, p. 53.

3. Chass M. Baseball; varied factors caused pitcher's death. *The New York Times*, February 19, 2003, p. D1.

4. Sheinin D. Bechler's widow plans to file suit; ephedra company would be focus. *The Washington Post*, February 25, 2003, p. D1.

5. Times wire services. In Brief/Utah: Company challenges FDA ban on ephedra. *Los Angeles Times*, May 5, 2004, p. A17.

6. Duenwald M. Despite FDA ban, ephedra won't go away. *The New York Times*, February 17, 2004, p. F5.

7. Costello D. Medicine; as ephedra ban takes effect, enforcement becomes the issue; FDA says it will monitor online availability, but critics contend people will be able to get the supplement. *Los Angeles Times*, April 12, 2004, p. F3.

8. Federal Trade Commission, Food and Drug Administration, National Association of Attorneys General. The facts about weight loss products and programs. Available at: http://vm.cfsan.fda.gov/~dms/wgtloss.html. Accessed March 25, 2004.

9. American Obesity Association Fact Sheets. Available at: http://www.obesity.org /subs/fastfacts/Obesity_Consumer_Protect.shtml. Accessed April 22, 2004.

10. CNN.com. Consumer Reports reveals successful diet tips. May 7, 2002. Available at: http://www.cnn.com/2002/HEALTH/05/06/diet/. Accessed May 23, 2004.

11. Burros M. National Briefing Washington: Group wants rules on food supplements. *The New York Times*, April 2, 2004, p. A17.

12. Pear R, Grady D. Government moves to curtail the use of diet supplement. *The New York Times*, March 1, 2003, p. A1.

13. Grady D. Seeking to fight fat, she lost her liver. *The New York Times*, March 4, 2003, p. F1.

14. Grady D. Quest for weight loss drug takes an unusual turn. *The New York Times*, April 15, 2003.

15. Morrow DJ. Fen-phen maker to pay billions in settlement of diet-injury cases. *The New York Times*, October 8, 1999, p. A1.

16. Anonymous. Diet drug firm accused of funding favorable articles. *Los Angeles Times*, May 24, 1999, p. A8.

17. Abelson R, Glater JD. A Texas jury rules against a diet drug. *The New York Times*, April 28, 2004, p. C1.

18. U.S. Department of Health and Human Services. Gastrointestinal surgery for severe obesity. NIH publication No. 01-4006, December 2001. Available at: www.niddk.nih.gov/health/nutrit/pubs/gastric/gastricsurgery.htm. Accessed May 23, 2004.

19. Langreth R. Operation! *Forbes*, October 27, 2003, p. 246.

20. Steinbrook R. Surgery for severe obesity. *N Engl J Med* 2004; 350: 1075–1079.

21. Grady D. Operation for obesity leaves some in misery. *The New York Times*, May 4, 2004, p. F1.

22. Davis R. Proliferation of obesity surgeries raises alarm. *USA Today*, May 5, 2004, p. 7D.

23. Narins RS. Liposuction. *Dermatol Clin* 2001; 19(3), 483–489, ix.

24. Schlosser E. *Fast Food Nation*. Boston: Houghton Mifflin Co., 2001.

25. Foster GD, Wyatt HR, Hill JO, McGuckin BG, Brill C, Mohammed BS, et al. A randomized trial of a low-carbohydrate diet for obesity. *N Engl J Med* 2003 348(21): 2082–2090.

26. Samaha FF, Iqbal N, Seshadri P, Chicano KL, Daily DA, McGrory J, et al. A low-carbohydrate as compared with a low-fat diet in severe obesity. *N Engl J Med* 2003 348(21): 2074–2081.

CHAPTER 17

1. Clemens S. *Mark Twain in Eruption; Mark Twain's Autobiography*, BA DeVoto ed. New York: Harper, 1940.

2. Brown D. First, do the trials. Then, do no harm. *The Washington Post*, August 4, 2002, p. B1.

3. Sackett DL, Rosenberg WMC, Gray JAM, Haynes RB, Richardson WS. Evidence-based medicine: What it is and what it isn't. *Br Med J* 1996; 312: 71–72.

4. Isaacs D, Fitzgerald D. Seven alternatives to evidence based medicine. *Br Med J* 1999; 319: 1618.

5. Chalmers I. The Cochrane collaboration: Preparing, maintaining, and disseminating systematic reviews of the effects of health care. *Ann NY Acad Sci* 1993; 703: 156–163.

6. Chalmers I, Haynes B. Reporting, updating, and correcting systematic reviews of the effects of health care. *Br Med J* 1994; 309: 862–865.

7. Naylor CD. Grey zones of clinical practice: Some limits to evidence-based medicine. *Lancet* 1995; 345: 840–842.

8. Lundberg GD. *Severed Trust: Why American Medicine Hasn't Been Fixed.* New York: Basic Books, 2000, pp. 162–183.

9. Barondess JA. Medicine and professionalism. *Arch Intern Med* 2003; 163: 145–149.

10. Brennan T, Blank L, Cohen J, et al. for the Medical Professionalism Project. Medical professionalism in the new millennium: A physician charter. *Ann Intern Med* 2002; 136: 243–246.

CHAPTER 18

1. Bufill JA. Patients need patience rather than the latest technology. *St. Louis Post-Dispatch*, March 20, 2000, p. D17.

2. Thomas L. *The Fragile Species*. New York: Collier Books, 1993, p. 44.

3. Detsky AS. Are clinical trials a cost-effective investment? *JAMA* 1989; 262: 1795–1800.

4. Brenner M, Jones B, Daneschvar HL, Triff S. New National Emphysema Treatment Trial paradigm of Health Care Financing Administration-sponsored clinical research trials: Advances and dilemmas. *J Invest Med* 2002; 50: 95–100.

5. Fishman A, Martinez F, Naunheim K, et al for the National Emphysema Treatment Trial Research Group. A randomized trial comparing lung-volume-reduction surgery with medical therapy for severe emphysema. *N Engl J Med* 2003; 348: 2059–2073.

6. Fishman A, Fessler H, Martinez F, et al for the National Emphysema Treatment Trial Research Group. Patients at high risk of death after lung-volume-reduction surgery. *N Engl J Med* 2001; 345: 1075–1083.

7. Ramsey SD, Berry K, Etzioni R, Kaplan RM, Sullivan SD, Wood DE, for the National Emphysema Treatment Trial Research Group. Cost effectiveness of lung-volume-reduction surgery for patients with severe emphysema. *N Engl J Med* 2003; 348: 2092–2102.

8. Stadtmauer EA, O'Neill A, Goldstein LJ, et al. Conventional-dose chemotherapy compared with high-dose chemotherapy plus autologous hematopoietic stem-cell transplantation for metastatic breast cancer. *N Engl J Med* 2000; 342: 1069–1076.

9. Antman K, Lagakos S, Drazen J. Designing and funding clinical trials of novel therapies. *N Engl J Med* 2001; 344: 762–763.

10. Crowley WF Jr, Sherwood L, Salber P, et al. Clinical research in the United States at a crossroads: Proposal for a novel public-private partnership to establish a national clinical research enterprise. *JAMA* 2004; 291: 1120–1126.

11. MacLean CH, Morton SC, Ofman JJ, Roth EA, Shekelle PG. How useful are unpublished data from the Food and Drug Administration in meta-analysis? J *Clin Epidemiol* 2003; 56: 44–51.

12. Psaty BM, Rennie D. Stopping medical research to save money: A broken pact with researchers and patients. *JAMA*, 289, 2003: 2128–2131.

13. Stern JM, Simes RJ. Publication bias: Evidence of delayed publication in a cohort study of clinical research projects. *Br Med J* 1997; 315: 640–645.

14. Krzyzanowska MK, Pintilie M, Tannock IF. Factors associated with failure to publish large randomized trials presented at an oncology meeting. *JAMA* 2003; 290: 495–501.

15. Dickersin K, Rennie D. Registering clinical trials. *JAMA* 2003; 290: 516–523.

16. Cowley AJ, Skene A Stainer K, Hampton JR. The effect of lorcainide on arrhythmias and survival in patients with acute myocardial infarction: An example of publication bias. *Int J Cardiol* 1993; 40: 161–166.

17. Braunholtz DA, Edwards SJL, Lilford RJ. Are randomized clinical trials good for us (in the short term)? Evidence for a "trial effect." J *Clin Epidemiol* 2001; 54: 217–224.

18. Earle CC, Weeks JC. Evidence-based medicine: A cup half full or half empty? *Am J Med* 1999; 106: 263–264.

19. Lansing S, Schwarzkopf N. Commentary; Greater clinical trail participation is crucial to fight cancer. *Los Angeles Times*, July 22, 2002, p. B11.

20. Sheingold SH. Technology assessment, coverage decisions, and conflict: The role of guidelines. *Am J Managed Care* 1998; 4: SP117–SP125.

21. Sabin JE, Daniels N. Making insurance coverage for new technologies reasonable and accountable. *JAMA* 1998; 279: 703–704.

22. Gruman J. A full partnership for the future. *Good Behavior!*, newsletter of the Center for the Advancement of Health, Washington, D.C., April 2004.

23. Clinton HR. Now can we talk about health care? *The New York Times Magazine*, April 18, 2004, p. 6-26.

24. Gruman J. Demography is destiny. *Good Behavior!*, newsletter of the Center for the Advancement of Health, Washington, D.C., March 2004.

CHAPTER 19

1. Toner R, Stolberg SG. Decade after health care crisis, soaring costs bring new strains. *The New York Times*, August 11, 2002, sec. 1, p.1.

2. Kelly K, Crowley J, Bunn PA Jr, et al. Randomized phase III trial of paclitaxel plus carboplatin versus vinorelbine plus cisplatin in the treatment of patients with advanced non-small-cell lung cancer: A Southwest Oncology Group trial. *J Clin Oncol* 2001; 19: 3210–3218.

3. Schiller JH, Harrington D, Belani CP, et al. Comparison of four chemotherapy regimens for advanced non-small-cell lung cancer. *N Engl J Med* 2002; 346: 92–98.

4. Ramsey SD, Moinpour CM, Lovato LC, et al. Economic analysis of vinorelbine plus cisplatin versus paclitaxel plus carboplatin for advanced non-small-cell lung cancer. *J Nat Cancer Inst* 2002; 94: 291–297.

5. Ramsey SD, Kessler LG. Does economics matter when treating advanced non-small cell lung cancer? *Oncologist* 2002; 7: 179–180.

6. Spiegel BM, Targownik L, Dulai GS, Gralnek IM. The cost-effectiveness of cyclooxygenase-2 selective inhibitors in the management of chronic arthritis. *Ann Intern Med* 2003; 138: 795–806.

7. Ramsey SD, Berry K, Etzioni R, Kaplan RM, Sullivan SD, Wood DE, for the National Emphysema Treatment Trial Research Group. Cost effectiveness of lung-volume-reduction surgery for patients with severe emphysema. *N Engl J Med* 2003; 348: 2092–2102.

8. Kolata G. New therapies pose quandary for Medicare. *The New York Times*, August 17, 2003, p. 1-1.

9. Pear R. Medicare overseers expect costs to soar in coming decades. *The New York Times*, March 24, 2004, p. A1.

10. Deyo RA, Nachemson A, Mirza SK. Spinal-fusion surgery—the case for restraint. *N Engl J Med* 2004; 350: 722–726.

11. Kuntz KM, Snider RK, Weinstein JN, Pope MH, Katz JN. Cost-effectiveness of fusion with and without instrumentation for patients with degenerative spondylolisthesis and spinal stenosis. *Spine* 2000; 25: 1132–1139.

12. Probstfield JL. How cost-effective are new preventive strategies for cardiovascular disease? *Am J Cardiol* 2003; 91(suppl): 22G–27G.

13. Lamm RD. Marginal medicine. *JAMA* 1998; 280: 931–933.

14. Eddy DM. Cost-effectiveness analysis: A conversation with my father. *JAMA* 1992; 267: 1669–1675.

15. Eddy DM. From theory to practice: Rationing resources while improving quality: How to get more for less. *JAMA* 1994; 272: 817–824.

16. Ginsburg PB, Nichols LM. The health care cost-coverage conundrum: The care we want vs. the care we can afford. Center for Studying Heath System Change, Annual Essay, Fall 2003. Available at www.hschange.org/content/616/. Accessed July 23, 2004.

CHAPTER 20

1. Petersen M. Vermont to require drug makers to disclose payments to doctors. *The New York Times*, June 13, 2002, p. C1.

2. Pear R. Drug makers battle a U.S. plan to curb rewards for doctors. *The New York Times*, December 26, 2002, p. A1.

3. Abelson R, Petersen M. An operation to ease back pain bolsters the bottom line, too. *The New York Times*, December 31, 2003, p. A1.

4. Kowalczyk L. Mass. General moves to curb drug vendors—concerns on influence spur hospital actions. *The Boston Globe*, August 1, 2002, p. C1.

5. Fletcher RH, Fletcher SW. Pharmaceutical advertisements in medical journals. *Ann Intern Med* 1992; 116: 951–952.

6. Lyles A. Direct marketing of pharmaceuticals to consumers. *Annu Rev Public Health* 2002; 23: 73–91.

7. American Health Line. Rx drugs: Bill would limit drug makers' tax breaks for ads. May 8, 2002. Available at: www.nationaljournal.com. Accessed May 8, 2002.

8. Shesgreen D. Bill would cap tax deductions for drug ads; senators seek to lower cost of medicine; industry calls proposal ineffective. *St. Louis Post-Dispatch*, May 8, 2002, p. A17.

9. American Health Line. Rx drugs: Senate democrats reintroduce bills that would lower prices. March 6, 2003. Available at: www.nationaljournal.com/pubs/healthline. Accessed March 6, 2003.

10. Milbank D. New drug rules aim to speed generics; FDA to limit industry tactics to stall release. *The Washington Post*, June 13, 2003, p. A27.

11. Schwartz J. Is FDA too quick to clear drugs? Growing recalls, side-effect risks raise questions. *The Washington Post*, March 23, 1999, p. A1.

12. Moore TJ, Psaty BM, Furberg CD. Time to act on drug safety. *JAMA* 1998; 279: 1571–1573.

13. Brewer T, Colditz GA. Postmarketing surveillance and adverse drug reactions: Current perspectives and future needs. *JAMA* 1999; 281: 824–829.

14. Wood AJJ, Stein CM, Woosley R. Making medicines safer—the need for an independent drug safety board. *N Engl J Med* 1998; 339: 1851–1854.

15. Sheingold SH. Technology assessment, coverage decisions, and conflict: The role of guidelines. *Am J Managed Care* 1998; 4: SP117–SP125.

16. Editorial. Let drugs duke it out. *Los Angeles Times*, September 7, 2003, p. M4.

17. Pear R. Congress weighs drug comparisons. *The New York Times*, August 24, 2003, sec. 1, p. 18.

18. The ALLHAT Officers and Coordinators for the ALLHAT Collaborative Research Group. Major outcomes in high-risk hypertensive patients randomized to angiotensin-converting enzyme inhibitor or calcium channel blocker vs. diuretic: The Antihypertensive and Lipid-Lowering treatment to prevent Heart Attack Trial (ALLHAT). *JAMA* 2002; 288: 2981–2997.

19. Echt DS, Liebson PR, Mitchell LB, et al. Mortality and morbidity in patients receiving encainide, flecainide, or placebo. The Cardiac Arrhythmia Suppression Trial. *N Engl J Med* 1991; 324: 781–788.

20. Gorelick PB, Richardson D, Kelly M, Ruland S, Hung E, Harris Y, et al. Aspirin and ticlopidine for prevention of recurrent stroke in black patients: A randomized trial. *JAMA* 2003; 289: 2947–2957.

21. Perry S. The brief life of the National Center for Health Care Technology. *N Engl J Med* 1982; 307: 1095–1100.

22. Herdman RC, Jensen JE. The OTA story: the agency perspective. *Technological Forecasting and Social Change* 1997; 54: 131–143.

23. National Public Radio. All things considered. July 18, 2001. Transcript produced by Burrelle's Information Services, Livingston, N.J.

24. Gray BH, Susmano MK, Collins SR. AHCPR and the changing politics of health services research. *Health Affairs*, June 25, 2003 (Web exclusive) W3-283–W3-307.

25. Ray WA, Griffin MR, Avorn J. Evaluating drugs after their approval for clinical use. *N Engl J Med* 1993; 329: 2029–2032.

26. Perry S, Thamer M. Medical innovation and the critical role of health technology assessment. *JAMA* 1999; 282: 1869–1872.

27. Diamond F. Making the case for a "Health Care Fed." *Managed Care*, January 2002: 26-33.

28. Reinhardt U. Harness information to make health care work. *Managed Care*, January 2002: 28.

29. Bimber B, Guston DH. Introduction: The end of OTA and the future of technology assessment. *Technological Forecasting and Social Change* 1997; 54: 125–130.

30. Wennberg JE. The more things change . . . : The federal government's role in the evaluative sciences. *Health Affairs*, June 25, 2003 (Web exclusive), W3-308–W3-310.

CHAPTER 21

1. Jefferson T. Letter to William Charles Jarvis, September 28, 1820.

2. Eysenbach G, Powell J, Kuss O, Sa ER. Empirical studies assessing the quality of health information for consumers on the world wide web: A systematic review. *JAMA* 2002; 287: 2691–2700.

3. Risk A, Petersen C. Health information on the Internet: Quality issues and international initiatives. *JAMA* 2002; 287: 2713–2715.

4. Holmberg L, Bill-Axelson A, Helgesen F, et al. A randomized trial comparing radical prostatectomy with watchful waiting in early prostate cancer. *N Engl J Med* 2002; 347: 781–789.

5. Kolata G. Perspectives: Dilemma on prostate cancer treatment splits experts. *The New York Times*, September 17, 2002, p. F5.

6. Braddock CH, Edwards KA, Hasenberg NM, Laidley TL, Levinson W. Informed decision making in outpatient practice: Time to get back to basics. *JAMA* 1999; 282: 2313–2320.

7. Coulter A, Entwistle V, Gilbert D. Sharing decisions with patients: Is the information good enough? *Br Med J* 1999; 318: 318–322.

8. O'Connor AM, Stacey D, Entwistle V, et al. Decision aids for people facing health treatment or screening decisions. (Cochrane Review). In: The Cochrane Library, Issue 2. Chichester, UK: John Wiley & Sons, Ltd., 2004.

9. Deyo RA, Cherkin DC, Weinstein J, Howe J, Ciol M, Mulley AG. Involving patients in clinical decisions: Impact of an interactive video program on use of back surgery. *Medical Care* 2000; 38: 959–969.

10. Kennedy ADM, Sculpher MJ, Coulter A, et al. Effects of decision aids for menorrhagia on treatment choices, health outcomes, and costs: A randomized controlled trial. *JAMA* 2002; 288: 2701–2708.

11. Man-Son-Hing M, Laupacis A, O'Connor AM, Biggs J, Drake E, Yetisir E, Hart RG. A patient decision aid regarding antithrombotic therapy for stroke prevention in atrial fibrillation: A randomized controlled trial. *JAMA* 1999; 282: 737–743.

12. Volk FJ, Cass AR, Spann SJ. A randomized controlled trial of shared decision making for prostate cancer screening. *Arch Fam Med* 1999; 8: 333–340.

13. Morgan MW, Deber RB, Llewellyn-Thomas HA, et al. Randomized, controlled trial of an interactive videodisc decision aid for patients with ischemic heart disease. *J Gen Intern Med* 2000; 15: 685–693.

14. Deyo RA. A key medical decision maker: The patient. *Br Med J* 2001; 323: 466–467.

15. Deyo RA. Tell it like it is: Patients as partners in medical decision making. *J Gen Intern Med* 2000; 15: 752–754.

16. Stolberg SG. On medicine's frontier: The last journey of James Quinn. *The New York Times*, October 8, 2002, p. D1.

17. Hanauer LB. Must medicine wait for science? When advocacy harms. *The New York Times*, April 20, 1999, p. A22.

18. Clark WF, Garg AX, Blake PG, Rock GA, Heidenheim AP, Sackett DL. Effect of awareness of a randomized controlled trial on use of experimental therapy. *JAMA* 2003; 290: 1351–1355.

19. Rampton S, Stauber J. *Trust Us, We're Experts.* New York: Jeremy P. Tarcher/Putnam, 2001.

20. Deyo RA, Walsh NE, Schoenfeld LS, Ramamurthy S. A controlled trial of transcutaneous electrical nerve stimulation (TENS) and exercise for chronic low back pain. *N Engl J Med* 1990; 322: 1627–1634.

21. Milne S, Welch V, Brosseau L, Saginur M, Shea B, Tugwell P, Wells G. Transcutaneous electrical nerve stimulation (TENS) for chronic low-back pain (Cochrane Review). In: The Cochrane Library, Issue 2. Chichester, UK: John Wiley & Sons, Ltd., 2004.

22. U.S. Preventive Services Task Force. Screening for prostate cancer: Recommendation and rationale. *Ann Intern Med* 2002; 137: 915–916.

23. Lenzer J. The grassroots are greener. Praxis Post, the webzine of medicine and culture. March 21, 2001. Available at: http://praxis.md/post/trends/032101. Accessed August 21, 2002.

24. Galewitz P. Pharmaceutical companies add celebrity to ad formula. *Houston Chronicle*, March 7, 1999.

25. Neergaard L. FDA warns faster drug bans possible; doctors, patients told to be wary. *The Arizona Republic (Phoenix)*, December 12, 2000, p. A1.

26. Ginsburg PB, Nichols LM. The health care cost-coverage conundrum: The care we want vs. the care we can afford. Center for Studying Health System Change, Annual Essay, Fall 2003. Available at www.hschange.org/content/616/. Accessed July 23, 2004.

INDEX

ABOUT THE AUTHORS

Richard A. Deyo, MD, MPH, is a Professor of Medicine and of Public Health at the University of Washington. As an academic general internist, he's involved with teaching, patient care, and research on new medical technology.

In 2004, he received the John M. Eisenberg Award for Career Achievement in Research from the Society of General Internal Medicine. Deyo is an elected member of the Association of American Physicians and a Fellow of the American College of Physicians. He is also a member of the Society of General Internal Medicine (formerly on its national council), and of the American Public Health Association, and is listed in *Who's Who in Medicine and Healthcare.*

Dr. Deyo has written more than 200 research publications and 50 invited editorials, review articles, and book chapters, and he recently co-edited a book entitled *Evidence-Based Clinical Practice.* In addition, he has lectured on special interests in medicine, and has been interviewed by ABC, CNN, and National Public Radio.

Best known for research on back pain, Deyo's interest in politics, profits, and the press arose when he was director of a research team on back surgery and member of a clinical guideline panel that came under attack from spine surgeons and implant manufacturers. Deyo described these events and their implications in the *New England Journal of Medicine,* the *New York Times, New Yorker,* and in an Australian television production entitled "Too Much Medicine."

Deyo is a graduate of Penn State School of Medicine and did his residency in internal medicine at the University of Texas in San Antonio.

Donald Patrick, PhD, MSPH, is Professor of Health Services in the School of Public Health and Community Medicine at the University of Washington. At UW, he directs the Social and Behavioral Sciences Program, the Seattle Quality of Life Group, and the Biobehavioral Cancer Training Program. He co-directs the End-of-Life Research Program.

His faculty career began at New York University and the University of California at San Diego, followed by appointments at Yale and St. Thomas's Medical School in London. He then returned to the U.S. to teach at the University of North Carolina, Chapel Hill, before moving to Seattle.

Patrick is a member of the Institute of Medicine, is inaugural president of the International Society for Quality of Life Research, and is a member of the American Sociological Association and the American Public Health Association, where he helped to found the Special Interest Group on Disability. He has been elected fellow of the Academy for Health Services Research and Policy.

Patrick has extensive experience with population health status assessment and outcomes research, and has applied his interests to working with vulnerable populations. His dissertation on measuring social preferences for health outcomes remains a classic in the field. In a previous book, *Health Status and Health Policy*, Patrick described the links between quality of life, cost-effectiveness, and health policy.

Also an expert in pharmacoeconomic outcomes research and its uses in regulatory approval and marketing, Patrick has authored more than 200 scientific articles, dozens of book chapters, and is editor of five books. He is frequently invited to speak on health policy, regulatory affairs, and disablement in the U.S. and Europe.

Dr. Patrick graduated from Northwestern University, and holds master's and doctoral degree from Columbia University.